Adverse Effects of Herbal Drugs

Volume 3

Editors
P.A.G.M. De Smet (Managing Editor)
K. Keller   R. Hänsel   R.F. Chandler

Springer
Berlin
Heidelberg
New York
Barcelona
Budapest
Hong Kong
London
Milan
Paris
Santa Clara
Singapore
Tokyo

Adverse Effects of Herbal Drugs 3

Edited by
P. A.G.M. De Smet (Managing Editor)
K. Keller   R. Hänsel   R. F. Chandler

Contributors
G. Abel R. Bos I.H.Bowen R.F.Chandler D.Corrigan
I.J. Cubbin P.A.G.M. De Smet N. Pras J.J.C. Scheffer
T.A.Van Beek W. Van Uden H.J. Woerdenbag

In collaboration with the Pharmaceuticals Programme
of the World Health Organization, Regional Office for Europe

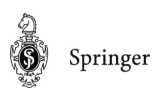 Springer

Dr. PETER A.G.M. DE SMET
Royal Dutch Association for the Advancement of Pharmacy
Alexanderstraat 11, 2514 JL The Hague
The Netherlands

Dr. KONSTANTIN KELLER
Bundesinstitut für Arzneimittel und Medizinprodukte
Seestraße 10, 13353 Berlin
Germany

Prof. Dr. RUDOLF HÄNSEL
Westpreußenstraße 71, 81927 München
Germany

Prof. Dr. R. FRANK CHANDLER
College of Pharmacy, Dalhousie University, Halifax B3H 3J5
Canada

ISSN 0942-2242

ISBN-13: 978-3-540-60181-4   e-ISBN-13: 978-3-642-60367-9
DOI: 10.1007/978-3-642-60367-9

Library of Congress Cataloging-in-Publication Data
92-219771

This work is subject to copyright. All rights are reserved, whether the whole or part of the material is concerned, specifically the rights of translation, reprinting, re-use of illustrations, recitation, broadcasting, reproduction on microfilm or in other way, and storage in data banks. Duplication of this publication or parts thereof is permitted only under the provisions of the German Copyright Law of September 9, 1965, in its current version, and permission for use must always be obtained from Springer-Verlag. Violations are liable for prosecution under the German Copyright Law.

Although great effort has been made to provide the reader with reliable data, the contributors, editors, and publisher cannot assume responsibility for the validity of all information in this book or for the consequences of its use.

© Springer-Verlag Berlin Heidelberg 1997
Reprint of the original edition 1997

The use of registered names, trademarks, etc. in this publication does not imply, even in the absence of a specific statement, that such names are exempt from the relevant protective laws and regulations and therefore free for general use.

SPIN: 10500557   13/3133-5 4 3 2 1 0 – Printed on acid-free paper

*Pour Valerie
qui m'enrubanne de nouveau*

Preface

This third contribution to our series has the same approach as the previous two volumes. The book opens with a general introductory chapter (this time on herbal postmarketing surveillance), which is followed by eighteen comprehensive monographs about specific medicinal herbs and important plant constituents. The herbs and constituents have been selected for several reasons, such as a prominent place in phytotherapy (e.g. *Valeriana* species), clinical expectations about therapeutic potential (e.g. *Tripterygium* species), and recent concern about a serious adverse reaction (e.g. *Teucrium chamaedrys*). Just as before, the result is a blend of new and old information.

December 1995   THE EDITORS

Contents

An Introduction to Herbal Pharmacovigilance................... 1
P. A.G. M. DE SMET

Artemisia Cina 15
H. J. WOERDENBAG, W. VAN UDEN and N. PRAS

Aspalathus Linearis..................................... 23
P. A.G. M. DE SMET

Citrullus Colocynthis 29
P. A.G. M. DE SMET

Fucus Vesiculosus and Allied Brown Algae................... 37
I. H. BOWEN and I. J. CUBBIN

Ginkgo Biloba 51
H. J. WOERDENBAG and T. A. VAN BEEK

Glycyrrhiza Glabra....................................... 67
R. F. CHANDLER

Linum Usitatissimum...................................... 89
H. J. WOERDENBAG, W. VAN UDEN and N. PRAS

Phoradendron Flavescens.................................. 99
P. A.G. M. DE SMET

Safrole – General Discussion 105
G. ABEL

Safrole – *Sassafras Albidum*............................. 123
G. ABEL

Spirulina Species 129
P. A.G. M. DE SMET

Teucrium Chamaedrys 137
P. A.G. M. DE SMET

Tripterygium Species 145
P. A.G. M. DE SMET

Valeriana Species 165
R. BOS, H. J. WOERDENBAG, P.A.G.M. DE SMET
and J. J. C. SCHEFFER

Yohimbe Alkaloids – General Discussion 181
P. A.G. M. DE SMET

Yohimbe Alkaloids – *Corynanthe* Species 207
P. A.G. M. DE SMET

Yohimbe Alkaloids – *Pausinystalia* Species 211
P. A.G. M. DE SMET

Zingiber Officinale 215
D. CORRIGAN

Notes Added in Proof 229
P. A.G. M. DE SMET

Subject Index 241

Contributors

Dr. GUDRUN ABEL
Plantamed Arzneimittel GmbH,
Kerschensteinerstraße 11-15,
Postfach 57, 92318 Neumarkt/Opf.,
Germany

Mr. REIN BOS
Department of Pharmaceutical Biology,
University Centre for Pharmacy,
University of Groningen, Antonius Deusinglaan 1,
9713 AV Groningen, The Netherlands

Dr. IAN BOWEN
School of Health Sciences,
University of Sunderland, Langham Tower, Ryhope Road,
Sunderland SR2 7EE
United Kingdom

Prof. Dr. R. FRANK CHANDLER
College of Pharmacy, Dalhousie University,
Halifax B3H 3J5,
Canada

Dr. DESMOND CORRIGAN
Department of Pharmacognosy, School of Pharmacy,
Trinity College, 18 Shrewsbury Road, Dublin 4
Ireland

Mr. IAN CUBBIN
School of Health Sciences,
University of Sunderland, Langham Tower, Ryhope Road,
Sunderland SR2 7EE
United Kingdom

Dr. PETER A.G.M. DE SMET
Royal Dutch Association for the Advancement of Pharmacy,
Alexanderstraat 11,
2514 JL The Hague
The Netherlands

Dr. NIESKO PRAS
Department of Pharmaceutical Biology,
University Centre for Pharmacy, University of Groningen,
Antonius Deusinglaan 1,
9713 AV Groningen,
The Netherlands

Prof. Dr. J. C. C. SCHEFFER
Division of Pharmacognosy,
LACDR, Leiden University, Gorlaeus Laboratories,
PO Box 9502,
2300 RA Leiden,
The Netherlands

Dr. TERIS A. VAN BEEK
Phytochemical Section,
Department of Organic Chemistry,
Wageningen Agricultural University,
Dreijenplein 8, 6703 HB Wageningen,
The Netherlands

Dr. WIM VAN UDEN
Department of Pharmaceutical Biology,
University Centre for Pharmacy,
University of Groningen,
Antonius Deusinglaan 1, 9713 AV Groningen,
The Netherlands

Dr. HERMAN J. WOERDENBAG
Department of Pharmaceutical Biology,
University Centre for Pharmacy,
University of Groningen,
Antonius Deusinglaan 1, 9713 AV Groningen
The Netherlands

An Introduction to Herbal Pharmacovigilance

P.A.G.M. De Smet

Introduction

To obtain a marketing authorization for a new drug, the manufacturer has to prove in well-designed clinical trials that his drug is efficacious as well as safe. These premarketing trials tend to be rather artificial, however, as they involve relatively small numbers of carefully selected patients, who are followed for relatively short periods of time in strictly controlled conditions. The patients are mostly treated by special health care professionals in special settings. They receive pre-fixed dose regimens and are submitted to frequent and thorough examinations. Moreover, certain subgroups, such as the elderly, children, pregnant women, patients with concomitant diseases and multiple drug users, are often excluded for ethical or statistical reasons. As a consequence, premarketing trials do not provide the ultimate answer to the question of how the drug is going to behave in everyday practice under everyday circumstances. To fill this void, premarketing trials have to be supplemented with pharmacoepidemiological studies performed after the drug has hit the market. This type of research has become generally known as postmarketing surveillance or pharmacovigilance [1,2].

Pharmacovigilance aims to assess the effects of the drug in the open, heterogeneous population, and can thus help to find out whether these effects are modified by factors such as uncontrolled dosage, pregnancy, lactation, genetics, concurrent pathology, additional drug taking, and so on. By monitoring much larger numbers of users than those investigated prior to marketing, pharmacovigilance also allows a more precise quantitation of the incidence of the effects that were observed in premarketing testing. Furthermore, pharmacovigilance can identify effects that have gone undetected in the premarketing phase. One reason may be that the effect needs a long period of use or a long latency period to become manifest. Another possibility is that the effect cannot be reliably detected in relatively small populations because of its low incidence [1,2].

There is a statistical "rule of three", which dictates that the number of studied subjects must be three times as high as the frequency of an adverse drug reaction to have a 95% chance that the reaction will actually occur in a studied population [3]. For example, when an adverse drug reaction occurs with a frequency of 1 in 2000, one needs to monitor 6000 users to have a 95% chance that the adverse reaction will be observed at least once (Table 1). To have a 95% chance that the reaction will occur twice or three times, one has to enroll 9600 and 13000 patients, respecti-

Table 1. Number of persons who need to be exposed to a drug to have a certain chance of detecting an adverse drug reaction occurring with a particular frequency [3]

Frequency of adverse drug reaction (ADR)	Probability that ADR occurs at least once			
	95%	90%	80%	63%
1 out of 100	300	231	161	100
1 out of 500	1 500	1 152	805	500
1 out of 1 000	3 000	2 303	1 610	1 000
1 out of 5 000	15 000	11 513	8 048	5 000
1 out of 10 000	30 000	23 026	16 095	10 000
1 out of 50 000	150 000	115 130	80 472	50 000

Table 2. Number of persons who need to be exposed to a drug to have a 95% chance of detecting an adverse drug reaction occurring with a particular frequency at least once, twice or three times [3]

Frequency of adverse drug reaction (ADR)	Number of ADR cases		
	1	2	3
1 out of 100	300	480	650
1 out of 200	600	960	1 300
1 out of 1 000	3 000	4 800	6 500
1 out of 2 000	6 000	9 600	13 000
1 out of 10 000	30 000	48 000	65 000

vely (Table 2). Since premarketing research usually involves a few thousands of patients or even less, it follows that it is not a reliable tool to discover uncommon effects of a drug. A recent example was the worldwide withdrawal of a synthetic antibacterial fluoroquinolone derivative, temafloxacin, following postmarketing detection of hemolytic anaemia and other serious adverse reactions. Before marketing, the drug had been studied in 4,261 patients, but apparently the hemolytic syndrome was rare enough to escape detection during this period [4].

Herbal Pharmacovigilance

Epidemiological surveillance of the drug market is not only useful to study the adverse effects of synthetic drugs. This methodology can also make a contribution to our knowledge about the adverse effects of herbal drugs. In contrast to newly marketed chemical drugs, herbal medicines often have a long history of traditional use, resulting in considerable experience with their effects in open populations. Such informal experience is a powerful tool, of course, for the identification of adverse effects, which occur commonly and develop rapidly after the start of therapy. Usually, it will also come to light, which ways of processing and which dosage regimens reduce the likelihood of acute adverse reactions. It can be questioned, however, whether empiricism will identify less conspicuous modifiers of toxicity, such as a concurrent disease, and whether delayed and uncommon adverse reactions will always be recognized.

Delayed Effects

When a herb has oxytocic properties (the capacity to cause contraction of the uterus), the risks of its unrestricted use during pregnancy will be readily discovered. However, when a sick baby is born, who will attribute the disease to maternal consumption of a herbal preparation many months before the baby's delivery? Herbal drugs containing pyrrolizidine alkaloids may have been used since prehistoric times [5], but the first case report about neonatal hepatotoxicity following the use of such a remedy during pregnancy did not appear until a few years ago [6,7]. There is a great need for more and better information about the embryotoxic and fetotoxic risks of herbal drugs, not in the least because herbal drug use during pregnancy is sometimes encouraged by uncritical publications [8]. This need for better information is illustrated by an Australian study, in which calls to a drug information center about drug use in pregnancy and lactation were analyzed. Herbal preparation calls numbered up to 10 per month and represented 2% of the overall calls [9]. It would seem useful to follow the pregnant women who call with questions about herbal drug therapy prospectively so that the outcome of any herbal drug use during their pregnancy can be documented.

Uncommon Effects

Not only delayed effects, but also infrequent events may go unnoted for a long time. In recent years, for instance, various Chinese formulae have been associated with serious bizarre reactions, such as hepatitis, pneumonitis, and cystitis. Although these medicines consist solely or largely of traditional herbal ingredients, their ability to cause such adverse effects was not known until they were documented in recent Japanese case reports (Table 3). The argument could be raised that such reports serve to prove that even uncommon adverse reactions to herbal drugs will be discovered sooner or later through spontaneous reporting. Later may not be soon enough, however, and the chance of spontaneous recognition will only be fair, when an adverse drug reaction falls outside the scope of normal disease patterns.

Even when an adverse drug reaction stands out as a distinct clinical entity, it may take many years before a mental connection with the responsible agent is made. An illustrative example is the so-called eosinophilia-myalgia syndrome. As indicated by its name, this syndrome is characterized by a high eosinophil blood count and intense generalized myalgia. Some years ago, an epidemic of the syndrome raged through the United States, causing hundreds of hospitalizations and several deaths. The epidemic was rapidly tied to the use of health food products containing the natural amino acid L-tryptophan. Subsequent investigations showed

Table 3. Recent Japanese case reports of hepatitis, pneumonitis and cystitis associated with herb-containing medicines

Preparation	Type and number of cases		Reported composition*
Juzentaiho-gan[11]	Pneumonitis	1x	Not specified
Kaigen[12,13]	Hepatitis	2x	Caryophylli oleum, Cinnamomi cortex, Glycyrrhizae radix, Hydrangeae dulcis folium, Zingiberis rhizoma; Acetoaminophen**, d-Borneol, Caffeine, l-Menthol, dl-Methylephedrine
Keimeigashin-san[14]	Hepatitis	1x	Only in Japanese (Gajutsu, Makonbu, Takugo)
Keishi-bukuryo-gan[11]	Pneumonitis	1x	Not specified
Kinshigan[13,15-19]	Hepatitis	8x	Arecae semen, Calumbae radix, Cinnamomi cortex, Coptidis rhizoma, Forsythiae fructus, Gardeniae fructus, Ginseng radix, Glycyrrhizae radix, Hydnocarpi semen, Paeoniae radix, Phellodendri cortex, Rhei rhizoma, *Saussurea lappa*, Scutellariae radix, Smilacis rhizoma, Sophorae flos, Sophorae radix
Kinshigyoku[13]	Hepatitis	1x	Not specified
MKsan[20]	Hepatitis	1x	Only in Japanese (Inyorai, Matsuba, Shakunage, Sohakuhi)
Rikkunshi-to[21]	Pneumonitis	1x	Atractylodis lanceae rhizoma, Aurantii nobilis pericarpium, Ginseng radix, Glycyrrhizae radix, Hoelen, Pinelliae tuber, Zingiberis rhizoma, Zizyphi fructus
Saiboku-to[22,23]	Pneumonitis Cystitis	1x 3x	Bupleuri radix, Ginseng radix, Glycyrrhizae radix, Hoelen, Magnoliae cortex, Perillae herba, Pinelliae tuber, Scutellariae radix, Zingiberis rhizoma, Zizyphi fructus
Sairei-to[11,23]	Pneumonitis Cystitis	1x 2x	Atractylodis lanceae rhizoma, Alismatis rhizoma, Bupleuri radix, Cinnamomi cortex, Ginseng radix, Glycyrrhizae radix, Hoelen, Pinelliae tuber, Polyporus, Scutellariae radix, Zingiberis rhizoma, Zizyphi fructus
Saiko-keishi-to[23]	Cystitis	1x	Bupleuri radix, Cinnamomi cortex, Ginseng radix, Glycyrrhizae radix, Paeoniae radix, Pinelliae tuber, Scutellariae radix, Zingiberis rhizoma, Zizyphi fructus
Sakaki Gachyagi[24]	Hepatitis	1x	Atractylodis lanceae rhizoma, Evodiae fructus, Ginseng, Magnoliae cortex, Phellodendri cortex; Medicinal carbon, Sodium hydrogen carbonate
Sho-saiko-to[11,18,23,25-27]	Hepatitis Pneumonitis Both Cystitis	1x 8x 1x 2x	Bupleuri radix, Ginseng radix, Glycyrrhizae radix, Pinelliae tuber, Scutellariae radix, Zingiberis rhizoma, Zizyphi fructus
Stronger-Neo-Minophagen C[28,29]	Hepatitis	2x	Glycyrrhizin; Cysteine, glycine

* Compositons were either taken from the case reports or derived from Tsumura [10]
** This ingredient is a well-known non-herbal hepatotoxin

a strong association between the epidemic and L-tryptophan material coming from one specific Japanese company. An intriguing aspect of the epidemic was that, although the major outbreak started around July 1989, a few percent of the reported cases had already occurred in the years 1981-1987. Their relationship with L-tryptophan consumption became only evident in 1989, however, after the attack rate among L-tryptophan users had gone up to more than 1 victim in 1000 users, following certain changes in the biotechnological manufacturing process of the Japanese company [30]. Thus the eosinophilia-myalgia syndrome illustrates that, without the support of epidemiological analysis, even a conspicuous adverse event may escape discovery for a prolonged period when it does not occur with a certain frequency. To put the recognizability of more than 1 reaction in 1000 users in perspective, it should be added that an incidence of 1 serious adverse reaction in 10,000 users may be considered unacceptable in official medicine when there is no clear therapeutic need for a drug [31].

Common Effects

Another obstacle to the detection of an adverse drug reaction can be that its signs and symptoms are not so rare in the general population. When the background noise of an adverse event is relatively high, it becomes difficult to discern a relationship between a traditional drug and the effect on the basis of isolated cases. An epidemiological approach will then be needed to establish the connection.

An illustrative example was reported by Traverso et al. [32] who performed a case-control study of risk factors predisposing to the development of neonatal tetanus. A systematic search covering 16,000 households in North Western Pakistan yielded 69 cases of neonatal tetanus death in a total of 5600 live births (i.e. about 12 cases per 1000 live births). For each case, three matching living infants were selected as controls. The comparison between cases and controls showed a significant difference in the application of ghee to the umbilical wound stump. Ghee is not a herbal product but the clarified butter from the milk of water buffaloes or cows. In the rural areas studied, it was mainly made at home from unpasteurized milk by a process that was unlikely to kill *Clostridium tetani* spores. Cases and controls did not significantly differ in the proportion of infants who had received a ghee dressing immediately after the cutting of the umbilical cord, but there was a significant difference in the proportion who had received subsequent applications, viz. 57% of the cases versus 33% of the controls (Table 4). The odds ratio for neonatal tetanus and subsequent applications of ghee was 3.3 (95% confidence interval of 1.8-6.3). By taking this odds ratio as a valid measure of relative risk, and by assuming that one-third of all newborn infants received subsequent applications of ghee, the researchers calculated that abandoning the practice in areas where home-made ghee is prevalent should reduce neonatal tetanus death rates by about 43%. At an observed rate of twelve cases per 1000 live births, 1 of every 200 infants born alive might thus be saved from an untimely tetanus death.

Table 4. Ghee dressing of the umbilical wound in rural Pakistan: cases of neonatal tetanus death versus controls [32]

Ghee application	Cases (n=69)	Controls (n=207)
initial only	1	20
initial + subsequent	26	51
initial overall	27 (39%)	71 (34%)
subsequent only	13	17
subsequent + initial	26	51
subsequent overall	39 (57%)	68 (33%)

Need for Quantitative Assessment

Pharmacoepidemiological research not only makes a contribution to the timely detection and corroboration of adverse drug reactions, but also helps to quantitate their incidence. While spontaneous case reporting can give good qualitative insight in the nature of an adverse drug effect, it does little to provide an accurate estimate of its incidence. Reliable data about the incidence of a serious adverse effect are essential for an unbiased assessment of the actual drug risk. On the one hand, the absence of reliable evidence of risk should not be mistaken for reliable evidence of the absence of risk, because this could lead to keeping relatively dangerous herbal drugs on the market. On the other hand, however, the conservative view that any serious health risk of a herbal drug is unacceptable, irrespective of its incidence, when there is insufficient clinical proof of efficacy could lead to the banning of herbal drugs with practically negligible health risks. This two-sidedness leads to the more general comment that pharmacoepidemiology is not a negative tool for the assessment of adverse drug effects, but a strictly neutral one. Certainly, when it identifies and quantitates a new serious drug risk, it can be the bringer of some bad news. Pharmacoepidemiology can also be reassuring, however, by providing evidence that certain drug risks are absent or negligible.

Available Approaches

Once one has decided to submit herbal drugs to pharmacovigilance, one is faced with the question which methodological approach should be used. The answer is, of course, that the choice of pharmacoepidemiological method should be tailored to the issue that needs to be addressed. If no single approach is sufficient to come up with good answers, it may be necessary to use more than one resource, simultaneously or successively [1]. Although a full presentation of the available methods would be outside the scope of this introductory chapter, some approaches and examples will be indicated briefly. For more detailed discussions, the interested reader is referred to general textbooks on pharmacoepidemiology [1,2].

Spontaneous Reporting

A classical type of pharmacoepidemiological data collection is the spontaneous reporting system. This system relies heavily on voluntary reports by health professionals, users or other individuals who spontaneously observe or experience a suspected or possible adverse reaction during daily practice. The collection and maintainance of such reports is relatively inexpensive, and the system can cover entire countries or large fractions thereof. The major strength of this approach lies in its ability to serve as a rapid warning mechanism that can signal the potential existence of hitherto unknown adverse reactions [1]. There is much to be said for the inclusion of herbal medicines in national and regional pharmacovigilance projects that are aimed at the collection and screening of adverse drug reactions in general. This has not only the advantage of obtaining epidemiological data on the adverse reaction potential of herbal drugs, but also offers the possibility that potential confounding of synthetic drug reactions by herbal drug use can be detected and accounted for.

Reporting Herbal Reactions

It goes without saying that reports of adverse reactions to herbal preparations have to fulfil the same general conditions that are required for reporting synthetic drug reactions. It should be realized, however, that herbal medicines are a special group of products, to which additional considerations apply.

A major difference between synthetic drugs and herbal medicines is that the quality assurance of the latter is sometimes much less stringent than that of synthetic preparations. As was extensively reviewed in the first volume of this book series, toxicity of herbal medicines not always results from the ingredients mentioned on the label, but can also be due to an undeclared toxic botanical, poisonous metal, potent synthetic drug substance, etc. [33]. As a consequence, any report about an adverse reaction to a herbal drug should make clear which efforts have been put into the exclusion of intentional and accidental substitution or contamination.

Another general point is that the toxicity of a herbal medicine may vary considerably with plant part and way of preparation. For instance, some parts (e.g. roots) of the forking larkspur (*Delphinium consolida*) contain poisonous diterpenoid alkaloids, which can elicit *Aconitum*-like symptoms. However, such alkaloids seem to be absent in the flowers, and there is no objection to the use of these flowers as ornamental admixture to herbal teas [34,35]. Another parameter which can have a profound impact on herbal drug toxicity is the exact way of processing the crude material. This was elegantly demonstrated by Hikino et al. [36], who investigated the influence of heating with and without water for up to 4 hours on the toxicity of *Aconitum* tubers. Raw tubers of *A.japonicum* and *A.carmichaeli* are highly toxic due to the presence of poisonous aconitines. However, heating at 100 °C in the presence of water (conditions employed for decoction) gradually transformed these toxic alkaloids into the much less poisonous benzoylaconines, and this was reflected by a reduction in the acute toxicity of the tubers in mice (Table 5). In other

Table 5. Changes in alkaloid composition and in acute toxicity in the mouse induced by heating *Aconitum* tubers at 100° C with and without a fourfold amount of water [36]

Source plant	Water added	Heating period	Level of aconitines	Level of benzoylaconines	LD$_{50}$ i.p.
A.japonicum	no	0 hr	0.33%	0.09%	0.09 g/kg
		1 hr	0.28%	0.12%	0.18 g/kg
		2 hr	0.24%	0.15%	0.51 g/kg
		4 hr	0.17%	0.25%	0.99 g/kg
A.japonicum	4-fold	0 hr	0.31%	0.10%	0.11 g/kg
		1 hr	0.19%	0.26%	1.6 g/kg
		2 hr	0.15%	0.31%	>10 g/kg
		4 hr	0.11%	0.33%	>10 g/kg
A.carmichaeli	4-fold	0 hr	0.21%	0.08%	0.18 g/kg
		1 hr	0.21%	0.13%	4.2 g/kg
		2 hr	0.19%	0.13%	7.9 g/kg
		4 hr	0.11%	0.17%	9.5 g/kg

words, reports about herbal drug toxicity should try to make clear which plant parts were actually used as source material and to which form of processing they were submitted.

Other Methods

The spontaneous reporting system may sometimes provide valuable information for case series studies which is not available from other sources [1]. For example, the recent identification and characterization of acute hepatitis following the use of wall germander (*Teucrium chamaedrys*) preparations was almost fully dependent on spontaneous reporting to regional French pharmacovigilance centers [37]. A spontaneous reporting system is especially useful for generating hypotheses, however, and other methods are preferable, when the need arises for strenghtening or testing hypotheses. For instance, initial signals in the United States that the eosinophilia-myalgia syndrome seemed to be related to the use of L-tryptophan products were followed by case-control studies, which established a statistically significant association between the use of L-tryptophan products and the development of the syndrome [38]. The Food and Drug Administration subsequently recalled all health food supplements containing at least 100 mg of L-tryptophan as their sole or major component [39].

A herbal example of epidemiological hypothesis exploration was recently reported by Siegers et al. [40]. These authors studied the relationship between colorectal cancer and abuse of anthranoid-containing laxatives (such as aloe, cascara, frangula, and rhubarb), because certain anthranoid laxatives show genotoxic potential in bacterial and mammalian test systems [41–43] and because two anthranoid derivatives (the synthetic laxative danthrone and the naturally occurring 1-hydroxyanthraquinone) had carcinogenic activity in rodents [44–46]. As a patient's recall of his drug consumption history over the years would be an unreliable method for establishing laxative abuse, Siegers et al. [40] took pseudomelanosis coli as a more reliable and anthranoid-specific indicator. In a retrospective study of 3049 patients, the incidence of pseudomelanosis coli was 3.13% in patients without abnormalities of the colorectal mucosa, compared to 8.64% in patients with colorectal carcinoma. In a prospective study of 1095 patients, however, these incidences were increased to 6.9% and 18.6%, respectively (Table 6). Statistical analysis showed that this latter incidence was significantly higher than the former, and it could be calculated that chronic abusers of anthranoid laxatives had an increased relative risk of 3.04 (95% confidence interval of 1.18–4.90) for colorectal cancer. The discrepancy between the retrospective and prospective results could have been due to incomplete documentation of pseudomelanosis coli in the retrospective cases of colorectal carcinoma. However, additional studies are still needed to clarify this point and to exclude the possibility that chronic constipation per se might increase the risk for colorectal cancer and thus would act as a confounding factor.

One of the greatest weaknesses of spontaneous reporting systems is their inability to provide reliable incidence rates, i.e., accurate measures of the proportion of users, who experience a given side effect. Reporting an adverse drug reaction requires detection of an adverse event, attribution of that event to drug exposure and, last but not least, going to the trouble of notifying the authorities [1]. Deficiencies in any of these steps will lead to underreporting, and there are no obvious reasons to presume that such deficiencies are less likely to occur with respect to herbal medicines. On the contrary, freely available botanical preparations enjoy a reputation of being generally harmless, and might thus come less easily under suspicion than conventional agents. Also, it takes quite some courage for unorthodox healers or their patients to report adverse consequences of a therapy that is still considered as controversial by others [47].

To overcome this disadvantage of underreporting, spontaneous reporting systems must be supplemented with more systematic studies. Illustrative is a recent report by Bruynzeel et al. [48], who evaluated the contact sensitization potential of 5 commercial herbal ointments in 1032 consecutive or randomly selected patients visiting their patch test clinics. Eleven patients reacted positively to one or more ointments. Two of these patients were sensitized by wool fat, a non-herbal consti-

Table 6. Occurrence of pseudomelanosis coli in patients undergoing diagnostic colorectal endoscopy [40]

Diagnosis	Retrospective study Patients	Pseud.coli	Prospective study Patients	Pseud.coli
No abnormalities	1151	36 (3.13%)	537	37 (6.9%)
Colitis	742	14 (1.89%)	221	5 (2.3%)
Diverticulosis	321	16 (4.98%)	110	10 (9.1%)
Adenoma	683	59 (8.64%)	225	22 (9.8%)
Carcinoma	152	6 (3.94%)	59	11 (18.6%)
Total	3094	130 (4.26%)	1095	77 (7.0%)

Table 7. Patch testing results for five commercial herbal ointments in 1032 dermatological patients seen for patch testing [48]

Trade name (Supplier)	Herbal ingredient	Patients with positive reaction (11 in total)
Arniflor (VSM)	Arnica tinct. 10%	no. 1[a] 2[a] 3
Kamillosan (Homburg)	Chamomile extr. 4%	no. 1[a] 2[a] 4[b] 5[b] 6[c]
Echinacea (VSM)	Echinacea tinct. 10%	no. 7 8
Hamametum (VSM)	Hamamelis extr. 25%	no. 1[a] 2[a] 9 10
Calendula (VSM)	Calendula tinct. 10%	no. 1[a] 11

[a] Also positive to woolfat
[b] Also positive to *Matricaria* leaf
[c] Also positive to colophony

tuent of the ointments, but the reactions in the nine remaining patients (8.7%) could very well have been herb-induced (Table 7). In two of the patients reacting positive to the chamomile ointment, this was verified by additional testing with the plant material itself (*Matricaria* leaf).

Concluding Remarks

In countries such as Germany and France, where herbal medicines are officially recognized as registered drugs [35], herbal pharmacovigilance already seems to profit from national and regional efforts to run pharmacovigilance schemes. The new requirement of the European Union that holders of marketing authorisations for pharmaceutical products are responsible for reporting suspected adverse reactions to the authorities of the Member States (and also to the European Evaluation Agency when a product is authorised under a centralised procedure) [49–51] will undoubtedly further these endeavours. In other countries, which still treat herbal products as non-registered unconventional items, there is also an increasing awareness of the need to monitor the safety of the herbal market. The American Food and Drug Administration (FDA) recently urged physicians to obtain information regarding dietary supplements as part of obtaining a complete medical history, and its newly implemented MEDWATCH programme, which monitors reports of adverse reactions to FDA-regulated products, specifically requests reports of adverse reactions to dietary supplements [52,53]. In the United Kingdom, the National Poisons Unit has performed a pilot study of adverse and toxic effects related to the use of traditional medicines and food supplements. The effects identified by this survey were considered serious enough to cause concern and to indicate a need for continuing this type of surveillance [54,55]. Last but not least, the European Scientific Co-operative for Phytotherapy (ESCOP) has taken the initiative for a pilot study in five countries of the European Union to start a special pharmacovigilance system for phytomedicines. This programme is aimed not only at the systematic collection of adverse reactions to herbal medicines, but also sets out to assess the perceptions of such adverse reactions among the consumers and suppliers of these products. This is considered an essential validation exercise, as the basic perceptions of what is an adverse effect could differ from those applied by users of conventional drugs or among different cultural groups within Europe [56].

References

1. Strom BL, red. (1989) Pharmacoepidemiology. New York: Churchill Livingstone
2. Hartzema AG, Porta MS, Tilson HH, red. (1991) Pharmacoepidemiology. An introduction. 2nd edition. Harvey Whitney Books Company, Cincinnatti
3. Loonen AJM (1989) Klinisch veiligheidsonderzoek van geneesmiddelen: methoden en instrumenten. Pharm Weekbl 124:1025–1031
4. Anonymous (1992) Temafloxacin – Anatomy of a withdrawal. Scrip no.1737, July 22nd, pp.20–21
5. Lietava J (1992) Medicinal plants in a Middle Paleolithic grave Shanidar IV? J Ethnopharmacol 35:263–266
6. Roulet M, Laurini R, Rivier L, Calame A (1988) Hepatic venoocclusive disease in newborn infant of a woman drinking herbal tea. J Pediatrics 112:433–436
7. Spang R (1989) Toxicity of tea containing pyrrolizidine alkaloids. J Pediatrics 115:1025
8. Bunce KL (1987) The use of herbs in midwifery. J Nurse-Midwifery 32:255–259
9. Hotham NJ (1990) Drug in pregnancy and lactation: analysis of an information service in South Australia. Austr J Hosp Pharm 20:153–159
10. Tsumura A (1991) Kampo – How the Japanese updated traditional herbal medicine. Tokyo: Japan Publications, Inc.
11. Takada N, Arai S, Kusuhara N, Katagiri M, Yanase N, Abe T, Tomita T (1993) A case of Sho-Saiko-to-induced pneumonitis, diagnosed by lymphocyte stimulation test using bronchoalveolar lavage fluid. Jap J Thorac Dis 31:1163–1169
12. Mizoguchi Y, Yoshiyasu K, Tsutsui H, Miyajima K, Sakagami Y, Higashimori T, Seki S, Yamamoto S, Morisawa S (1985) A case of drug-induced allergic hepatitis by herbal medicine. Acta Hepatol Jap 26:376–379
13. Tazawa J, Mae S, Sakai H, Nishimura M, Hasumura Y, Takeuchi J (1985) A case of herb drug-induced liver injury showing the different morphological findings during the disease course of two years. Acta Hepatol Jap 26:1669–1674
14. Satake I, Maeda M, Koyama W, Sakamoto S, Koizumi S, Kanayama M (1986) A case of hepatic injury caused by an herb drug. Acta Hepatol Jap 27:238–241
15. Mizoguchi Y, Miyajima K, Sakagami Y, Yamamoto S (1986) A serious case of drug-induced allergic hepatitis by a herbal medicine. Nippon Naika Gakkai Zasshi (J Jap Soc Int Med) 75:1453–1456
16. Yamazaki K, Suzuki K, Sato K, Ouchi K, Yoshinari H, Isozaki I, Nakadata I, Madarame T, Yoshida T, Kashiwabara T, Sato S, Murakami A (1991) Herbal drug-induced fulminant hepatitis. Acta Hepatol Jap 32:724–729
17. Sato E, Maeta H, Honda K, Ito T, Tsukioka S, Shibasaki K, Yoshimasu H, Ichida F (1984) A case report of herb medicine induced hepatic injury. Acta Hepatol Jap 25:674–681
18. Kubo K, Watanabe F, Sakuma K, Abe A, Kutsukake S, Shimano K, Abe M, Kuribayashi N (1986) Hypersensitive hepatic injury induced by Shosaikoto, a liver-supporting herb medicine. IRYO (Jap J Nat Med Serv) 40:205–206,257–260
19. Ikeda R, Kanaoka M, Fujisawa T, Doi Y, Kumamoto I, Onji M (1994) A case of drug induced liver injury caused by Kinshigan. Gastroenterological Endoscopy 36:1445–1451
20. Tozuka S, Tsutsui H, Sakamoto S, Kanayama M (1983) A case of drug-induced liver injury caused by a herb drug. Acta Hepatol Japon 24:1032–1035
21. Maruyama Y, Maruyama M, Takada T, Haraguchi M, Uno K (1994) A case of pneumonitis due to Rikkunshi-to. Jap J Thorac Dis 32:84–89

22. Soda R, Takahashi K, Tada S, Takahashi H, Okamoto S, Katagi S, Mifume T, Kajimoto K, Kimura I (1992) A case of pulmonary infiltration with eosinophilia (PIE) syndrome induced by Saiboku-To (TJ96). Detection of ECF activity in lymphocytes stimulated with TJ96. Jap J Thoracic Dis 30:662–667
23. Anonymous (1993) Chinese herbal medicines (Saiboku-to, Sairei-to, Sho-saiko-to and Saikokeishi-to) and cystitis-like symptoms. Information on adverse reactions to drugs. No.123. Safety Division Pharmaceutical Affairs Bureau, Ministry of Health and Welfare, Japan. November 1993, pp.3–6
24. Goto M, Komatsu M, Ishida S, Goto T, Masamune O, Segawa Y (1990) A case of drug induced liver injury showing potato-like liver caused by herb drug. Gastroenterological Endoscopy 32:2427–2432
25. Daibo A, Yoshida Y, Kitazawa S, Kosaka Y, Bando T, Sudo M (1992) A case of pneumonitis and hepatic injury caused by a herbal drug (Sho-saiko-to). Jap J Thoracic Dis 30:1583–1588
26. Tsukiyama K, Tasaka Y, Nakajima M, Hino J, Nakahama C, Okimoto N, Yagi S, Soejima R (1989) A case of pneumonitis due to Sho-saiko-to. Jap J Thoracic Dis 27:1556–1561
27. Imokawa S, Sato A, Taniguchi M (1992) A case of Sho-saiko-to induced pneumonitis and the review of literature. Jap J Chest Dis 51:53–58
28. Akashi K, Shirahama M, Iwakiri R, Yoshimatsu H, Nagafuchi S, Hayashi J, Ishibashi H (1988) Drug-induced allergic hepatitis caused by glycyrrhizin, or extract of licorice root. Acta Hepatol Jap 29:1633–1637
29. Sugiyama T, Sugaya T, Chiba S, Suga M, Yabana T, Yachi A (1992) A case of drug-induced allergic hepatitis by glycyrrhizin. Jap J Gastroenterol 89:1450–1453
30. De Smet PAGM (1991) Drugs used in non-orthodox medicine. In: Dukes MNG, Aronson JK, red. Side Effects of Drugs Annual 15. Elsevier, Amsterdam, pp.514–531
31. Offerhaus L (1987) Metamizol: een honderdjarige treurnis. Ned Tijdschr Geneeskd 131:479–481
32. Traverso HP, Bennett JV, Kahn AJ, Agha SB, Rahim H, Kamil S, Lang MH (1989) Ghee applications to the umbilical cord: a risk factor for neonatal tetanus. Lancet 1:486–488
33. De Smet PAGM (1992) Toxicological outlook on the quality assurance of herbal remedies. In: De Smet PAGM, Hänsel R, Keller K, Chandler RF, red. Adverse Effects of Herbal Drugs. Volume 1. Heidelberg: Springer-Verlag pp.1–72
34. Czygan F-C (1989) Rittersspornblüten. In: Wichtl M, red. Teedrogen. Ein Handbuch für die Praxis auf wissenschaftlicher Grundlage. 2. Auflage. Stuttgart: Wissenschaftliche Verlagsgesellschaft, pp.403–404
35. De Smet PAGM (1993) Legislatory outlook on the safety of herbal remedies. In: De Smet PAGM, Hänsel R, Keller K, Chandler RF, red. Adverse Effects of Herbal Drugs. Volume 2. Heidelberg: Springer-Verlag pp.1–90
36. Hikino H, Yamada C, Nakamura K, Sato H, Ohizumi Y, Endo K (1977) Change of alkaloid composition and acute toxicity of *Aconitum* roots during processing. Yakugaku Zasshi 97:359–366
37. Castot A, Larrey D (1992) Hépatites observées au cours d'un traitement par un médicament ou une tisane contenant de la germandrée petit-chêne. Bilan des 26 cas rapportés aux Centres Régionaux de Pharmacovigilance. Gastroenterol Clin Biol 16:916–922
38. Anonymous (1989) Eosinophilia-myalgia syndrome and L-tryptophan-containing products – New Mexico, Minnesota, Oregon, and New York, 1989. Morbid Mortal Weekly Rep 38:785–788
39. Anonymous (1990) Risk with L-tryptophan. JAMA 263:202
40. Siegers C-P, Von Hertzberg-Lottin E, Otte M, Schneider B (1993) Antrhanoid laxative abuse - a risk for colorectal cancer? Gut 34:1099–1101
41. De Smet PAGM, Vulto AG (1988) Drugs used in non-orthodox medicine. In: Dukes MNG, Beeley L, red. Side Effects of Drugs Annual 12. Elsevier: Amsterdam, pp.402–415
42. Westendorf J, Marquardt H, Poginsky B, Dominiak M, Schmidt J, Marquardt H (1990) Genotoxicity of naturally occurring hydroxyanthraquinones. Mutat Res 240:1–12

43. Siegers C-P (1992) Anthranoid laxatives and colorectal cancer. Trends Pharmacol Sci 13:229–231
44. Mori H, Sugie S, Niwa K, Takahashi M, Kawai K. Induction of intestinal tumours in rats given chrysazin (1985) Br J Cancer 52:781–783
45. Mori H, Sugie S, Niwa K, Yoshimi N, Tanaka T (1986) Carcinogenicity of chrysazin in large intestine and liver of mice. Jpn J Cancer Res (Gann) 77:871–876
46. Mori H, Yoshimi N, Iwata H, Mori Y, Hara A, Tanaka T, Kawai K (1990) Carcinogenicity of naturally occurring 1-hydroxyanthraquinone in rats: induction of large bowel, liver and stomach neoplasms. Carcinogenesis 11:799–802
47. De Smet PAGM (1992) Gezondheidsrisico's van voedingssupplementen. In: Anema PJ, Bemelmans K, Pieters JJL, red. Voedingssupplementen. Aktueel Gezondheidsbeleid 14. Rijswijk: Ministerie van Welzijn, Volksgezondheid en Cultuur, pp.23–34
48. Bruynzeel DP, Van Ketel WG, Young E, Van Joost Th., Smeenk G (1992) Contact sensitization by alternative topical medicaments containing plant extracts. Contact Dermatitis 27:278–279
49. Working Party on Pharmacovigilance (1993) Guideline on adverse reaction reporting by marketing authorisation holders. Draft No.4. Brussels, Committee for Proprietary Medicinal Products, Commission of the European Communities, December 1993
50. Working Party on Pharmacovigilance (1993) Guideline for marketing authorisation holders on periodic drug safety update reports. Draft No.4. Brussels, Committee for Proprietary Medicinal Products, Commission of the European Communities, December 1993
51. Working Party on Pharmacovigilance (1993) Guideline for marketing authorisation holders on on-going pharmacovigilance evaluation during the post-marketing period. Draft No.4. Brussels, Committee for Proprietary Medicinal Products, Commission of the European Communities, December 1993
52. Nightingale SL (1993) Dietary supplement use: significant information in the medical history. JAMA 270:454
53. Kessler DA (1993) Introducing MEDWATCH: a new approach to reporting medication and device adverse effects and product problems. JAMA 269:2765–2768
54. Perharic L, Shaw D, Murray V (1993) Toxic effects of herbal medicines and food supplements. Lancet 342:180–181
55. Perharic L, Shaw D, Colbridge M, House I, Leon C, Murray V. Toxicological problems resulting from exposure to traditional remedies and food supplements. Drug Safety 1994;11:284–94
56. Anonymous (1993) Determining European standards for the safe and effective use of phytomedicines. A concerted action for the Biomedical and health research programme of the European Community. Biomed No: PL 931238

Artemisia Cina

H.J. Woerdenbag, W. Van Uden and N. Pras

Botany

Artemisia cina O.C. Berg et C.F. Schmidt, a member of the Asteraceae family, belongs to the large genus *Artemisia* that comprises over 100 species. Synonyms are *A. cina* Berg, *A. cina* (Berg) Willkomm., and *A. mogoltavica* Poljak [3]. *A. cina* is a shrubby aromatic plant, a xerophyte, growing in semi-desert areas where extremes of temperature, both high and low, prevail. This species prefers a saline sandy soil. *A. cina* is native to the steppe-areas East of the Caspic Sea, in Afghanistan and in the Southern Ural region [1,2]. Vernacular names for *A. cina* are wormwood, levant wormseed (E); Wurmsaat, Zitwersamen, Wurmsamen, Zitwerbeifuß (G); semencine and barbotine (F) [3,4]. The unexpanded flowerheads of the plant have been used medicinally because of the anthelmintic action of santonin (see below), and are known as santonica, Cinae anthodia, semen contra, semen Cinae, Santonica semen, flos Cinae, Zitwersemen and Zitwerblüte [3,5].

In addition to *A. cina*, particularly *A. maritima* (sea mugwort), that is widely distributed all over the northern hemisphere of the Old World, has been used as a source of santonin. Further santonin-containing *Artemisia* species are *A. absynthium*, *A. alba*, *A. brevifolia* Wall., *A. camphorata* Vill., *A. gallica* Willd., *A. kurramensis*, *A. mexicana* Willd. ex Spreng., *A. monogyna*, *A. neo-mexicana* Greene ex Rydb., *A. pauciflora* Weber, and *A. wrightii* Gray [1,6–9].

Chemistry

The main anthelminthic constituent of *A. cina* is the bicyclic sesquiterpene lactone α-santonin (synonyms: santolactone, L-santonin) [4,10]. Other sesquiterpenes, closely related to santonin, are artemisin (8-hydroxysantonin), monogynin (dihydrosantonin), mibulactone, pseudosantonin and desoxypseudosantonin. These compounds are by-products when santonin is extracted [11]. The santonin content of the plant varies considerably between the different seasons of the year [11]. Sesquiterpene lactone contents between 1 and 7% have been reported [3]. *A. cina* is richer in santonin than *A. maritima* [2,12]. From *A. maritima* 0.4 - >1% santonin has been isolated [12]. According to the Deutsches Arzneibuch Ed. 6 (DAB 6) and the Österreichisches Arzneibuch Ed. 9 (ÖAB9) (older pharmacopoeias containing the unexpanded flowerheads of *A. cina* as an official drug) [3,5], these flowerheads should not contain less than 2 or 2.5% santonin, respectively. The santonin contents decrease rapidly after the flowerheads have opened. In other aerial parts of the plant very low santonin concentrations are present, while roots are devoid of this sesquiterpene lactone [6,13].

The unexpanded flowerheads of *A. cina* contain 2–3% essential oil, with cineole as the main constituent. Furthermore, terpineol, pinene and terpinene are present in the oil. In addition, resin-like compounds, fat, pectin, gum, betain, mucilage, cholin and free fatty acids have been found [14].

Pharmacology and Uses

Formerly, santonin has been used extensively as an anthelmintic in the treatment of roundworm (*Ascaris*) infection in doses of 60 to 200 mg daily for 3 days. Santonin does not kill worms in the host organism, but stimulates the muscles of the worms, causing convulsions, thereby expelling them alive from the bowels. This process is facilitated by using a laxative. Against other worms, such as oxyures and taenia, santonin is not effective [1,2]. Low concentrations of santonin have a selective toxic action on the ganglion located in the nerve ring of ascaris [15]. For the anthelmintic properties of santonin the lactone functionality and the oxynaphthalin ring with the angular methyl group are held responsible [1].

Santonin has now been superseded by other anthelmintics because of its potential toxicity [5,16]. The toxicity of santonin might be reduced by administering it together with kainic acid, since lower doses of santonin could then be used to give the same effect [5]. However, kainic acid is known to have neurotoxic effects [17]. A combination of santonin with chenopodium oil has been shown more effective in treating roundworm infections than the individual drugs, given separately [2].

Santonica, the crude drug, has been administered as a decoction or infusion for the expulsion of roundworms and threadworms [18,19]. When using the unexpanded flowerheads, the essential oil is said to support the action of santonin [1]. The crude drug is no longer official.

Pharmacological studies with flowerheads of *A. cina* are not known, because isolated santonin was already available and used as from 1830. However, because of the high santonin contents in the plant material, the same pharmacological and toxicological profile may be expected as for santonin [3].

Dried, unexpanded flowerheads of *A. cina* are also used in homeopathy to treat fever, intestinal worms, intestinal and stomach cramps, and certain central nervous disorders [20,21]. In traditional Chinese medicine, *A. cina* fruits are used under the name 'Heshi' [22].

Santonin (in its α- and β-form) has been found to cause a decrease in the body temperature of rats, made febrile by subcutaneous injection of beer yeast. The decrease was dose-dependent and antagonized by pretreatment with haloperidol. As this agent also opposes the antipyretic activity of dopamine, the investigators suggested that santonin acts on rectal temperature in a way similar to dopamine [23]. Santonin has been used clinically in diabetes, but with little success [15]. Finally, antibacterial activity of santonin has been reported [24].

Pharmacokinetics

After ingestion, santonin is dissolved in the intestine as sodium santoninate, and the greater part is eliminated unchanged in the faeces. A smaller amount is absorbed, oxidized, and the derivatives (especially santogenin) and a coloured product (oxysantonin) are excreted in the urine [15]. After doses of 0.5 g santonin, traces of unchanged santonin have also been found in the urine [25].

Following oral administration of santonin, the absorbed part gives rise to the occurrence of frequent side effects (see below) [4]. In order to reduce the absorption, it is recommended to administer santonin within a few hours after the patient has eaten [13,15], but the effectiveness of this practice remains to be established. Fasting, in contrast, increases absorption [15]. Fats must be excluded from the diet for 12 hours before treatment, because it enhances the absorption of santonin [26].

Poisoning with santonin may not only occur as a result of an excessive single dose, but also when santonin has been administered for too long a period. The elimination of santonin from the body takes place slowly, and it acts as a cumulative poison [27].

After subcutaneous injection, santonin has been found in the small intestine, indicating that part of the santonin that is absorbed from the stomach and intestine is excreted into the bowels [28].

Adverse Reaction Profile

General Animal Data

In mice, the LD_{50} values for santonin are 900 mg/kg for oral application, 130 mg/kg for intraperitoneal injection, and 180 mg/kg for intravenous administration [3].

In the rat, β-santonin has been shown to produce a marked central depressive action [23]. A single oral dose of 0.2 mg/kg bodyweight induced hemolysis in rabbits [3].

General Human Data

Santonin has a narrow therapeutic window [17]. The susceptibility to side effects of santonin varies greatly, with many idiosyncrasies, especially with infants [15]. A lethal dose of santonin in humans of 15 mg/kg body weight, most probably taken orally, has been reported [3].

In children, 60 mg santonin has produced serious poisoning and two such doses have been fatal [18]. In other cases, 180 mg caused only light symptoms, and recovery has occurred after 720 mg. By adults, 0.5 to 1 g and more have been taken without damage [28]. Consumption of almost 10 g flos Cinae has led to a fatal ending after two days [28]. In 1940, autopsy findings of a 21-year-old man who had taken santonin for a longer period (total ingested amount unknown) were published [27]. The body showed great emaciation. The skin was tough and harsh, and of a dull brownish shade, especially over the abdomen. The lungs were healthy. The right side of the heart was slightly dilated but otherwise it was normal. The tongue was furred and brownish in colour; the lips were normal. The oesophagus was whitened and blistered throughout its length and some of the mucous membrane hung in shreds. The stomach was greatly dilated and contained a small amount of milky fluid; the mucous membrane was atrophic and coated with yellow mucus, the cardiac end being blistered like the oesophagus. The duodenum was congested in its first and second parts. The small and large intestines were empty and apparently normal except that the walls were very thin. All other organs were normal [27].

Santonin may cause headache, apathy, profuse sweating, disorders of hearing. Death may occur from cardiac and respiratory failure [2]. After ingestion of santonin painful micturition, albuminuria, hematuria, swelling of the spleen and paralysis of the lowest extremities have been reported [4]. The drug may cause a reduction of the body temperature [20]. Disturbance of taste and smell due to santonin are known [14]. An inadequate dose of santonin may result in migration of the worms into the appendix, biliary tract, etcetera, with inflammatory sequelae [26]. Anticholinesterase action of santonin has been described [26].

An oxidation product of absorbed santonin colours acid urine bright yellow or orange and alkaline urine purplish-red [5].

Allergic Reactions

Artemisia species are wind pollinated and some are important causes of hayfever [29]. However, it seems that up to now *A. cina* has not been specifically associated with such reactions.

Auricular Reactions

Anomalities of hearing occur frequently after intake of santonin, even when there are no other symptoms of poisoning [15].

Central Nervous System Reactions

Santonin acts on the central nervous system (brain, spinal cord), where it causes stimulation of motoric centers [4]. In many individuals santonin causes general restlessness [28]. Large doses may give rise to epileptiform convulsions followed by coma. Santonin may cause hyperemia of the brain, leading to hallucinations, stupefaction, dizziness, giddiness, delirium, mental sluggishness, mydriasis, flood of tears, sickness with vomiting, and abundant secretion of saliva, dyspnoea, and convulsions of the facial muscles [4,20,26].

Dermatological Reactions

Santonin may act as an irritant on mucous membranes [17]. It may produce abnormal nail pigmentation. A yellow colour of the nail plate has been observed after treatment with santonin [30].

Gastrointestinal Reactions

Santonin may cause nausea, vomiting and diarrhoea. Severe irritation and inflammation of the mucosa of the mouth, oesophagus, stomach and small intestine may occur [27,28]. Enhanced bile formation has been reported as a result of ingestion of santonin [4].

Haematological Reactions

The use of unknown amounts of santonin has caused severe haemolytic anemia in a 2.5-year-old negro-girl [3].

Hepatic Reactions

The use of santonin may cause icterus [4].

Ocular Reactions

Poisoning with santonin affects vision. Doses slightly exceeding the normal range cause xanthopsia persisting for some hours, with white objects looking green, blue or yellow. Xanthopsia is an early and characteristic symptom of santonin overdosing [26]. The capacity of seeing in the dim light is also reduced [15]. Santonin-induced xanthopsia is probably caused by an action on the retinal violet receptors, first stimulant, then depressant [5,15,31]. The minimal dose for inducing xanthopsia in one individual has been reported to be 0.2 g santonin [31].

Several cases of temporary blindness due to santonin intoxication are mentioned by Lewin [28].

A relationship between xanthopsia and the excretion of a yellow coloured metabolite of santonin in the urine has been established by Marshall [25].

Toxic doses of santonin may lead to mydriasis, and may thus impair traffic participation [3].

Respiratory Reactions

Fatal respiratory failure is mentioned in a secondary handbook as a symptom of intoxication [32] but this statement is not backed up with a primary reference.

Drug Interactions

There seems to be clinical evidence that santonin combined with kainic acid is more effective in the treatment of ascariasis than santonin alone [5]. Formerly, santonica was combined with a laxative, but when castor oil was used, the side effects became more pronounced because of increased absorption [26,33].

Fertility, Pregnancy, and Lactation

After taking santonin by a pregnant woman at a dose of 0.3–0.5 g in order to induce abortion, the drug could be detected in the fetus 45 min later [3]. The detection of santonin in the fetus could imply that santonin may indeed have been effective as an abortifacient. According to Lewin [28], santonin is excreted into the mothermilk. No further data on a possible effect of santonin on fertility, pregnancy, and lactation could be retrieved from the literature.

Mutagenicity and Carcinogenicity

It is known that a basic structural requirement for high cytotoxicity of sesquiterpene lactones is an exocyclic methylene group, fused to the lactone ring, which has alkylating properties [34]. In santonin, this reactive functionality is absent.

At concentrations between 0.78 and 100 ppm no cytotoxic effects or chromosomal aberrations have been found in in vitro cultured CHO (Chinese Hamster Ovary) cells [3].

Santonin has been found to be efficient as a curing agent in eliminating specifically small, multicopy, relaxed ColE$_1$ group plasmids (pBR322 and pBR329) in *Escherichia coli* strains. This indicates that santonin is, in principle, able to cause changes in the DNA. The mechanism of action on DNA and DNA synthesizing enzymes is as yet unknown [35].

References

1. Steinegger E, Hänsel R (1972) Lehrbuch der Pharmakognosie. 3. Auflage. Berlin: Springer-Verlag, pp 450–451
2. Anonymous (1948) The Wealth of India. A Dictionary of Indian Raw Materials and Industrial Products. Vol. I. New Delhi: Council of Scientific & Industrial Research, pp 121–122
3. Hänsel R, Keller K, Rimpler H, Schneider G, eds. (1992) Hagers Handbuch der Pharmazeutischen Praxis. 5th edn. Vierter Band: Drogen A-D. Berlin: Springer-Verlag, pp 368–370
4. Roth L, Daunderer M, Kormann K (1984) Giftpflanzen - Pflanzengifte. Landsberg, München: Ecomed Verlagsgesellschaft mbH, pp IV-1A, 49–50; IV–3S, 4–5
5. Reynolds JEF, Prasad AB, eds. (1982) Martindale The Extra Pharmacopoeia. 28th edn. London: The Pharmaceutical Press, p 105
6. Younken HW (1948) A Textbook of Pharmacognosy, 6th edn. Philadelphia, Toronto: The Blakiston Company, pp 885–887

7. Kern W, Roth HJ, Schmid W, List PH, Hörhammer L, eds. (1967) Hagers Handbuch der Pharmazeutischen Praxis. Band I. 4th edn. Berlin, Heidelberg, New York: Springer-Verlag, pp 927–932
8. Hoppe HA (1975) Drogenkunde. Band 1. Angiospermen. 8. Auflage. Berlin: Walter de Gruyter, pp 121–125
9. Perez-Souto N, Lynch RJ, Measures G, Hann JT (1992) Use of high-performance liquid chromatographic peak deconvoltion and peak labelling to identify antiparasitic components in plant extracts. J Chromatogr 593: 209–215
10. Moffat AC, Jackson JV, Moss MS, Widdop B, eds. (1986) Clarke's Isolation and Identification of Drugs, 2nd edn. London: The Pharmaceutical Press, p 967.
11. Evans WC (1989) Trease and Evans' Pharmacognosy. 13th edn. London: Ballière Tindall, p 532
12. Gessner O, Orzechowski G (1974) Gift- und Arzneipflanzen von Mitteleuropa. 3. Auflage. Heidelberg: Carl Winter Universitätsverlag, p 261
13. Pratt R, Younken HW (1951) Pharmacognosy. Philadelphia, London, Montreal: J.B. Lippincott Company, p 433
14. Jaretzky R (1949) Lehrbuch der Pharmakognosie. Drogen aus dem Pflanzen und Tierreich. Braunschweig: Friedrich Vieweg & Sohn, pp 355–356
15. Sollmann T (1957) A Manual of Pharmacology and its Applications to Therapeutics and Toxicology. 8th edn. Philadelphia: W.B. Saunders Company, pp. 230–231
16. Tyler VE, Brady LR, Robbers JE (1988) Pharmacognosy, 9th ed. Philadelphia: Lea & Febiger, p 75
17. Steinegger E, Hänsel R (1992) Lehrbuch der Pharmakognosie, 5. Ausgabe. Berlin: Springer-Verlag, pp 167–168; 445
18. Blacow NW, Wade A, eds. (1972) Martindale The Extra Pharmacopoeia. 26th edn. London: The Pharmaceutical Press, p 156
19. Weiß RF (1980) Lehrbuch der Phytotherapie. 6. Auflage. Stuttgart: Hippokrates Verlag, pp 99–100
20. Madaus G (1938) Lehrbuch der Biologischen Heilmittel. Leipzig: Georg Thieme Verlag, pp 988–994
21. Wiesenauer M (1989) Homöopathie für Apotheker und Ärzte. Stuttgart: Deutscher Apotheker Verlag, pp 3/34; 4/38
22. Chen J, Chen C (1991) Some herbal textual comments on tianmingjing (*Carpesium abrotanoides* L.). China J Chin Mat Med 16: 67–99, 125
23. Martín ML, Morán A, Carrón R, Montero MJ, San Roman L (1988) Antipyretic activity of α- and β-santonin. J Ethnopharmacol 23: 285–290
24. Naik U, Mavuinkurve S (1987) α-Santonin 1,2-reductase and its role in the formation of dihydrosantonin and lumisantonin by *Pseudomonas cichorii* S. Can J Microbiol 33: 658–662
25. Marshall W (1927) Santonin excretion and its relation to santonin xanthopsia. J Pharmacol Exp Ther 30: 389–405
26. Osol A, Farrar GE (1955) The Dispensatory of the United States of America. 25th edn. Philadelphia: J.B. Lippincott Company, pp 1211–1212
27. Cookson HA, Stock CJH (1940) Santonin poisoning; a fatal case. Lancet 2: 745
28. Lewin L (1962) Gifte und Vergiftungen. Lehrbuch der Toxikologie. Fünfte, unveränderte Ausgabe. Ulm/Donau: Karl F. Haug Verlag, pp 758–762
29. Mitchell J, Rook A (1979) Botanical dermatology. Plants and plant products injurious to the skin. Greengrass: Vancouver, pp 176–177
30. Ellenhorn MS, Barceloux DG (1988) Medical Toxicology. New York, Amsterdam, London: Elsevier, p 35
31. Marshall W (1927) A study of santonin xanthopsia. J Pharmacol Exp Ther 30: 361–388
32. Wade A, Reynolds JEF, eds. (1977) Martindale The Extra Pharmacopoeia. 27th edn. London: The Pharmaceutical Press, p 111
33. Van Hellemont J (1985) Fytotherapeutisch Compendium. Brussels: APB Wetenschappelijke Dienst, pp 77–78

34. Kolodziej H (1993) Sesquiterpenlactone. Biologische Aktivitäten. Dtsch Apoth Ztg 133: 1795–1805
35. Bharathi A, Polasa H (1990) Elimination of ColE$_1$ group (pBR322 and pBR329) plasmids in *Escherichia coli* by α-santonin. FEMS Microbiol Lett 68:213–216

Aspalathus Linearis

P.A.G.M. De Smet

Botany

Aspalathus linearis (Burm.fil.) R.Dahlgr. belongs to the Fabaceae. Latin synonyms are *Aspalathus contaminatus* Druce, *Aspalathus corymbosus* E. Mey., *Borbonia pinifolia* Marl. and *Psoralea linearis* Burm. The plant is the botanical source of rooibos tea. Some references specify that this tea comes from the subspecies *linearis* [1–3].

To obtain commercial rooibos tea, the young, green shoots are harvested, finely cut, moistened, bruised and placed in heaps to ferment. The material is then sun-dried to a moisture content of 8 to 10%, and course material is removed [2]. During the bruising, the leaves change from green to brick red due to the release of a red pigment from the leaves and stems [4]. Rooibos tea is also called red bush tea, rooibosch tea, rooitea, or red tea in English; it is known as roter Busch Tee or Massai Tee in German [1,5].

Chemistry

Early investigators reported that rooibos tea contains traces of caffeine, but this has not been confirmed by more modern research methods [6]. Theaflavins are also absent [7]. Another difference with ordinary black tea is a low tannin content of 4.4% or less [6].

Koeppen and co-workers [8] isolated 20 g of crude polyphenols from 250 g of dried leaves of *Aspalathus linearis*. In this polyphenolic fraction, they identified the flavone-*C*-glycosides orientin and homo-orientin [8–10], the *C*-glucopyranosyl-dihydrochalcone aspalathin [8,11,12], and the quercetin glycosides isoquercitrin and rutin [8]. Aspalathin was by far the major flavonoid constituent of the fresh plant, but as it is rather unstable, it does not survive the manufacturing process of commercial rooibos tea [13]. Snyckers and Salemi [14] extracted quercetin and luteolin from commercial rooibos tea; the former was by far the major component. A cup of finished rooibos tea yielded an average amount of 1.5 mg of quercetin.

Van Wijk and Verdoorn [15] isolated the quinolizidine alkaloid spartein from *Aspalathus linearis*, but the total alkaloid yield was extremely low (3 µg/g). No evidence was found for the presence of pyrrolizidine alkaloids [15], which are known to occur in other genera (*Crotalaria, Lotononis*) of the tribe Crotalarieae [16].

Vacuum steam distillation of rooibos tea yields approximately 1 mg of volatile oil from 100 g of material. As much as 99 different components have been identified, the major ones being guaiacol (24.0%), 6-methyl-3,5-heptadien-2-one (5.2%), damascenone (5.0%), geranylacetone (4.2%), β-phenylethylalcohol (4.1%), 6-methyl-5-hepten-2-one (4.0%) and 2,4-heptadienal (two isomers, 2.8% and 2.5% respectively) [17].

Rooibos tea also contains ascorbic acid; reported levels vary considerably from 0.16 mg/g to 94 mg/g [1,4]. Brewed rooibos tea can provide 21–27 mg/l of ascorbic acid [18] and 0.14–0.57 mg/l of fluoride [19].

Pharmacology and Uses

Rooibos tea is used as a caffeine-free alternative to ordinary tea, in particular in South Africa, where it constitutes 15% of total tea consumption [7]. A cup of tea brew is normally prepared by adding boiling water to one teaspoon of tea and by steeping for a few minutes. Unlike ordinary tea, the same rooibos tea leaves can be used more than once, without loss of taste and flavour [2].

Rooibos tea allegedly has health giving properties [4], such as improving appetite, calming digestive disorders, reducing nervous tension, and promoting sound sleep [1]. Some sources claim that it has mild spasmolytic as well as anti-allergic properties [3]. Snyckers and Salemi [14] found that an ether extract showed marked acetylcholine and histamine antagonism in the guinea pig ileum, and they identified quercetin as major antispasmodic component. However, there is no clinical evidence for the spasmolytic or anti-allergic usefulness of rooibos tea. In a human study, local application or ingestion of rooibos tea failed to inhibit allergic type I skin reactions in adult volunteers [20].

Yoshikawa et al. [21] studied the anti–oxidant action of a hot water extract from *Aspalathus linearis* in vitro and found evidence to suggest that this extract scavenges superoxide radicals. Sasaki et al. [22] reported that rooibos tea reduced the frequency of chromosomal aberrations induced by mitomycin C and benz(*a*)-pyrene, while Komatsu et al. [23] observed that it suppressed the radiation–induced oncogenic transformation of mouse C3H10T1/2 cells. These findings have raised the suggestion that antioxidant compounds in rooibos tea may have an inhibitory effect on carcinogenesis [23]. It should be noted, however, that after a long series of increasingly optimistic reports about the preventive effects of dietary antioxidants on cancer and cardiovascular disease, recent randomized trials have shown conflicting results. One reason may be that the substantial differences in the biological properties of specific antioxidants are likely to influence their ability to prevent a specific disease [24,25].

An evaluation of repellent activity against German cockroaches (*Blatella germanica*) detected no significant activity for either processed rooibos tea or its vacuum steam distillate [17].

Adverse Reaction Profile

Rooibos tea is claimed to be devoid of undesirable effects and there are no clinical reports of toxicity [1,4,5].

Du Plessis and Roos [26] showed that the number of coliform bacteria in harvested rooibos tea is increased by processing (i.e. cutting, bruising and fermentation). They demonstrated that 40% of 384 batches of processed tea samples were contaminated with *Escherichia coli* type I, and they also recovered *Salmonella enteridis* or *S.lindrick* from three different fermentation heaps. The *Salmonella* bacteria could only be found at the end of fermentation, which indicated that this process increased their number. Treatment of the tea in a 5 mm layer at 99.5° C for 2 min in a steam cabinet effectively reduced coliform numbers, and eliminated *Salmonella greiz* five out of six times.

General Animal Data

According to Snyckers and Salemi [14], an oral LD_{50} of 160 mg/kg has been reported for quercetin. However, they did not see any toxic effects in animals (species not specified) following repeated administration of quercetin in oral doses up to 3 g/kg. When the animals were sacrificed, extensive deposits of unabsorbed material were found in the gastrointestinal tract.

Drug Interactions

Hesseling et al. [18] found that freshly prepared rooibos tea did not significantly affect iron absorption, in contrast to ordinary tea. They gave 200 ml of rooibos tea, ordinary tea or water, immediately after iron ingestion, to three groups of volunteers (each consisting of 10 healthy young men). The mean iron absorption was 7.25%, 1.70% and 9.34%, respectively.

The level of free fluoride in the brewed tea is reduced by the addition of milk [19].

Fertility, Pregnancy and Lactation

No data have been recovered from the literature.

Mutagenicity and Carcinogenicity

Neethling et al. [27] reported that only highly concentrated hot water extracts of rooibos tea (148–260x the normal concentration) showed some mutagenic activity in *Drosophila melanogaster*. These authors concluded that rooibos tea of normal strength is unlikely to have a mutagenic effect.

References

1. Morton JF (1983) Rooibos tea, *Aspalathus linearis*, a caffeineless, low-tannin beverage. Econ Bot 37:164–173
2. Joubert E (1988) Effect of batch extraction conditions on yield of soluble solids from rooibos tea. Int J Food Sci Technol 23:43–47
3. Wannenmacher R (1990) Rooibos – ein Wundertee? Österr Apoth Ztg 44:346–347
4. Cheney RH, Scholtz E (1963) Rooibos tea, a South African contribution to world beverages. Econ Bot 17:186–194
5. Anonymous (1990) Red bush tea. Lawrence Rev Nat Prod, August issue
6. Blommaert KLJ, Steenkamp J (1978) Tannien- en moontlike kafeïeninhoud van rooibostee, *Aspalathus* (subgen. *Norteria*) *linearis* (Burm. fil.) R. Dahlgr. Agroplantae 10:49
7. Joubert E (1990) Chemical and sensory analyses of spray-and freezedried extracts of rooibos tea (*Aspalathus linearis*). Int J Food Sci Technol 25:344–349
8. Koeppen BH, Smit CJB, Roux DG (1962) The flavone C-glycosides and flavonol O-glycosides of *Aspalathus acuminatus* (Rooibos tea). Biochem J 83:507–511
9. Koeppen BH (1962) Flavone C-glycosides: the periodic acid oxidation of orientin and homoorientin tetramethyl ethers. Chem Ind (London), p.2145
10. Koeppen BH (1964) Structure and interrelationship of orientin and homo-orientin. Z Naturforsch B (Anorg Chem, Org Chem, Biochem, Biophys, Biol) 19:173
11. Koeppen BH (1963) Isolation and partial characterization of aspalathin, the principal phenolic constituent of unfermented rooibos tea (*Aspalathus acuminatus*). S Afr J Lab Clin Med 9, 141–142
12. Koeppen BH, Roux DG (1965) Aspalathin: a novel C-glycosylflavanoid from *Aspalathus linearis*. Tetrahedron Lett 39, 3497–3503
13. Anonymous (1970) C-glycosyl compounds in rooibos tea. Food Industries of South Africa 22(april):49
14. Snyckers FO, Salemi G (1974) Studies of South African medicinal plants. I. Quercetin as the major *in vitro* active component of rooibos tea. J South Afr Chem Inst 27:5–7
15. Van Wyk B-E, Verdoorn GH (1989) Alkaloids of the genera *Aspalathus*, *Rafnia* and *Wiborgia* (Fabaceae – Crotalarieae). S Afr J Bot 55:520–522
16. Van Wyk B-E, Verdoorn GH (1990) Alkaloids as taxonomic characters in the tribe Crotalarieae (Fabaceae). Biochem Syst Ecol 18:503–515
17. Habu T, Flath RA, Mon TR, Morton JF (1985) Volatile components of rooibos tea (*Aspalathus linearis*). J Agric Food Chem 33:249–254
18. Hesseling PB, Klopper JF, van Heerden PD (1979) Die effek van Rooibostee op ysterabsorpsie. S Afr Med J 55:631–632
19. Hanekom M, Snyman WD (1982) Fluoride ingestion in tea consumers. J Dent Res 61:606
20. Hesseling PB, Joubert JR (1982) The effect of rooibos tea on the type I allergic reaction. S Afr Med J 62:1037–1038
21. Yoshikawa T, Naito Y, Oyamada H, Ueda S, Tanigawa T, Takemura T, Sugino S, Kondo M (1990) Scavenging effects of Aspalathus linealis (Rooibos tea) on active oxygen species. Adv Exp Med Biol 264:171–174
22. Sasaki YF, Yamada H, Shimoi K, Kator K, Kinae N (1993) The clastogen-suppressing effects of green tea, Po-lei tea and Rooibos tea in CHO cells and mice. Mutat Res 286:221–232
23. Komatsu K, Kator K, Mitsuda Y, Mine M, Okumura Y (1994) Inhibitory effects of Rooibos tea, *Aspalathus linealis*, on X-ray-induced C3H10T1/2 cell transformation. Cancer Lett 77:33–38
24. Hennekens CH, Buring JE, Peto R (1994) Antioxidant vitamins - benefits not yet proved. N Engl J Med 330:1080–1081
25. Hankinson SE, Stampfer MJ (1994) All that glitters is not beta carotene. JAMA 272;1455–1456

26. Du Plessis HJ, Roos IMM (1986) Recovery of coliforms, *Escherichia coli* type I and *Salmonella* species from rooibos tea (*Aspalathus linearis*) and decontamination by steam. Phytophylactica 18:177–181
27. Neethling HS, Theron HE, Geerthsen JMP (1988) Die mutagenisiteit van rooibostee. S Afr J Sci 84:278–279

Citrullus Colocynthis

P.A.G.M. De Smet

Botany

Citrullus colocynthis (L.) Schrad. belongs to the Cucurbitaceae or squash family. The plant is cultivated in Europe for ornamental purposes. Vernacular names are colocynth, bitter gourd, bitter apple, and bitter cucumber (English); Koloquinthe (German); and coloquinte (French). The principal medicinal part of the plant is the fruit pulp [1,2].

Chemistry

Phytochemical investigations have shown that various parts of the colocynth contain cucurbitacins. Darwish-Sayed et al. [3] reported the presence of cucurbitacins B, E, I, and L and their glycosides in the fruit pulp, fruit peel, seeds, stem, and leaves and the presence of cucurbitacin E in free and glycosidal form in the roots. They found the highest level of cucurbitacin E glycoside (= α-elaterin glycoside) in the fruit pulp (0.21%) and the lowest concentration in the roots (0.05%). Müller and Auterhoff [4] studied ripe and unripe seeds and recorded cucurbitacin concentrations of 2.2% and 9.1%, respectively, corresponding to 2.8% and 12% of cucurbitacin glycoside. This suggests that the cucurbitacin content of fruit material, from which the seeds have not been removed, will vary depending on ripeness. Hatam et al. [5] obtained four cucurbitacin glycosides from the dried fruit and identified them as the 2-O-β-D-glucopyranosides of cucurbitacin E, cucurbitacin I, (22-27)-hexanorcucurbitacin I, and cucurbitacin L. Contrary to previous studies, they could not recover free cucurbitacin aglycones, which is in accordance with the reported absence of elaterase, the enzyme capable of hydrolysing the glycosides. Gamlath et al. [6] described the isolation of cucurbitacins I, J and T from the fruit of *Colocynthis vulgaris* (= *Citrullus colocynthis*).

Darwish-Sayed et al. [7] isolated choline and two unidentified alkaloids from various plant parts; a third alkaloid was detected only in the fruit pulp, seeds, leaves and roots.

Heptacosan-1-ol, hentriacontane, n-octacosanol, 1,26-hexacosan-diol and sterols have been found in the fruit [8-10], and the fruit peel reportedly contains alkanes, an aliphatic unsaturated ketone, free hydroxyl and carbonyl compounds, docosan-

1-ol acetate, 10,13-dimethylpentadec-13-en-1-al, 11,14-dimethyl-hexadecan-14-ol-2-one and 10,14-dimethyl-hexadecan-14-ol-2-one [9,11-13].

Reported oil contents of the seeds vary from 13% to 36%; in one study, colocynth seeds yielded 26.6% of oil, together with 52.9% of crude fiber and 13.5% of protein, on a dry weight basis [14]. The crude seed oil was found to consist mainly of triglycerides and yielded free fatty acids, phospholipids and sterols as minor fractions. Further analysis of the fatty acid methyl esters revealed that the degree of unsaturation was over 75%, and the oil showed relatively low peroxide values upon storage [15]. The chemistry of protein from Nigerian colocynth seeds was studied in detail by King and Onuora [16-18]. According to Sawaya et al. [14], the protein of colocynth seeds has an adequate content of essential amino acids. Two ribosome-inactivating glycoproteins, named colocin 1 and colocin 2, are present in the seeds in trace amounts of 5 and 4 mg per 50 g, respectively [19]. The aromatic constituents of the roasted seeds have been characterized by Soliman et al. [20].

Pharmacology and Uses

The fruit pulp has been primarily applied as a powerful laxative, producing copious watery evacuations within 2-3 hours [21]. However, it has been superseded now by less drastic and less toxic purgatives [1,2,22]. In the nineteenfifties, the fruit was suggested to possess antitumour potential [8,23] but follow-up studies appear to be unavailable. The fruits are used for purgation and various other purposes in traditional Arab medicine [24,25] and Ayurvedic medicine [26, 27]. In the Sudan, the plant serves as a purgative and as an insecticide [28], and Sahelian nomads employ tar prepared from colocynth seeds to flavour drinking water, as a preservative, and as a topical traditional medicine for camels and humans [29].

The cucurbitacins are held responsible for the cathartic effect [2]. According to Banerjee and Dandiya [27], the purgative properties of α-elaterin-2-D-glucopyranoside (= coloside A) are only apparent upon oral ingestion and not after intraperitoneal administration. These authors were unable to demonstrate a spasmogenic effect of coloside A on isolated rabbit intestine or guinea pig ileum. Coloside A produced a negative chronotropic and a negative inotropic effect on isolated mammalian and amphibian hearts but in dogs doses up to 5 mg/kg intravenously had no effect on the heart in situ or on blood pressure.

The colocins which occur in the seeds belong to a group of glycoproteins, which inhibit protein synthesis by inactivating ribosomes in a catalytic manner and which modify rRNA in a similar manner as the A-chain of ricin [19].

Colocynth seeds are under investigation as a possible source of edible oil and protein [14-18]. The seeds are reported to be heavily consumed by humans in some African countries [14]. For instance, they are popular in Egypt as a roasted edible substitute for nuts [20]. In Nigeria, the seed kernel has traditionally been used as the basis for soups and stews, in which it performs thickening, emulsifying, fat binding and flavouring functions [16,18].

Pharmacokinetics

Early textbooks claim that colocynth is excreted by the kidneys [21,30,31], but it is unclear how this was established.

Adverse Reaction Profile

General Animal Data

Shah et al. [24] evaluated the acute and chronic toxicity of an alcoholic extract of the colocynth fruit in mice. Single oral doses of 0.5-3 g/kg produced mortality rates of 40-100%. Death was preceded by stimulation, piloerection, increased motor activity, tremors, convulsions, diarrhoea and rapid irregular respiration. Treatment with daily oral doses of 0.1 g/kg body weight for 3 months killed 45% of the animals. Among the observed signs and symptoms were inflammation in the hind leg, hind paw and tail, eye lesions, leucocytosis, and spermatotoxicity.

Weber et al. [32] reported that dietary feeding of powdered colocynth seeds to weanling mice produced 100% mortality within 5 days.

Ickert [33] treated rats for 4 weeks with a herbal product prepared from colocynth fruit, quince apple, buckthorn bark and sage leaves. Daily doses corresponding to 1.3 or 6.5 mg/kg of colocynth extract (i.e. 10 and 50 times the recommended human dose, respectively), did not produce evidence of systemic toxicity.

Sawaya et al. [14,15] performed feeding trials with colocynth seed preparations in chicks from day 1 until day 19 to 21 of their lives. At a dietary level of 15%, a colocynth seed meal (prepared by extracting the seeds with petroleum ether at 60-80° C and then drying under a hood for 2 days) significantly depressed body weight and feed efficiency, but dietary feeding of 5-10% of the seed oil or 5-20% of the whole seeds did not compromise growth.

Sheep treated with daily oral doses of 1-10 g/kg of fresh colocynth fruits died after 5 hours to 25 days, whereas sheep fed with daily amounts of 0.25-10 g/kg of fresh colocynth leaves succumbed after 4 hours to 15 days. The main signs of poisoning were diarrhoea, dyspnoea, anorexia, and loss of condition. Necropsy examinations revealed areas of haemorrhages and congestion in the kidneys, lungs, heart, liver and gall bladder as well as catarrhal enteritis. Major histopathological changes were fatty cytoplasmic vacuolation of the centrilobular hepatocytes, the cells of the renal tubules and some cardiac muscle fibers. Also observed were congestion of the hepatic sinusoids and of the renal and cardiac vessels and pulmonary alveolar capillaries [28]. Similar results were obtained by feeding colocynth fruits to Nubian goats and Zebu calves, the latter being less susceptible than the former [34].

When colocins and other ribosome-inactivating proteins were administered intraperitoneally to mice in lethal doses, necrotic alterations in the liver were the main histological finding [19].

General Human Data

Colocynth pulp has a narrow therapeutic window, with therapeutic doses ranging from 0.12 to 0.3 g and 0.6-1 g already constituting a toxic dose. Although 15 g was reputedly survived, 3-4 g could be fatal [22,30,31,35,36]. The intake of 0.6-1 g has been associated with gastrointestinal pain, watery or bloody stools with tenesmus, vomiting, increased diuresis and later urinary retention, and a weak pulse. Larger doses of 2 g or more may cause weakness, fainting, sensory disturbances, dizziness, fear, and raving, which can be followed by circulatory collapse and finally by death [35].

Central Nervous System Reactions

Confusion and loss of consciousness can be clinical signs of colocynth poisoning [2,36].

Dermatological Reactions

When colocynth was still a component of brilliantine and of denaturated spirits frequently used by hairdressers, eczema localised on hairdresser's hands could sometimes be traced to this ingredient [37-39].

Gastrointestinal Reactions

Berrut et al. [2] described a 61-year-old woman who developed a reversible acute colitis (presenting as abdominal cramps and bloody diarrhoea) and confusion after the accidental ingestion of colocynth instead of zucchini. Goldfain et al. [40] reported acute colitis in three Moroccan men who had taken milk mixed and incubated with colocynth fruit pulp for the ritual purpose of purification and vitalisation. Dysenteric diarrhoea, abdominal pain and deshydration developed 8-12 hours after ingestion and resolved within 3-6 days. Colonoscopy revealed congestion and hyperaemia of the colonic musoca with abundant exudates but without ulceration or pseudopolyp formation. Colonic biopsies showed erosions with fibrino-purulent exudate, early fibrosis of the lamina propria, and hyaline thickening of the superficial epithelial basal membrane. On the 15th day after the colocynth ingestion, the colonic mucosa had almost returned to normal in all three cases.

Rawson [41] reported on cathartic colon (characterized sigmoidoscopically by a pale, oedematous mucosa) in four women with a long history of ingestion of a vegetable laxative that contained a colocynth extract. Podophyllin resin was among the other ingredients of the product, however, and this substance is believed to have been an important cause of carthartic colon following laxative abuse [42].

Haematological Reactions

Leucocytosis has been observed in animal experiments [24,28, 34] as well as in a human case [43].

Hepatic Reactions

Hepatotoxicity has been observed in animal experiments (see the section on general animal data). There is one human case reported from Sweden, in which a 20-year-old woman developed a reversible icterus some days after the ingestion of approximately 50 ml of a composite colocynth tincture to induce abortion [43]. The tincture consisted of Fructus Anisi stellati (1 part), Fructus Colocynthidis (10 parts), and Spiritus concentratus (100 parts) [44].

Nasal Reactions

Powdered colocynth pulp causes severe pain if it comes into contact with the nasal mucous membrane [22,39].

Ocular Reactions

The dried fruit pulp is irritating to the eye [39].

Renal Reactions

Renal toxicity has been observed in animal experiments [43] (see also the section on general animal data). Moeschlin [36] reproduces a case where a woman who had taken a colocynth decoction for suicidal purposes suffered not only from transient loss of consciousness, bloody diarrhoea, and abdominal cramps but also from an oliguria that lasted for 4 days.

Fertility, Pregnancy and Lactation

In Ayurvedic medicine, the fruit pulp has a reputation of causing miscarriage, when administered to pregnant women [27], and colocynth has also been used for this purpose in Europe [35,43]. Such activity could arise indirectly from congestion in the pelvic region as a manifestation of the cathartic action [27]. It should be added, however, that on several occasions colocynth was ineffective as an abortive agent, even though it produced serious poisoning [35]. To see whether the pulp contained a principle with direct uterus-stimulating properties, Banerjee and Dandiya [27] tested the effects of α-elaterin-2-D-glucopyranoside on the isolated rat uterus. The compound did not produce any contractions in concentrations up to 0.1

mg/ml and it failed to alter the responses produced by uterine stimulants, such as oxytocin and ergometrine.

An ethanolic extract of colocynth seeds, administered at an oral dose of 200 mg/kg for 2 days, did not inhibit copper acetate induced ovulation in rabbits to such an extent that further research seemed warranted [45]. Prakash et al. [26] screened different colocynth extracts for anti-implantation activity by feeding female rats with each extract from day 1 to day 7 of their pregnancy. Acetone and methanolic root extracts in doses of 150 mg/kg prevented implantation in 3 and 4 of 7 test animals, respectively, whereas 200 mg/kg of an ethanolic leaf extract and 150 mg/kg of a benzene leaf extract inhibited implantation in 4 of 6 rats.

Shah et al. [24] observed spermatotoxicity in mice treated with an alcoholic extract of colocynth fruit in daily oral doses of 0.1 g/kg body weight for 3 months.

Early textbooks claim that colocynth is excreted into breast milk, and should therefore not be given to nursing women [21,30,31]. It is unclear, however, whether this was established in a reliable way.

Mutagenicity and Carcinogenicity

To screen for cytotoxic activity, Shah et al. [25] treated mice for 5 days with an ethanolic extract of colocynth fruit in daily oral amounts of 500 mg/kg. This treatment significantly increased mitotic activity and the percentage of chromosomal aberrations in the bone marrow cells of the mice, which suggested that colocynth may represent a mutagenic hazard.

The colocynth seed tar which is traditionally used by Sahelian nomads contains a large number of polycyclic aromatic hydrocarbons, including known carcinogens such as benzo(*a*)pyrene, benz(*a*)anthracene, benzo(*b*)fluoranthene and benzo(*j*)fluoranthene. A dose-related carcinogenic activity has been observed after chronic epicutaneous application of the tar to mouse skin. This implies that the traditional preparation and application of colocynth seed tar may entail the risk of cancer development [29].

References

1. List PH, Hörhammer L (1973) Hagers Handbuch der Pharmazeutischen Praxis. Vierte Neuausgabe. Vierter Band. Chemikalien und Drogen (Cl-G). Berlin: Springer-Verlag, pp.79–83
2. Berrut C, Bisetti A, Widgren S, Tissot J-D, Loizeau E (1987) Colite pseudomembraneuse causée par l'ingestion de coloquinte. Schweiz Med Wschr 117:135138
3. Darwish-Sayed M, Balbaa SI, Afifi MS (1974) The glycosidal content of the different organs of *Citrullus colocynthis*. Planta Med 26:293–298
4. Müller R, Auterhoff H (1968) Über Inhaltsstoffe der pharmazeutisch verwendeten Koloquinthen. Dtsch Apoth Ztg 108:1191–1192
5. Hatam NAR, Whiting DA, Yousif NJ (1989) Cucurbitacin glycosides from *Citrullus colocynthis*. Phytochemistry 28:1268–1271
6. Gamlath CB, Gunatilaka AAL, Alvi KA, Atta-Ur-Rahman, Balasubramaniam S (1988) Cucurbitacins of *Colocynthis vulgaris*. Phytochemistry 27:3225–3229

8. Faust RE, Cwalina GE, Ramsted E (1958) The antineoplastic action of chemical fractions of the fruit of *Citrullus colocynthis* and Sarcoma-37. J Am Pharm Assoc Sci Ed 47:1–5
9. Hussein Ayoub SM, Yankov LK (1981) On the constituents of the peels of *Citrullus colocynthis* - Part 1. Fitoterapia 52:9–12
10. Hatam NAR, Whiting DA, Yousif NJ (1990) Lipids and sterols of *Citrullus colocynthis*. Int J Crude Drug Res 28:183–184
11. Hussein Ayoub SM, Yankov LK (1981) On the constituents of the peels of *Citrullus colocynthis* - Part 2. Fitoterapia 52:13–16
12. Hussein Ayoub SM, Yankov LK (1981) On the constituents of the peels of *Citrullus colocynthis* - Part 3. Fitoterapia 52:17–18
13. Hussein Ayoub SM, Yankov LK (1981) On the constituents of the peels of *Citrullus colocynthis* - Part 4. Fitoterapia 52:19–20
14. Sawaya WN, Daghir NJ, Khalil JK (1986) *Citrullus colocynthis* seeds as a potential source of protein for food and feed. J Agric Food Chem 34:285–288
15. Sawaya WN, Daghir NJ, Khan P (1983) Chemical characterization and edibility of the oil extracted from *Citrullus colocynthis* seeds. J Food Sci 48:104–106,110
16. Onuora JO, King RD (1984) Thermal transitions of melon (colocynthis citrullus) seed proteins. Food Chem 13:309–316
17. King RD, Onuora JO (1984) Aspects of melon seed protein characteristics. Food Chem 14:65–77
18. King RD, Onuora JO (1984) Effect of processing factors on some properties of melon seed flour. J Food Sci 49:415–418
19. Bolognesi A, Barbieri L, Abbondanza A, Falasca AI, Carnicelli D, Battelli MG, Stirpe F (1990) Purification and properties of new ribosome-inactivating proteins with RNA N-glycosidase activity. Biochim Biophys Acta 1087:293–302
20. Soliman MA, El Sawy AA, Fadel HM, Osman F, Gad AM (1985) Volatile components of roasted *Citrullus colocynthis* var. *colocynthoides*. Agric Biol Chem 49:269–275
21. Osol A, Farrar GE (1955) The Dispensatory of the United States of America. 25th edn. Philadelphia: J.B. Lippincott Company, pp.359–360
22. Blacow NW, Wade A, red. (1972) Martindale The Extra Pharmacopoeia. 26th edn. London: The Pharmaceutical Press, p.1627–1628
23. Belkin M, Fitzgerald DB (1952) Tumor-damaging capacity of plant materials. I. Plants used as cathartics. J Nat Cancer Inst 13:139–149
24. Shah AH, Qureshi S, Tariq M, Ageel AM (1989) Toxicity studies on six plants used in the traditional Arab system of medicine. Phytother Res 3:25–29
25. Shah AH, Tariq M, Ageel AM, Qureshi S (1989) Cytological studies on some plants used in traditional Arab medicine. Fitoterapia 60:171–173
26. Prakash AO, Saxena V, Shukla S, Tewari RK, Mathur S, Gupta A, Sharma S, Mathur R (1985) Anti-implantation activity of some indigenous plants in rats. Acta Eur Fertil 16:441–448
27. Banerjee SP, Dandiya PC (1967) Smooth muscle and cardiovascular pharmacology of α–elaterin-2-D-glucopyranoside glycoside of *Citrullus colocynthis*. J Pharm Sci 56:1665–1667
28. Elawad AA, Abdel Bari EM, Mahmoud OM, Adam SEI (1984) The effect of Citrullus colocynthis on sheep. Vet Hum Toxicol 26:481–485
29. Habs M, Jahn SAA, Schmähl D (1984) Carcinogenic activity of condensate from coloquint seeds (*Citrullus colocynthis*) after chronic epicutaneous administration to mice. J Cancer Res Clin Oncol 108:154–156
30. Anonymous (1941) The Extra Pharmacopoeia - Martindale. 22th edn. Volume 1. London: The Pharmaceutical Press, p.450
31. Sollmann T (1957) A Manual of Pharmacology and its Applications to Therapeutics and Toxicology. 8th edn. Philadelphia: W.B. Saunders Company, p.216
32. Weber CW, Berry JW, Philip T (1977) Citrullus, Apodanthera, Cucurbita, and Hibiscus seed protein. Food Technol 31:182–183

32. Weber CW, Berry JW, Philip T (1977) Citrullus, Apodanthera, Cucurbita, and Hibiscus seed protein. Food Technol 31:182–183
33. Ickert G (1979) Zur Toxikologie der Koloquinthe (*Citrullus colocynthis* L.). Zentralbl Pharm 118:1159–1166
34. Barri MES, Onsa TO, Elawad AA, Elsayed NY, Wasfi IA, Abdul Bari EM, Adam SEI (1983) Toxicity of five Sudanese plants to young ruminants. J Comp Pathol 93:559–575
35. Lewin L (1962) Gifte und Vergiftungen. Lehrbuch der Toxikologie. Fünfte unveränderte Ausgabe. Ulm/Donau: Karl F. Haug Verlag, pp.722–723
36. Moeschlin S (1972) Klinik und Therapie der Vergiftungen. 5. Auflage. Stuttgart: Georg Thieme Verlag, p.418
37. Haxthausen H (1930) Fall von Koloquintemekzem. Dermatol Wschr 91:1391
38. Tulipan L (1938) Cosmetic irritants. Arch Dermatol Syph 38:906–917
39. Mitchell J, Rook A (1979) Botanical dermatology. Plants and plant products injurious to the skin. Greengrass: Vancouver, p.237
40. Goldfain D, Lavergne A, Galian A, Chauveinc L, Prudhomme F (1989) Peculiar acute toxic colitis after ingestion of colocynth: a clinicopathological study of three cases. Gut 30:1412–1418
41. Rawson MD (1966) Cathartic colon. Lancet 1:1121–1124
42. Müller-Lissner SA (1993) Adverse effects of laxatives: fact and fiction. Pharmacology 47 (Suppl.1):138–145
43. Hammarsten G, Lindgren G (1941–43) Ein Fall von Koloquinten-Vergiftung. Vergiftungsfälle 12, A919, 107–110
44. Anonymous (1901) Svenska Farmakopén (Pharmacopoea Svecica, Ed.VIII). Stockholm: Kungl. Boktryckeriet P.A. Norstedt & Söner, p.327
45. Vohora SB, Khan MSY, Afaq SH (1973) Antifertility studies on Unani herbs. Part 2. Antiovulatory effects of '*hanzal*', '*halun*', '*kalonji*' and '*sambhalu*'. Indian J Pharm 35:100–102

Fucus Vesiculosus and Allied Brown Algae

I.H. Bowen and I.J. Cubbin

Botany

The term 'fucus' was originally used in a non-specific sense to describe the higher algae [1]. This has led to misleading accounts in the literature whereby several distinct genera have been referenced under the same term. A considerable amount of the botanical confusion can be traced to one of the commercial uses of these algae, viz : the production of kelp, which is the residue obtained after drying and incineration [2]. Since different botanical sources have been used to produce kelp over three centuries, in attempts to obtain higher yields of iodine, bromine, potassium and sodium salts, it is not surprising that taxonomic difficulties have arisen [3]. Accordingly, this monograph includes those products which have been used medicinally, but excludes the Rhodophyta (red seaweeds) and the lichen *Cetraria islandicus*, commonly referred to as Iceland moss but which has been known as fucus in Europe [4].

Within the family Fucales, the species which have been most commonly used in medicine are *Fucus vesiculosus* L., which is known as bladderwrack, but which has also been referred to as cut-weed, black-tang, kelp-ware and *Quercus marina* [5]; *F. serratus* L., the blackwrack; *F. spiralis* L.; and *Ascophyllum nodosum* LeJol. (formerly *F. nodosum* L.), the knobbed-wrack. These seaweeds are small plants 30–100 cm long, the thallus being flat and branching dichotomously. The branches all lie in the same plane and are approximately 2 cm wide. The thallus is attached to the rock by a cord-like portion, the base of which is expanded into a disc [6]. All of these algae grow on the shore-line within the tidal range and are frequently referred to in the United States as 'rockweeds' to distinguish them from the larger brown algae, e.g. *Macrocystis pyrifera* (L.) C.Ag. which are there termed 'kelps' [7]. The other family of the Phaeophyta which is of importance is the Laminariaceae. Three species are commonly used, namely, *Laminaria digitata* (Huds.) Lamour, the seagirdle or sea-tangle; *L. cloustoni* Edm. and *L. saccharina* (L.) Lamour. These are collectively known as kelps in Europe. They are olive-green to brown in colour and grow up to 4 m in length, although they are commonly between 1–2 m. They consist of a stalk attached to the rocks by a branching basal portion and carrying a large flattened thallus which is a single leafy frond in *L. saccharina*, but consists of several fronds in the other species. They can thrive up to a depth of 10 fathoms although they are commonly found near low water mark [8]. Japanese seaweeds of the genus *Laminaria*, principally *L. japonica* Aresch.

(Japanese: Makombu), *L. ochotensis* (Rishirikombu or Hosome–kombu) and *L. longissima* (Nagakombu), are sometimes encountered in western health food stores for use in macrobiotic diets [9–11].

Chemistry

There have been several investigations into algal constituents and a number of reviews are available in the literature [12, 13]. This section is confined to those compounds which are thought to exert some therapeutic action. Brown algae all contain chlorophylls and α– and β-carotene, the brown colouring being due to the presence of the xanthophyll, fucoxanthin [14].

The various species all contain phycocolloids, which are polysaccharide complexes forming colloids when dispersed in water; the amount and composition of these compounds varying with geographical source and reproductive stage of the seaweed, as well as with the season and presence and type of pollutants in the environment [15]. Alginic acid, algin or alginate is a complex mixture of varying amounts of guluronic and mannuronic acids and forms the major constituent of cell walls in most Phaeophyta, occurring to the extent of 15–35% dry weight in *L. saccharina* and up to 40% in *L. digitata*, both of which are commercial sources [16]. Fucoidan which is a high viscosity polysaccharide, containing between 30–70% of L-fucose, is also widely distributed, forming 6–8% in *A. nodosum*, 9–11% in *Fucus* species and between 5–20% in Laminariaceae. Ascophyllan, which is similar to fucoidan, represents 6% in *A. nodosum* and *F. spiralis*. Laminaran (1–3 β-glucan) which exists in both a soluble and insoluble form is found only in the fronds and not the stipes of *Laminaria* and other brown algae. In *L. saccharina*, it is present up to 33%. All of these are the storage polysaccharides for the seaweeds [17].

Brown seaweeds contain up to 3% of lipids, which are mainly highly unsaturated fatty acids. Included in this fraction are the sterols, the most common being fucosterol, first isolated from *F. vesiculosus*, but which is now known to be widely distributed. Cholesterol is also a frequent constituent. Fucinic acid has been isolated from *A. nodosum* [18]. In addition, sugar alcohols, of which mannitol is the most common, are present up to 20–30% in some species. Volatile oils, tannins and a large variety of vitamins have also been reported [7].

The constituents of kelp, and its yield, are very variable, the usual yield obtained being 4–10% of the dry weight of seaweed used. Kelp was formerly the principal source of sodium carbonate (present at approximately 5%), and was also used to obtain potassium salts, in particular the sulphate (10%) and the chloride (20%). The development as a source of iodine came later, and it was always a low yield. Drift weed kelp, obtained from *Laminaria* species yields up to 0.8% iodine whilst cut-weed kelp (from *Fucus* species) gives a maximum of 0.2% [19]. Muller et al. [20], in a comparative study of *Fucus vesiculosus*, *F. serratus*, *F. spiralis* and *Ascophyllum nodosum*, found that *A. nodosum* contained more alginic acid (29.9% vs 23.5–26.3%) and iodine (0.07% vs 0.02–0.03%) than the *Fucus* species, but less total mineral and potassium [20]. The iodine content of kelp tablets can vary considerably, even within the same brand [21] and it may decline on storage.

Tablets from surface layers of packages contained as little as 200 mg/kg of iodine compared with as much as 2500 mg/kg in tablets from the lower layers. After one and a half years storage no iodine could be detected [22]. In the Japanese brown seaweeds, iodine content varied from 0.012% to 0.26% [9,10,23,24]. *Macrocystis pyrifera* is the source for at least one Dutch kelp product, which is said to contain 0.2 mg iodine per tablet [25].

The ability of algal polysaccharides to form complexes with heavy metal ions, and thus concentrate them, is well-known, and is being investigated as a possible environmental marker to monitor marine pollution [26]. It should be borne in mind that it is possible for seaweed products to contain more than trace amounts of elements such as lead, arsenic, cadmium and mercury, and that the possibility of the presence of radioisotopes should not be excluded [9,27-29].

Pharmacology and Uses

Algae have enjoyed a long usage in the materia medica of Europe and Asia (the Chinese employing them at least 4000 years ago) particularly in coastal areas, and it is not surprising that claims for their efficacy are diverse and sometimes contradictory. The main uses of seaweeds have traditionally involved them as gelling agents in foods, as applications and decoctions in rheumatism and in the control of obesity; this last use being attributable to the iodine content which makes the oral preparations effective where weight gain is due to hyperthyroidism (see endocrine reactions below). French authorities appear to accept the use of fucus as an aid to slimming [30] and as a laxative [31] but medicinal uses are not, apparently, accepted by German authorities [32]. The literature does not provide convincing evidence for the use of seaweed products as weight control agents [33,34] with rare exceptions where overweight is due to an iodine deficiency which is reversed by the iodine content of the product [35].

Fucus species have been prescribed for prophylactic use against sclerosis, against scrofulosis and goitre, and to reduce plasma cholesterol levels [36]. Recent screening has shown that they possess some antifungal and antibacterial activity [37]. *Laminaria*, which is an important dietary principle in Japan, has been implicated in the low level of breast cancer in the Japanese, particularly post-menopausal women, where the incidence is only 11% of that in the USA and Britain [38]. In traditional Japanese medicine, *Laminaria* has been used as an antihypertensive, whilst in China it is employed for the treatment of menstrual disorders. Its use on the Indian subcontinent has been in the treatment of syphilis [39]. *Laminaria* tents have been widely employed in gynaecological operations. *Laminaria* tents (0.4 cm diameter, 6 cm length) have been inserted into the cervical canal to induce pretreatment dilatation of the cervix during terminations in both the first and second trimester [40,41]. These have been found to be as effective as prostaglandin pretreatment, and caused fewer gastrointestinal disturbances [42]. It has been shown that this pretreatment is reversible, and that normal term pregnancy can continue without side effects once the tents are removed [43]. This same pretreatment has been used to remove myomas without recourse to hysterectomy or myomectomy [44].

Alginates from *Fucus* and *Laminaria* have been widely employed in several areas of formulation. The rapid hydration of alginic acid has enabled the production of tablets with high disintegration rates, whilst other alginates have shown useful controlled release properties. Most commercial dental impression powders now use alginate salts because of their high strength, elasticity and dimensional stability [45].

Alginates also have a haemostatic action and have lately found application in wound management [46], particularly for ulcers and surgical lesions, where their ability to absorb moisture and still retain their structure has meant that wounds are prevented from drying out; healing is then enhanced [47].

The use of a widening variety of seaweed preparations in foods and health food supplements, e.g. kelp tablets, has increased the exposure of the population to algal metabolites, and it is to be expected that further reports of both beneficial and toxic effects will appear in the literature if this trend continues.

Adverse Reaction Profile

General Human Data

Few references have been recovered from the literature on the general toxicity of seaweeds. Relevant information has been incorporated into the sections below. Since this monograph focuses on iodine-containing kelp products, however, it will be useful to consider iodine toxicity generally.

The WHO has recommended dietary levels of 0.10–0.14 mg iodine/day for an adult [48] which compares with the French requirement that adult daily iodine exposure should not exceed 0.12 mg [31]. The Joint FAO/WHO Expert Committee on Food Additives considers that 1 mg/day or less of iodine is probably safe for the majority of people but may cause adverse effects in some individuals. In considering safety, the Committee has set a provisional maximum tolerable daily intake of 1 mg of iodine (0.017 mg/kg body weight) from all sources [48]. The average western diet provides up to 0.3–0.4 mg/day of iodine [49,50], which implies that any iodine from non-dietary sources should be restricted to a maximum of 0.6–0.7 mg/day. Some currently available kelp preparations may exceed such a limit [21].

The effects of seaweed can be considered in two categories viz: extra- and intra-thyroidal. The extrathyroidal effects, which one would expect to find in sensitive individuals exposed unknowingly to the compounds, include allergenic reactions such as oedema, iodine fever and eosinophilia. It is also possible for cutaneous iodism to manifest itself as well as transitory inflammation of both the parotid and sub-maxillary glands which is usually referred to as "iodine mumps" [51,52]. The intrathyroidal effects are more serious, and include thyroiditis, hypothyroidism and thyrotoxicosis (see Endocrine Reactions). Becker et al. [53], in a report of the use of iodine as a thyroidal blocker to prevent uptake of radioactive iodine in the event of a reactor accident, summarized both extrathyroidal and intrathyroidal effects of higher than normal doses of iodine. These are summarized in Table 1, but it must be emphasised that iodine levels even from iodine-rich

Table 1. Extrathyroidal and intrathyroidal effects of iodine [53]

Dose level	Extrathyroidal effects	Intrathyroidal effects
Low (< 25 mg/day)	Ioderma, periarteritis, dermatitis herpatiformis, and allergies such as oedema and nasal polyps (all rare)	Iodide-induced thyrotoxicosis
High (50–500 mg/day)	Sialadenitis (iodide mumps), iodide fever (rare)	Iodide goitre and/or hypothyroidism
Very High (> 1 g/day)	Upper GIT disturbances	Thyroiditis (rare)

dietary sources and supplements such as seaweed products are unlikely to be higher than the lower end of the "low dose" range quoted in the table.

The adverse reaction potential of relatively low doses of iodine is supported by case reports. A 24-year-old woman developed thyroid goitre after taking a proprietary blood mixture, which included 0.4–0.5 mg/day of iodine, for three months. The thyroid gland reduced after withdrawal of the iodine preparation but some swelling was still evident after 1 year possibly due to a gland defect which made her susceptible to iodide goitre [54]. Thyroid autoantibodies developed in patients given 0.15–0.3 mg of potassium iodide per day. It is not known how long the autoantibodies persist or whether or not they are harmful [55]. In a group of patients with pre-existing conditions characterized by the presence of autonomous thyroid tissue, maintained on a daily supplement of 0.5 mg iodide per day over a period of 3–10 months, modified thyroid function was observed in several subjects by measurement of PBI values and thyroxine levels which indicated hyperthyroidism. Clinical symptoms of hyperthyroidism did not appear until several months later [56]. These finding are similar to those of Livadas et al. [57], where supplementation was in the range 0.1–0.4 mg iodine per day, and of Paul et al. [58], who investigated the effects of supplements of 0.1–1.0 mg/day. It would appear that the vast majority of the population can tolerate relatively large amounts of iodine in the diet but adverse effects may rarely be encountered in a small number of susceptible subjects (see also the section on endocrine reactions).

The presence of arsenic in seaweed and kelp preparations, and the associated toxicology, has been discussed by De Smet [59]. Studies of levels of urinary arsenic have indicated that considerable elevation can occur in patients who routinely selfadminister kelp supplements [60]. Most of the arsenic in the seaweeds is present in a bound form and has not been shown to give rise to the toxicity problems associated with inorganic arsenic. Urinary levels of arsenic were found to return to normal within 90 days of cessation of the supplements. The tolerable daily intake of inorganic arsenic is 0.002 mg/kg body weight [61]. Norman et al. [21] found that the total daily intake of arsenic from kelp products varied according to manufacturer's recommended dosage and the source of the kelp. In one instance, an Australian brand gave rise to an intake of 1.6 mg/day (bound form) [21]. Inorganic arsenicals are established human carcinogens and their presence in foods and food additives needs to be monitored [62–64]. In the United States, arsenicals are listed as risky substances only under 'inorganic substances' and not under 'organic substances'. This is supported by work of Sabbioni et al. [65], who investigated the carcinogenic potential of seafood arsenic and found that the main form, arsenobetaine, failed to induce cytotoxic effects or neoplastic transformations. The carcinogenic potential of the organoarsenic substances would appear to be negligible (see also the section on mutagenicity and carcinogenicity].

Severe dyserythropoiesis and autoimmune thrombocytopenia in a 54-year-old woman was attributed to arsenic ingestion of 2.2 µg arsenic daily from a six-week course of vitamin and kelp tablets with a calcium supplement. Withdrawal of the kelp product followed by treatment with intravenous immunoglobulin, prednisolone and azathioprine reversed the condition [66].

Cardiovascular Reactions

There are only sparse references in the literature to cardiac activity although several workers have carried out screening procedures [67,68] and various other marine organisms have shown cardiac activity. The amino acid laminine (trimethyl-(5-amino-5-carboxypentyl)-ammonium) which is commonly found in these genera is known to be weakly hypotensive [69].

Work by a Japanese group on commercial preparations of *Laminaria* species has resulted in the isolation of histamine. Attempts to isolate it from authenticated samples have been unsuccessful, despite acid digestion to release bound forms of the compound. The commercial samples exhibited a hypotensive activity equivalent to 0.02 mg/kg histamine [70]. Fatty acids with a stimulant effect on the frog heart and histamine dihydroiodate, which caused acceleration of the guinea pig atrium, have been isolated from "nekombu", a Japanese member of the Laminariaceae [71].

Dermatological Reactions

There are many references in the literature to contact dermatitis due to swimmers touching seaweeds. In all cases these have been shown to be toxic rather than allergenic reactions and usually they refer to the blue-green alga *Lyngbya majuscala*, which is outside the scope of this monograph [72,73]. It is, however, well-known that halides can exacerbate pre-existing acne and other related acneiform conditions and the presence of iodine and bromine within seaweed preparations may cause pustular inflammation of previously well-controlled cases. Harrell and Rudolph reported two cases of kelp tablet supplements producing such a reaction [74].

Endocrine Reactions

These arise from the presence of iodine in the seaweeds, and in particular in kelp preparations. Iodine is known to exert an effect on the thyroid gland and the literature is well supplied with reviews on the subject [75,76]. American estimates suggest that between 1–3% of the population is iodine-sensitive, and the increasing popularity of kelp diets as slimming aids has produced a greater incidence of reports of adverse reactions [77]. Effects on the thyroid gland include thyroiditis, hypothyroidism and hyperthyroidism (thyrotoxicosis or Jod-Basedow). Thyroiditis, which is a painful enlargement of the thyroid gland, usually subsides rapidly with discontinuation of the iodine-containing compounds. This condition has frequently been reported in Japan where seaweed is part of the staple diet [10,24,78,79] and occasionally the iodine-induced thyroiditis may be accompanied by immunological changes [78]. The other two conditions may take rather longer to reverse.

Thyrotoxicosis is more usually encountered when exogenous thyroid hormone is ingested, and of 147 cases investigated by Fradkin and Wolff [80], only 3 were found to be related to seaweed and these are included below. The risk of iodine-induced hyperthyroidism is more frequent in areas where there is iodine deficiency [53] and comparisons have been made of incidence of endemic goitre in people groups from areas where there is mandatory iodine prophylaxis and from areas where no iodine prophylaxis programme currently exists [81]. Seasonal variations in dietary iodine may also affect the prevalence of thyrotoxicosis [49]. Transient thyrotoxicosis, thought to be iodine-induced due to excessive intake of Japanese kombu, has been reported in Japan [82]. Two Japanese women, aged 42 and 59 years, developed thyrotoxicosis one month and one year respectively, after ingestion of foods containing 28–140 mg/day of iodine calculated from their daily diet. Both patients had abnormal levels and ratios of the normal thyroid hormones, and high concentrations of serum inorganic iodine. Thyrotoxic signs and symptoms disappeared and hormone levels returned to normal one month after removal of kombu from their diets.

De Smet et al. [83] reported a case where a patient ingested six tablets with 200 mg of kelp each on a daily basis to lose weight. After two months she had developed hyperthyroidism, which remitted on discontinuation of the tablets [83]. Another patient admitted to hospital because of goitre and hypothyroidism was discovered to have been taking six seaweed tablets per day for a prolonged period of time, during which she had ingested "a few mg of iodine daily". Initial symptoms (2 years earlier) of hyperthyroidism were thought to be hyperthyroid episodes of chronic thyroiditis, the thyroiditis possibly being the result of iodine-induced hypothyroidism [22]. A 35-year-old woman with a pre-existing thyroid disorder developed hypothyroidism and enlargement of multinodular goitre following the daily use of two kelp tablets [84]. A 38-year-old female patient who ingested four seaweed tablets per day over a 2–3 year period (estimated iodine intake was 1–2 mg daily) developed hyperthyroidism and goitre. There was spontaneous remission of both goitre and the hyperthyroidism on discontinuation of the source of excess iodine. This case illustrates that iodine-induced hyperthyroidism can occur even when neither iodine deficiency nor goitre pre-exist [85]. Similarly, in a 72-year-old woman without pre-existing thyroid disease, ingestion of kelp tablets caused hyperthyroidism which had disappeared 6 months after stopping the tablets [86]. Two male patients aged 36 and 52 years developed thyrotoxicosis after ingesting 2–10 mg/day of iodine for 2–12 months in the form of a seaweed preparation. All clinical and biochemical symptoms had returned to normal 11 weeks after withdrawal of the seaweed preparation. No evidence of pre-existing thyroid abnormality was found but both had a family history of thyroid disease which might indicate a latent abnormality in their glands [87]. It would appear that kelp-induced hyperthyroidism, therefore, may occur in the absence of a pre-existing thyroid disorder [85–87], whereas hypothyroidism has only been reported in patients with an underlying thyroid disease [22,84]. Poor remission rates in patients receiving antithyroid drugs for the treatment of Graves disease (diffuse toxic goitre) were attributed to high levels of dietary iodine [88] and it may be more difficult to control Graves disease with antithyroid preparations if patients are concurrently (and perhaps inadvertently) ingesting higher than normal levels of iodine [89], whether from their diet or from a non-dietary source such as kelp.

Haematological Reactions

Considerable work has been carried out on algal extracts in relation to their effect on erythrocytes. Ferreiros and Criado [90] isolated and characterized a lectin-type agglutinin from *Fucus vesiculosus* which produced powerful agglutination in sheep erythrocytes. They also found that the same compound had an immunomodulatory effect in mice. It was able to stimulate lymphocytes, possibly working as a polyclonal activator, although it did not agglutinate them [91]. Human erythrocytes were unaffected by this. Rogers and Loveless [92] reported strong hemagglutination with the polyphenol fraction rather than the lectin fraction of extracts of *Fucus* species.

A crude fucoidan from the edible brown seaweed *Laminaria religiosa* was found to have anticoagulant and fibrinolytic activities and also to inhibit platelet aggregation if injected prior to blood drawing. A significant inhibition of tumour growth (Sarcoma-180) in mice was also noted [93].

Dyserythropoiesis and autoimmune thrombocytopenia associated with the presence of arsenic in kelp supplements has already been mentioned in the section on general human data [66].

Drug Interactions

Both amiodarone and benziodarone have been used in the management of angina pectoris, but amiodarone is nowadays used in the treatment of tachycardia associated with Wolff-Parkinson-White syndrome, whilst benziodarone is sometimes used as a uricosuric. They contain respectively 37.2% and 46% by weight of iodine and the usual dosage range is 0.2–1.2 g/day. It has been shown that a 300 mg dose of amiodarone gives rise to 9 mg of free iodine per day [94]. The drug has a half life in excess of 5 days and there is a danger of iodine-induced thyrotoxicosis [95]. This risk could obviously be increased if these or other iodine-containing drugs were taken in conjunction with seaweed products rich in iodine, but since most non-dietary kelp products will add less than 1 mg/day of iodine the additional effect of the kelp will be minimal.

Lithium carbonate potentiates the hypothyroid action of iodides and iodide-containing products should be avoided by patients receiving lithium carbonate therapy [96].

Fertility, Pregnancy and Lactation

No information has been recovered from the literature concerning the effect of *Fucus* or related algae on fertility.

It is known that iodine can cross the placenta and there are cases of goitre and hypothyroidism in infants born to mothers taking iodides during pregnancy. Martindale cites a Collaborative Perinatal Project report from 1977, where, of the 50,282 children studied, 489 had been exposed to halides through their mothers. Four children had cateracts [97].

Independent confirmation of possible teratogenicity has not been recovered from the literature. Although there are no reports on seaweed, it would seem prudent to avoid iodine-rich preparations during pregnancy.

Iodides appear to be concentrated in breast milk and it would be a wise precaution for nursing mothers to discontinue seaweed preparations from their diets while they are feeding their children [98].

Mutagenicity and Carcinogenicity

The available literature does not suggest carcinogenic effects, and on the contrary, anticarcinogenic effects have been reported.

Ohno [99] has reported a tentative link between reduced incidence of prostate carcinoma in men aged 50–70 years and seaweed ingestion. He unsuccessfully attempted to establish the causal agent as β-carotene. Similarly the findings of Teas [38] have indicated that low levels of breast carcinoma in post-menopausal women may be linked to the *Laminaria* intake in the rural Japanese diet. She has published experimental work on rats in support of this theory [100].

It has been reported by Yamamoto et al. [101,102] that Sarcoma-180 cells in mice and mammary tumours in rats are inhibited by dietary seaweed. Yamamoto et al. [103] also performed partial purification of the seaweeds and worked with a crude fucoidan extract which led them to propose that in sulphated polysaccharides, e.g. laminaran, the ester sulphate content might be the determining factor as to whether or not the compounds cause tumour inhibition. An antitumour fucoidan, active against Sarcoma-180, has also been isolated from *Fucus* species [93,104].

As discussed under general human data, there is no concrete evidence that organoarsenic constituents of seaweeds have carcinogenic potential [65].

References

1. Grieve M (1974) A Modern Herbal. London: Jonathan Cape, pp.111–114
2. Kraemer H (1920) Scientific and Applied Pharmacognosy. London: Chapman and Hall Ltd, pp.5–8
3. Levring T, Hoppe HA, Schmid OJ (1969) Marine Algae – a survey of research and utilization. Hamburg: Cram de Gruyter & Co. pp.5–22
4. Frohne D (1989) Tang. In: Wichtl M, red. Teedrogen. Ein Handbuch fur die Praxis auf wissenschaftlicher Grundlage. 2. Auflage. Stuttgart: Wissenschaftliche Verlagsgesellschaft, pp.483–484
5. Anonymous (1986) British Herbal Pharmacopoeia. London: British Herbal Medical Association, p.89
6. Wallis TE (1960) A Text Book for Pharmacognosy. 4th ed. London: Churchill, pp.284–286
7. Hoppe HA, Levring T, and Tanaka Y, red. (1979) Marine Algae in Pharmaceutical Science. New York: Walter de Gruyter, pp.28–85
8. Newton L (1931) A Handbook of British Seaweeds. London: British Museum Press, pp.202–204
9. Luten JB (1983) Spoorelementen in voor de consumptie bestemde zeewieren. Voeding 44:232–236
10. Wolff J (1967) Iodide goiter and the pharmacologic effects of excess iodide. Am J Med 47:101–124
11. Ohsawa G (1971) Macrobiotics, an invitation to health and happiness. San Francisco: G Ohsawa Macrobiotic Foundation
12. Glombitza K-W, Koch M (1989) Secondary metabolites of pharmaceutical potential. In: Cresswell RC, Rees TAV, Shah N, red. Algal and Cyanobacterial Biotechnology. Harlow: Longman, pp.101–238
13. Baker JT (1984) Seaweeds in pharmaceutical studies and applications. Hydrobiologia 116/117:29–40
14. Trease GE, Evans WC (1983) Pharmacognosy. 12th ed. Eastbourne: Balliere Tindall, pp.158–159
15. Matveega EG (1986) Changes in the basic photosynthetic pigment contents of *F.vesiculosus* and *C.glomerata* under the influence of petrochemical products. Dokl Bolg Akad Nauk 39:133–136
16. Cardinal A, Breton-Provencher M (1977) Variations de la tenour en acide alginique des laminariale de l'estuaire maritime du Saint-Laurent. Botanica Marica 20:243–245
17. Ordin CG, Greenwood Y, Hail FJ, Patterson IW (1985) The rumen microbiology of seaweed digestion in Orkney sheep. J Appl Bacteriol 59:585–596
18. Springer R, Middendorf L (1961) Acid functions of several algae polysaccharides. Arch Pharm 294:693–699
19. Newton L (1931) A Handbook of British Seaweeds. London: British Museum Press, p.IX
20. Muller D, Carnat A, Lamaison JL (1991) Comparative study of *Fucus vesiculosus*, *Fucus serratus* L. and *Ascophyllum nodosum* Le Jolis. Plantes Med Phytother 5:194–201
21. Norman JA, Pickford CJ, Sanders TW, Waller M (1987) Human intake of arsenic and iodine from seaweed based food supplements and health foods available in the UK. Food Add Contam 5:103–109
22. Liewendahl K, Turula M (1972) Iodine-induced goitre and hypothyroidism in a patient with chronic lymphocytic thyroiditis. Acta Endocrinol (Copenh) 71:289–296
23. Funazo K, Tanaka M, Morita K, Kamino M, Shono T (1986) Pentafluorobenzyl-p-toluenesulfonate as a new derivatizing reagent for electron-capture gas chromatographic determination of trace inorganic anions. J Chromatogr 354:259–267
24. Suzuki H, Higuchi T, Sawa K, Ohtaki S, Horiuchi Y (1965) "Endemic coast goitre" in Hokkaido, Japan. Acta Endocrinol (Copenh) 50:161–176

25. De Lang AC (1993) Anders beter worden volgens de inzichten van A. Vogel. 9e druk. Utrecht: Kosmos, p.496
26. Baxter MS, Aston SR (1983) Deep ocean radioactive waste disposal. An evaluation of the seaweed critical pathway. Health Physics 45:139–144
27 Sharp GJ, Samant HS, Vaidya OC (1988) Selected metal levels of commercially valuable seaweeds adjacent to and distant from point sources of contamination in Nova Scotia and New Brunswick. Bull Environ Contam Toxicol 40:724–730
28. Ray S, McLeese DW, Burridge LE, Waiwood BA (1980) Distribution of cadmium in marine biota in the vicinity of Belledure. In Can Tech Rep Fish Aquat Sci 963:12–27
29. Bowen IH, Cubbin IJ, Sharpe DJ (1990) A survey of uses of seaweeds, and an investigation of arsenic levels in British seaweed species. Unpublished results. Undergraduate research project, School of Health Sciences, University of Sunderland
30. Thromm S (1987) Leitfaden fur Hersteller zur Formulierung von Zulassungsantragen für Arzneispezialitäten auf pflanzlicher Basis. Pharm Ind 49:1264–1274
31. Anonymous (1989) Leitfaden fur Hersteller von Phytopharmaka mit abführender Wirkung, die Gegenstand eines vereinfachten Zulassungsverfahrens sein können. Pharm Ind 51:858–863
32. Anonymous (1990) Monographie: Fucus (Tang). BAnz nr.101 from 01.06.1990
33. Bjorvell H, Roessner S (1987) Longterm effects of commonly available weightreducing programmes in Sweden. Int J Obes 11:67–71
34. Hayes Jr AH, Schweiker RS (1982) Weight control drug products for over-the-counter human use; establishment of a monograph. Fed Reg 47:8466–8484
35. Tyler VE (1987) The New Honest Herbal. A sensible guide to herbs and related remedies. 2nd edn. Philadelphia: George F. Stickley Company, pp.139–140
36. Reiner E, Topliff J, Wood JD (1962) Hypocholesterolemic agents derived from sterols of marine algae. Can J Biochem Physiol 40:1401–1406
37. Biard JF, Verbist JF, et al (1980) Seaweeds of the French Atlantic coast with anti-bacterial and anti-fungal compounds. Planta Medica (Suppl):136–151
38. Teas J (1983) The dietary intake of *Laminaria*, a brown seaweed, and breast cancer prevention. Nutr Cancer 4:217–222
39. Chopra RN, Nayer SL, Chopra IE (1956) Glossary of Indian Medicinal Plants. New Delhi: Council of Scientific & Industrial Research New Delhi, p.149
40. Blumenthal PD (1988) Prospective comparison of DILAPAN and *Laminaria* for pre-treatment of the cervix in 2nd-trimester abortion. Obst Gyn 72:243–246
41. Herczeg J, Sas M, Szabo J, Vajda GY (1986) Pre-evacuation dilation of the pregnant uterine cervix by *Laminaria japonica*. Acta Med Hung 43:145–154
42. Krishna U, Gupta AN, HoKei Ma, et al. (1986) Randomised comparison of different prostaglandin analogues and *Laminaria* tent for pre-operative cervical dilation. Contraception 34:237–251
43. Van Le L, Darney PD (1987) Successful pregnancy outcome after cervical dilation with multiple *Lamanaria* tents in preparation for 2nd-trimester elective abortion – a report of two cases. Am J Obst Gyn 156:612–613
44. Goldrath MH (1957) Vaginal removal of the pedunculated submucous myoma: the use of *Laminaria*. Obst Gyn 70:670–672
45. McDowell RH (1986) Properties of Alginates. 5th Ed. London: Kelco International
46. Barnett AH, Odugbesan O (1988) Seaweed based dressings in the management of leg ulcers and other wounds. Intensive therapy and clinical monitoring, Unpublished data
47. Gilchrist T, Martin AM (1983) Wound treatment with Sorbsan – an alginate fibre dressing. Biomaterials 4:317–320
48. Anonymous (1989) Evaluation of certain food additives and contaminants. 33rd Report of the Joint FAO/WHO Expert Committee on Food Additives. Technical Report Series 776. Geneva: World Health Organisation, pp.32–33
49. Nelson M, Phillips DI (1985) Seasonal variations in dietary iodine intake and thyrotoxicosis. Hum Nutr Appl Nutr 1985; 213–216

50. Van Dokkum W, De Vos RH, Muys Th, Wesstra JA (1989) Minerals and trace elements in total diets in The Netherlands. Br J Nutr 61:7-15
51. Peacock L, Davison H (1958) Observations of iodide sensitivity. Ann Allergy 16:158
52. Talbot JM, Fisher KD, Carr CJ (1976) FDA 223-75-2090. Bethesda, Maryland: Life Sciences Research Office, Federation of American Societies for Experimental Biology, p.11
53. Becker DV, Braverman LE, Dunn JT, et al. (1984) The use of iodine as a thyroidal blocking agent in the event of a reactor accident. Report of the Environmental Hazards Committee of the American Thyroid Association. JAMA 252:659-661
54. Dimitriadou A, Fraser R (1961) Iodine goitre. Proc Royal Soc Med 54:345-346
55. Koutras DA, Karaiskos KS, Evangelopoulou K, et al. (1986) Thyroid autoantibodies after iodine supplementation. In: Drexhage HA, Wiersinga WM, red. The thyroid and autoimmunity. Amsterdam: Elsevier Science Publishers, pp.211-212
56. Ermans AM, Camus M (1972) Modifications of thyroid function induced by chronic administration of iodide in the presence of "autonomous" thyroid disease. Acta Endocrinol (Copenh) 70:463-475
57. Livadas DP, Koutras DA, Souvatzoglou A, Beckers C (1977) The toxic effects of small iodine supplements in patients with autonomous thyroid nodules. Clin Endocrinol (Oxford) 7:121-127
58. Paul T, Meyers B, Witorsch RJ, Pino S, Chipkin S, Ingbar SH, Braverman LE (1988) The effect of small increases in dietary iodine on thyroid function in euthyroid subjects. Metabolism 37:121-124
59. De Smet PAGM (1991) Toxicological outlook on the quality assurance of herbal remedies. In: De Smet PAGM, Hänsel R, Keller K, Chandler RF, red. Adverse Effects of Herbal Drugs. Volume 1. Heidelberg: Springer-Verlag pp.1-72
60. Walkin O, Douglas DE (1974) Health food supplements prepared from kelp – a source of elevated urinary arsenic. Can Med Assoc J 111:1301-1302
61. Anonymous (1981) Environmental Health Criteria 18. Arsenic. Geneva: World Health Organisation
62. Anonymous (1987) Arsenic and arsenic compounds. IARC Monographs. Suppl 7:100-106
63. Ahmed FE, Hattis D, Wolke RE, Steinman D (1993) Risk assessment and management of chemical contaminants in fishery products consumed in the USA. J Appl Toxicol 13:395-410
64. Anonymous (1989) Evaluation of certain food additives and contaminants. 33rd eport of the Joint FAO/WHO Expert Committee on the Food Additives. Technical Report Series 776. Geneva: World Health Organisation, pp.27-28
65. Sabbioni E, Fischbach M, Pozzi G, Pietra R, Gallorini M, Piette JL (1991) Cellular retention, toxicity and carcinogenic potential of seafood arsenic. I. Lack of cytotoxicity and transforming activity of arsenobetaine in the BALB/3T3 cell line. Carcinogenesis 12:1287-1291
66. Pye KG, Kelsey SM, House IM, Newland AC (1992) Severe dyserythropoiesis and autoimmune thrombocytopenia associated with ingestion of kelp supplements. Lancet 339:1540
67. Carlyle RF (1968) The occurrence of catecholamines in sea anemone *Actinia equina*. Br J Pharmacol 36:182P
68. Searl PB, Norton TR, Lum BKB (1981) Study of a cardiotonic fraction from an extract of the seaweed *Undaria pinnatifida*. Proc West Pharmacol Soc 24:63-65
69. Ozawa H, Gomi Y, Otsuki H (1967) Pharmacological studies on laminine monocitrate. Yakugaku Zasshi 87:935-939
70. Funayama S, Hikino H (1981) Hypotensive principle of *Laminaria* and allied seaweeds. Planta Med 41:29-33
71. Kosuge T, Nukaya H, Yamamoto T, Tsuji K (1983) Isolation and identification of cardiac principles from *Laminaria*. Yakugaku Zasshi 103:683-685
72. Izumi AK, Moore RE (1987) Seaweed (*Lyngbya majuscula*) dermatitis. Clin Dermatol 5:92-100

73. Sims JK, Zandee Van Rilland RD (1981) Escharotic stomatitis caused by the stinging seaweed *Microleus lyngbyaceus* (formerly *Lyngba majuscula*). Hawaii Med J 40:743–748
74. Harrell BL, Rudolph AH (1976) Kelp diet: a cause of acneiform eruption. Arch Derm 112:560
75. WHO Study Group on Endemic Goitre (1953) Final report. Bull WHO 9:293
76. Wolff J (1976) Iodine homeostasis. In: Klein E, Reinwein D, red. Regulation of thyroid function. Stuttgart: Schattauer Verlag, pp.65–78
77. Anonymous (1975) Kelp diets can produce myxedema in iodide-sensitive individuals. JAMA 273:9–10
78. Okamura K, Inoue K, Omae T (1978) A case of Hashimodo's thyroiditis with thyroid immunological abnormality after habitual ingestion of seaweed. Acta Endocrinol 88:703–712
79. Tajiri J, Higashi K, Morita M, Umeda T, Sata T (1986) Studies of hypothyroidism in patients with high iodine intake. J Clin Endocrinol Metab 63:412–417
80. Fradkin JE, Wolff J (1983) Iodide-induced thyrotoxicosis. Medicine (Baltimore) 63:1–20
81. Subcommittee for the Study of Endemic Goitre and Iodine Deficiency of the European Thyroid Association (1985) Goitre and iodine deficiency in Europe. Lancet i:1289–1293
82. Ishizuki Y, Yamauchi K, Miura Y (1989) Transient thyrotoxicocis induced by Japanese kombu. Fol Endocrinol Jap 65:91–98
83. De Smet PAGM, Stricker BHCh, Wilderink F, Wiersinga WM (1990) Hyperthyreoïdie tijdens het gebruik van kelptabletten. Ned T Geneeskd 134:1058–1059
84. Leemhuis MP, Quarles van Ufford (1980) Jodium-struma en hypothyreoïdie tijdens het gebruik van een zeewierpreparaat. Ned T Geneesk 124:1119
85. Liewendahl K, Gordin A (1974) Iodine-induced toxic diffuse goitre. Acta Med Scand 196:237–239
86. Shilo S, Hirsch HJ (1986) Iodine-induced hyperthyroidism in a patient with a normal thyroid gland. Postgrad Med J 62:661–662
87. Skare S, Frey HMM (1980) Iodine induced thyrotoxicosis in apparently normal thyroid glands. Acta Endocrinol (Copenh) 94:332–336
88. Wartofsky L (1973) Low remission after therapy for Graves disease. Possible relation of dietary iodine with antithyroid therapy results. JAMA 226:1083–1088
89. Hall R, Lazarus JH (1987) Changing iodine intake and the effect on thyroid disease. Br Med J 294:721–722
90. Ferreiros CM, Criado MT (1983) Purification and partial characterisation of a *Fucus vesiculosus* agglutinin. Rev Espan Fisiol 39:51–60
91. Criado MT, Ferreiros CM (1983) Immunomodulatory effect produced in mice by a complex carbohydrate specific lectin-like muco-polysaccharide from *Fucus vesiculosus*. IRCS Med Sci 11:286–287
92. Rogers DJ, Loveless RW (1985) Haemagglutinins of the Phaeophyceae and non-specific aggregation phenomena by polyphenols. Botanica Marina 28:135–137
93. Maruyama H, Nakajima J, Yamamoto I (1987) A study on the anticoagulant and fibrinolytic activities of a crude fucoidan from the edible brown seaweed *Laminaria religiosa*, with special reference to its inhibitory effect on the growth of Sarcoma-180 ascites cells subcutaneously implanted into mice. Kitasata Arch Exp Med 60:105–121
94. Broekhuysen J, Larvel R, Sion R (1969) Recherches dans la serie de benzofurannes. Études comparée du transit et du metabolisme de amiodarone chez diverses espèces animales et chez l'homme. Arch Int Pharmacodyn 177:340
95. Anonymous () British National Formulary. London: British Medical Association and The Pharmaceutical Press, p.66
96. Li Wan Po A (1982) Non Prescription Drugs. Oxford: Blackwell Scientific Publications p.7
97. Reynolds JEF, red. (1989) Martindale: The Extra Pharmacopoeia. 29th ed. London: The Pharmaceutical Press, p.1184
98. Briggs GG, Freeman RH, Yaffe SJ (1986) Drugs in Pregnancy and Lactation. 2nd ed. Baltimore: Williams and Wilkins, pp.364–365

99. Ohno Y, Yoshida O, Oishi K, Okada K, Yamabe H, Schroeder FH (1988) Dietary beta-carotene and cancer of the prostate: a case-control study in Kyoto, Japan. Cancer Res 48: 1331–1336
100. Teas J, Harbison ML, Gelman RS (1984) Dietary seaweed (*Laminaria*) and mammary carcinogenesis in rats. Cancer Res 44:2758–2761
101. Yamamoto I, Maruyama H, Takahashi M, Komiyama K (1986) The effect of dietary or intraperitoneally injected seaweed preparations on the growth of Sarcoma-180 cells subcutaneously implanted into mice. Cancer Lett 30:125–131
102. Yamamoto I, Maruyama H, Moriguchi M (1987) The effect of dietary seaweeds on 7,12-dimethyl-benz(a)anthracene-induced mammary tumorgenesis in rats. Cancer Lett 35:109–118
103. Yamamoto I, Takahashi M, Suzuki T, Seino H, Mori H (1984) Antitumour effect of seaweeds IV. Enhancement of antitumour activity by sulphation of a crude fucoidan action from *Sargassum kjellmannianum*. Jap J Exp Med 54:143–151
104. Chida K, Yamamoto I (1987) Antitumour activity of a crude fucoidan prepared from the roots of kelp (*Laminaria* species). Kitasato Arch Exp Med 60:33–39

Ginkgo Biloba

H.J. Woerdenbag and T.A. Van Beek

Botany

Ginkgo biloba L. belongs to the Ginkgoaceae family and is the only living representative of the Ginkgoales. Other plants of this order became extinct in the past few million years and are only known as fossils. Before the 18th century, *G. biloba* was solely represented in East Asia. Nowadays this tree is rather commonly distributed in temperate regions of the northern hemisphere [1-5].

Incorrect Latin synonyms for *G. biloba* are *Salisburia adiantifolia* Smith and *Pterophyllus salisburiensis* Nelson [6,7]. Vernacular names include maidenhair tree (English), Elefantenohr, Fächerblattbaum, Japanbaum (German), noyer du Japon, arbre aux quarante écus (French), ginkyo (silver apricot) (Japanese) and yin-hsing (silver apricot), ya chio (duck's foot), pei kuo (white fruit), kung sun shu (grandfather-grandson tree) (Chinese) [8,9].

Seeds of *G. biloba* have been and are still used in Chinese traditional medicine. Nowadays acetone-water extracts from ginkgo **leaves** take a prominent place in phytotherapy in several western countries, especially in Germany and France [3,10,11].

Chemistry

In the leaves of *G. biloba* a large number of different metabolites has been identified [8,12-14]. Characteristic compounds for this species are found among the terpenoids and flavonoids. Ginkgolides are irregularly built methylmononorditerpene trilactones with a bitter taste. They consist of six five-membered rings, in a cage-shaped configuration, and possess as the only natural products so far a tert-butyl group. Naturally occurring ginkgolides include ginkgolide A, B, C, J, and M (root only), which differ in the number and position of their hydroxyl groups [15-17]. These substances are also termed BN 52020, BN 52021, BN 52022, BN 52024, and BN 52023, respectively [18]. Besides in leaves, ginkgolides have also been found in the root bark of the tree [15]. In addition, a characteristic sesquiterpene trilactone (cage) molecule, named bilabolide, has been isolated from the leaves [19,20] and from the roots [21]. Dried leaves contain between 0.000% and 0.50% ginkgolides and between 0.005% and 0.4% bilobalide [21-26].

Flavonoids are abundant in ginkgo leaves. Nearly 40 different structures have been identified so far [12,27-35]. They include catechins (e.g. (epi)catechin, (epi)gallocatechin), dehydrocatechins (proanthocyanidins, prodelphinidin), flavones (e.g. luteolin, delphidenone (tricetin), delphidenone glucoside), and biflavones (e.g. (iso)ginkgetin, amentoflavone, bilobetin, sciadopitysin). The flavonols may occur as aglycones or as mono-, di-, and triglycosides, and are in some cases esterified with coumaric acid [36,37]. In most cases, they can be regarded as derivatives of the aglycones kaempferol, quercetin or isorhamnetin [36]. The total concentration of flavonol glycosides varies from 0.5-1% [37,38].

Further constituents of ginkgo leaves are 2-hexenal (the main volatile component), steroids (sitosterol, sitosterol glycoside, stigmasterol), polyprenols, simple organic acids (shikimic, chlorogenic, vanillic, p-hydroxybenzoic, protocatechuic, quinic, ascorbic and p-coumaric acid), long-chain benzoic acid derivatives (ginkgolic acids), long-chain phenols, lower aliphatic acids, carbohydrates (glucose, fructose, saccharose, as well as water- and alkali-soluble polysaccharides with low and high molecular weight), cyclitols (pinitol, sequoyitol), straight-chain hydrocarbons, alcohols and ketones, (Z,Z)-4,4'-(1,4-pentadiene-1,5-diyl)diphenol, the nitrogen containing 6-hydroxykynurenic acid, cytokinine, β-lecitine, and carotenoids [2,5,8,11,29-52].

From the heartwood of the ginkgo tree the sesquiterpene bilobanone, E- and Z-10,11-dihydroatlantone, E-10,11-dihydro-6-oxo-atlantone, β- and γ-eudesmol, and elemol have been isolated [53-55].

Seeds of *G. biloba* contain 38% carbohydrates, 4.3% proteins and 1.7% fat [56]. The lipid fraction is mainly composed of neutral lipids, but polar lipids and glycolipids are present as well [2]. The major protein of ginkgo seeds has a legumin-like structure [57]. The sarcotesta of the seeds contains high concentrations of butanoic and hexanoic acids, with lesser amounts of octanoic acid and methyl hexanoate. These account for the malodour [58]. In this foul-smelling fleshy part of the seed, the alkylbenzoic acid derivatives and alkylphenol derivatives with a long, unbranched C_{15}, C_{17} or C_{19} hydrocarbon chain, ginkgolic acid, hydroginkgolic acid, hydroginkgolinic acid, ginkgol and bilobolol are found [2,59,60]. In addition, 4-O-methylpyridoxine has been isolated from the seeds [61,62].

When the pharmacological action and the clinical efficacy of phytotherapeutic ginkgo preparations are considered, it should be taken into account that their composition is highly determined by the applied extraction method and the subsequent purification and concentration steps [11]. An even more important factor is the variation in the basic flavonoid and terpenoid content of the leaves. The ginkgo terpene trilactone content is both tree and season dependent [22-25,63]. The variation in flavonoid content appears to be smaller [34,37,38]. It is clear that quality control is a necessity [38,64]. A monograph in the European Pharmacopoeia for Ginkgo Folium is currently in preparation.

The majority of the pharmacological experiments and all clinical studies have been conducted with standardized, enriched extracts, containing a higher concentration of active principles (flavonoids, terpenoids) and minimal concentrations of undesired compounds, especially ginkgolic acids. Of the components initially extracted from the leaves, ca. 90% is removed by technological processes while manufacturing these preparations [65]. A well-known preparation is EGb 761, until

1989 patented by the Dr. Wilmar Schwabe company. The chemical composition of this particular preparation has been summarized by Jaggy [66] (see further below).

A fact to which, according to our knowledge, no attention has so far been paid in all the clinical trials with standardized extracts, is that the standardized extracts show a significant variation in composition. A higher concentration of bilobalide (not a PAF-antagonist) with a constant 6% of ginkgo terpene trilactones, automatically means less ginkgolides. This may have clinical consequences. A recent investigation of two different batches of Tanakan showed percentages of 1.9 and 2.3% respectively for ginkgolides A and B combined [67].

Such enriched extracts, further designated as GBE in this monograph, are standardized to contain 24% ginkgo flavone glycosides and 6% terpene lactones (ginkgolide A, B, C and J, and bilobalide combined). Furthermore, they contain 5-10% oligomeric proanthocyanidins and ca. 9% organic acids. Ginkgolic acids and ginkgols are limited to a maximum of 0.0005% (5 ppm), because they are potent contact allergens. The concentration of biflavones is less than 0.1%, because they tend to form poorly soluble precipitations. The presence of condensed tannins (proanthocyanidins) is limited because they may disturb the absorption of other compounds [65,68]. The large amount of acids present in the extract plays a role in increasing the solubility of both the flavones and terpenes, which are poorly water-soluble on their own. This property significantly increases the bioavailability of these compounds in the extract [69].

Other available phytotherapeutic preparations include among others extracts that are prepared with ethanol-water, but that are not further processed, e.g. homeopathic mother tinctures. They are not standardized, and analyses revealed that such preparations contain 10-15 times less flavonoids and terpene lactones than GBE if good quality ginkgo leaves are used as starting material [11,22]. A possible complication of full extracts is the presence of unknown quantities of anacardic acids which are very irritant toxins [45].

Pharmacology and Uses

In Chinese folk medicine, the leaves of *G. biloba* are used for the treatment of cardiovascular diseases [2]. Inhalation of a decoction of the leaves is used to alleviate asthma [18,70,71]. Far more popular than the leaves are the seeds. Peikuo, the dry ripe seed of the tree, is officially listed in the Chinese Pharmacopoeia and has been used in traditional medicine for centuries, as an antiasthmatic drug and expectorant, as well as against polyuria, tuberculosis, leukorrhoea, miction problems, pollakiuria and spermatorrhea. The seeds are roasted prior to use [2,8,13,72]. Next to this, ginkgo seed has been a component of certain cosmetics, soaps and the base of certain fine oriental lacquerware [73]. In Japan the seeds and its albumin are still used as food, under the name gin-nan [61]. Also in many other East Asian countries ginkgo seeds are nowadays a highly esteemed food.

In Europe, ginkgo has never been used traditionally [8], but in Western European phytotherapy, extracts from ginkgo leaves are nowadays used to treat cerebral insufficiency and peripheral arterial vascular diseases in elderly [37,38,74,75]. These extracts are available for self-medication, but they are also used on physician's prescription, depending on the country. Cerebrovascular insufficiency may cause forgetfulness, dizziness, hearing impairment, difficulties with concentration, memory impairment, tinnitus, depressive mood, anxiety, absent mindedness, lack of energy and confusion [76,77]. Disturbance of the peripheral arterial blood circulation, as a result of degenerative vascular diseases, may cause a cold feeling and tingling in the extremities (so called 'pins and needles'), and, in a further stage, intermittent claudication. These symptoms are claimed to be relieved by treatment with ginkgo leaf extract [8,11,39,78-80]. In addition, eye problems are mentioned as an indication for ginkgo [81].

The flavonoids (ginkgo flavone glycosides) and terpenoids (ginkgolides and bilobalide) are held responsible for most of the pharmacological action. Summarizing the broad spectrum of pharmacological activities of ginkgo leaf extract, it has been shown that tolerance to hypoxia is increased in the brain and that cerebral metabolism remains normal for a longer period under hypoxic and ischemic conditions. The blood circulation, in cerebral as well as in peripheral tissue, increases and the rheological properties of the blood improve. It causes reduction of edemas. Furthermore, free radical scavenging properties, platelet-activating factor (PAF)-antagonism and interaction with neurotransmitters have been reported. These mechanisms of action have recently been reviewed in detail by Tang and Eisenbrand [2], Sticher et al. [11], Herrschaft [81] and Krieglstein and Oberpichler [80,82].

Flavonoids are able to scavenge free radicals, that may be generated to a higher extent under pathological conditions, such as hypoxia, ischemia and metabolic disturbances. Free radicals may damage the wall of blood vessels, cause lipid peroxidation and disturb a variety of cellular processes. This may eventually result in enhanced thrombocyte aggregation, vasoconstriction, thrombosis, damage to arteries, veins and capillaries, metabolic disturbances, reduced blood circulation and edema. Flavonoids may offer protection here. Due to membrane stabilizing properties, the flavonoids may protect erythrocytes against hemolysis [11,34,36]. Myricetine and quercetin have been shown to greatly induce oxidative metabolism in both resting and Ca^{2+}-loaded brain neurons. Such an antioxidant action may be responsible for part of the beneficial effects of GBE on brain neurons subject to ischemia [83].

Ginkgolides are potent PAF-antagonists. They act by competitive displacement of the PAF molecule from the receptor binding site. The liberation of PAF, playing a role in allergic reactions and inflammation, causes thrombocyte aggregation, vasodilatation, enhanced vascular permeability, formation of edema and bronchoconstriction. PAF receptors are present in both peripheral tissue and in the brain. Receptor binding studies have revealed that the more apolar ginkgolide B is the most potent PAF-antagonist of all ginkgolides. PAF-antagonism appears to decrease with increasing polarity [11,18,80].

For bilobalide a protecting action against neurotoxic myeline damage has been described [75]. Moreover, this sesquiterpene lactone has been held responsible for the lowering effect of ginkgo leaf extract on postischemic cerebral edema [8]. Bruno et al. [84] have described the regeneration of motor nerves in bilobalide-treated rats. Ginkgolide B has been found to be inactive against brain damage in dogs, induced by complete cerebral ischemia. In these experiments the drug was given at 20 mg/kg, i.v., 5 min prior to ischemia [85].

It has been shown that ginkgolide B prevents the acute pulmonary edema by scorpion venom in rats [86]. Shortening of the sleeping time, induced in mice by anesthetics, has been described for bilobalide and ginkgolide A [87]. In the cerebral cortex of rats an increased concentration of normetanephrin, a physiological metabolite of noradrenaline, as well as a reduced amount of β_2-receptors has been found under the influence of ginkgo leaf extract [80].

Hundreds of pharmacological and clinical investigations have been carried out with GBE and its specific constituents. They are, a.o., described in special issues of La Presse Medicale [88], of the Münchener Medizinische Wochenschrift [89], in books on this subject [90-93], and in several recent reviews [39,76,77,81,82,94].

The clinical efficacy of ginkgo preparations is often judged controversially, due to an apparent lack of well-performed and detailed clinical trials [94-101]. Indeed, according to an epidemiological study, 15 controlled studies focusing on the indication intermittent claudication, were performed with GBE between 1975 and 1991 [76,77]. In the same period, 40 controlled studies were directed to cerebral insufficiency [76]. For the first indication, only two studies were found to be of reasonable quality; for the second indication eight. In almost all cases positive results were obtained with a daily dose of 120-160 mg GBE, given for at least 4-6 weeks. This means that the use of such extracts to treat cerebral insufficiency is better proven than their effectiveness against intermittent claudication [76,77]. The latter should be considered a promising indication under investigation [77]. Marketing authorizations are given in France and Germany for the above mentioned symptoms with ginkgo preparations (Kommission E). In contrast, ginkgo preparations have not been accepted by countries with an Anglo-Saxon tradition in drug registration. Serious reservations against ginkgo preparations have been expressed in the literature concerning their effectiveness [97,103-106].

Shortcomings of most studies were the limited number of patients included, incomplete description of randomization procedures, patient characteristics, effect measurement and data presentation. In no trial double blindness was checked. However, these are problems related to the therapeutic group of "nootropics" and are found with piracetam as well. Despite this, all trials indicated positive effects of GBE [76,77], suggesting a publication bias. Ginkgo preparations should not be taken prophylactically. They only appear to act if circulatory disturbances exist [102]. However, from experiments with rats it has become clear that they recovered better from artificially induced cerebral ischemia when they were pretreated with GBE [82].

In addition, complaints of dizziness, tinnitus and learning impairment have been found to be positively influenced by GBE [11]. Next to trials performed with patients, studies with healthy volunteers are known, giving evidence for a positive effect of GBE on reaction and memory [76,77,107,108]. Effects of ginkgo extracts on human EEG profiles have been described [109]. In rats, improved memory effects have been found following administration of standardized ginkgo extracts [110]. As to other ginkgo leaf extracts, that are not enriched, evidence for their efficacy lacks so far. It has even been stated that such preparations are probably underdosed [8,39].

At present, attention is given to a possible therapeutic application of pure ginkgolides as PAF-antagonists in the treatment of asthma, allergical and immunological reactions, shock, ischemia and thrombosis [18,111-113]. In pharmacological models they have been shown to be highly effective in protecting against a diverse range of pathologies, such as thrombosis, atherosclerosis, cardiac and cerebral ischemia, graft rejection, immune impairments, airway hyperreactivity, and various inflammatory syndromes. Clinical trials are currently being undertaken [18,111-123].

In homeopathy, D2, D3, D4 and D6 potencies of a mother tincture prepared from fresh ginkgo leaves are used against tonsillitis, headache and writer's cramp [124,125]. The use of homeopathic preparations for the usual allopathic indications, i.e. problems with central and peripheral blood circulation has been severely questioned and criticised [125]. This would suggest that the allopathic action is largely independent of the dosage, which would be truly unique. More likely, the use of homeopathic mother tinctures for these indications should be considered underdosed phytotherapy [8,39]. Suppliers of homeopathic ginkgo preparations are urged to proof the efficacy and safety of their extracts and preparations [38]. Mother tinctures might pose a higher health risk due to the presence of ginkgolic acids.

Extracts from ginkgo seeds possess antibacterial and antifungal activity [126]. This activity has been ascribed to the characterisitc phenol and benzoic acid derivatives substituted with long-chain alkyl groups. Furthermore, these long-chain phenols showed antitumor activity against Sarcoma 180 ascites and P388 leukemia in mice, as well as cytotoxicity to Chinese hamster V-79 cells [60,127].

Pharmacokinetics

From the amount of radioactivity in the expired air, urine and faeces of rats that were given ^{14}C-labeled GBE, it was deduced that the absorption is at least 60%. After 72 hours, 38% of the radioactivity was excreted through the lungs. During the first 3 h after administration the radioactivity was mainly present in the plasma. After 48 h, radioactivity was also found in the erythrocytes and equalled the plasma level. Especially glandular and neuronal tissue as well as the eyes showed a high uptake of the labeled material [128].

The bioavailablility and pharmacokinetics of flavonoids from GBE have been studied in humans. After oral administration of 400 mg extract, rapid absorption was seen. The maximum blood concentration was attained after 1 h, being ca. 20 ng/ml for kaempferol. The elimination half-life ranged between 1.5 and 4 h. For film-coated tablets, almost complete bioavailability was found [39,129].

In a recent article, Kleijnen and Knipschild [77] summarized the pharmacokinetics of *Ginkgo biloba* extract as listed in Table 1.

Table 1. Pharmacokinetics of *Ginkgo biloba* extract. After Kleijnen and Knipschild [77].

	Ginkgo flavone glycosides	Ginkgolide A	Ginkgolide B	Bilobalide
Oral bioavailability (%)	> 60	> 98	> 80	70
Time to peak plasma concentration (h)	1.5-3	1-2	1-2	1-2
Volume of distribution (l)	unknown	40-60	60-100	170
Protein binding	unknown	unknown	unknown	unknown
Clearance (ml/min)	unknown	130-200	140-250	600

Adverse Reaction Profile

General Animal Data

Acute toxicity (LD_{50}) after oral application of GBE has been determined in mice and rats. Mouse: 7,725 mg/kg p.o.; 1,900 mg/kg i.p.; 1,100 mg/kg i.v. Rat: 2,100 mg/kg i.p. and 1100 mg/kg i.v. Up to 10 g/kg p.o. no lethal effect was seen. Higher doses could not be administered [4,69].

Chronic toxicity studies have been done with dogs and rats during a period of 6 months. Each day, GBE was administered orally at doses up to 500 mg/kg (rat) and 400 mg/kg (dog). Dogs were more sensitive for GBE than rats. At 100 mg/kg light and transient vasodilatory effects were seen in the head; following the highest dose of 400 mg/kg these disturbances were stronger and occurred after 35 days of treatment. No biochemical, hematological or histological damage was observed. Liver and kidney function remained unaltered [4,39,69].

The acute LD_{50} in mice of bilobol, which has not been detected in leaves, has been established at 761 mg/kg [2]. Bilobol produced a transitional hypotensive effect in rabbits [2].

An aqueous extract of ginkgo seed given orally at 11 mg/kg to guinea pigs of eather sex, caused paralysis of legs, opisthotonus, clonic convulsions, and auditory hyperalgesia, for which 4-O-methylpyridoxine has been held responsible [61,62].

General Human Data

The toxicity of oral phytotherapeutic preparations from leaves of *G. biloba* is generally considered to be low. Taken orally, at the recommended dose, hardly any adverse effects should be expected [8,69,77,81]. Side effects that became apparent from clinical trials with a daily dose of 120-160 mg GBE for 4-6 weeks did not differ from the placebo group [77]. However, the German health authorities list headache, dizziness, heart palpitations, gastrointestinal problems and allergic skin reactions as possible side effects [130]. Vertigo, nausea and heart palpitations are mentioned in Meyler's Side Effects of Drugs [131].

Parenteral application of GBE, however, seems to be less safe. Circulatory disturbances, allergic skin reactions and phlebitis may occur [132]. Injectable GBE is still available in Germany, but not allowed in Switzerland [11]. The Bundesgesundheitsamt (BGA) warns for the possible risk of proteins, peptides, nucleic acids, pyrogens and toxins present in GBE for parenteral administration [130]. Recently, the German health authorities have announced at first to abstain from the registration of ginkgo preparations for parenteral use, because of the severe side effects that have been reported [133]. Further investigations are deemed necessary and should give clarity as to the balance between usefulness and risk. Recently, the Willmar Schwabe company has withdrawn the preparations Tebonin® p.i. and Tebonin® p.i. 175 from the market, because of the severity of the side effects that happen to occur after intravenous administration [134].

In Japan the so-called 'gin-nan food poisoning' sometimes occurred after ginkgo seeds had been taken to excess during food shortages. The main symptoms of this poisoning were convulsions and loss of consciousness. According to about 70 reports from the period between 1930 and 1960 dealing with this poisoning, the sequelae were not serious to survivers, but about 27% lethality was found. Infants were particularly vulnerable. It has been stated that 4-O-methylpyridoxine, also named ginkgotoxin, is the toxic substance responsible for this poisoning. 4-O-Methylpyridoxine is a potent convulsive agent, with vitamin B_6 antagonizing activity in man and in several experimental animals. In addition, it inhibits the formation of 4-aminobutyric acid (GABA) from glutamate in the brain. A deficiency of GABA in the brain may induce seizures [61,62].

Doses of 720 mg pure ginkgolide A, B or C gave no observable adverse effects in humans. Doses of 360 mg pure ginkgolide per day during one week gave no toxic effects [135].

Allergic Reactions

The ginkgols and ginkgolic acids, as present in the raw seeds of *G. biloba*, may provoke strong allergic reactions [136]. It has been stated that the concentration of these allergens in preparations of ginkgo leaves, such as GBE, is so low that allergic reactions are not to be expected [11,68]. In a recent Alarmtelegramm, however, the authors pointed to the fact that flavonoids possess a possible immunogenic action, and that GBE may provoke heavy immunoallergic reactions after parenteral administration [99]. For oral ginkgo preparations light allergic reactions of the skin and gastrointestinal tract, as well as headache rarely occur [137]. Following parenteral administration also cardiovascular disturbances (hypotension, dizziness, arrythmia) may occur [137]. Allergy to ginkgo preparations is a contraindication for their use [8].

Cross-reactivity between ginkgo fruit pulp and several *Rhus*-species (poison ivy family, Anacardiaceae) has been demonstrated. The allergens are chemically similar and belong to the class of alkylphenols [1,138]. In addition, cross-reactivity between the ginkgo fruit pulp and cashew nut shell oil (*Anacardium occidentale*) has been reported [73]. Pollens of *G. biloba* have been found to act as allergens, causing pollinosis [139].

Cardiovascular Reactions

In a clinical trial, performed in Germany, 112 patients of both sexes suffering from chronic cerebral insufficiency and aged between 55 and 94 years, were treated for one year with 120 mg GBE daily. During the period of the trial no heart rate and blood pressure modifications could be detected and blood cholesterol and triglyceride levels remained practically unchanged [140].

In patients that were treated with ginkgo leaf extracts before, severe circulatory disturbance (fall of blood pressure, dizziness and eventually shock) may develop after injection of GBE (intramuscular, intravenous, but especially intra-arterial) [130]. Local irritation of the vein into which ginkgo preparations are injected sometimes occur [137].

In June 1993 anaphylactic shock has been reported after parenterally administered Tebonin® in four patients. Dizziness, sickness and faintness were seen. All patients showed high fever and leucocytosis. As a sign of impaired circulation, metabolic acidosis and an increase of liver enzymes were found. In one case life-threatening heart arrythmia occurred [133].

Dermatological Reactions

The fleshy part of the seeds of *G. biloba* has been known from ancient times to irritate the skin. The alkylbenzoic acid derivatives and the alkylphenol derivatives are very irritant and responsible for the dermatitis that occurs after contact with the skin [68], and may be compared with the allergic effects caused by *Rhus* species. Erythema, edema, papules and vesicles are seen, complicated by intense itching. The irritation disappears after 7-10 days following the contact [138]. The dermatitic action of these compounds is consistent with oxidation of the allergen to a quinone, which then binds covalently to a protein nucleophile, yielding an antigenic complex [1]. To provoke an allergic reaction, the fleshy part of the seed should be crushed first [73].

After taking ginkgo preparations, both full extracts and GBE, orally as well as parenterally, allergic skin reactions rarely occur [137].

Gastrointestinal Reactions

Allergens causing skin sensitization, such as ginkgols and ginkgolic acids, can also cause allergic contact reactions of mucous membranes, resulting in cheilitis, stomatitis, proctitis and pruritis ani [136]. After ingestion of preparations containing allergens from the ginkgo tree, reactions of the mouth mucosa have been described, as well as stomatitis, gastroenteritis and proctitis [68].

Slight gastric symptoms have been reported from a trial with 112 patients receiving 120 mg GBE per day at the start of the treatment, but these repressed spontaneously as treatment continued [140].

The central kernel of the ginkgo seed is edible when roasted, but the fleshy fruit pulp is toxic, even after roasting [73].

After taking ginkgo preparations, orally as well as parenterally, gastrointestinal reactions rarely occur [137].

Hematological Reactions

Although pharmacological studies with ginkgo leaf extract have demonstrated distinct effects on hemorheological parameters, such as a decreased blood viscosity, PAF-antagonism and vasoregulatory activity, no clinical reports exist on hematological adverse effects or interactions with antithrombotic drugs. However, a theoretical risk on this point may not be excluded.

Oral Reactions

See the section on gastrointestinal reactions.

Fertility, Pregnancy, and Lactation

In experimental animals no indications were found for embryotoxic, mutagenic or teratogenic effects [81]. Oral administration of up to 1600 mg/kg/day of standardized ginkgo extract to rats and 900 mg/kg/day to rabbits did not produce teratogenic effects. In addition, reproduction was not affected [69]. Human data on adverse effects of ginkgo preparations with respect to fertility, pregnancy and lactation are not available [4].

The pathophysiological phenomena for which ginkgo leaf extracts are indicated, typically occur in elderly people. Ginkgo preparations are sometimes regarded as geriatric drugs [78]. Therefore, possible risks concerning fertility, pregnancy and lactation are of limited significance here.

Mutagenicity and Carcinogenicity

No carcinogenic effects could be detected in experiments with rats, fed with kernels of ginkgo seed for almost a year [141]. In a study in which GBE was given orally to rat for 104 weeks at doses of 4, 20 and 100 mg/kg, no carcinogenic effects were found [4].

For GBE no mutagenic potential was found in the Ames-test, using the *Salmonella typhymurium* strains TA 1535, 1537, 1538, 98 and 100, with and without metabolic activation using rat liver S9-mix; in the host-mediated-assay (mouse, *S. typhymurium* strain TA 1537, GBE doses up to 20 g/kg p.o.); in the micronucleus test (mouse, GBE doses up to 20 g/kg p.o.); and in the chromosome aberration test (human lymphocytes, GBE concentrations up to 100 μg/ml) [4].

References

1. Evans WC (1988) Trease and Evans' Pharmacognosy, 13th ed. London: Ballière Tindall, pp 163, 750
2. Tang W, Eisenbrand W (1992) *Ginkgo biloba* L. Chinese Drugs of Plant Origin. Berlin: Springer-Verlag, pp 555–565
3. Spegg H (1990) *Ginkgo biloba* – Ein Baum aus Urzeiten, ein Phytopharmakon mit Zukunft. PTA Heute 4:576–583
4. Spieß E, Juretzek W (1993) Ginkgo. In: Hänsel R, Keller K, Rimpler H, Schneider G, eds. Hager's Handbuch der Pharmazeutischen Praxis. 5th edn. Vol. 5. Berlin: Springer-Verlag, pp 269–292
5. Huh H, Staba EJ (1992) The botany and chemistry of *Ginkgo biloba* L. J Herbs Spices Med Plants 1:91–124
6. Penso G (1983) Index Plantarum Medicinalium Totius Mundi Eorumque Synonymorum. Milano: Organizzazione Editoriale Medico Farmaceutica, p 442
7. Melzheimer V (1992) *Ginkgo biloba* L., aus Sicht der systematischen und angewandten Botanik. Pharm unserer Zeit 21:206–214
8. Jaspersen-Schib R (1990) *Ginkgo biloba* L. – Magische Droge oder modernes Therapeutikum? Schweiz Apoth Ztg 128:123–128
9. Li H-L (1956) A horticultural and botanical history of ginkgo. Morris Arboretum Bull 7:3–12
10. Drieu K (1986) Préparation et définition de l'extrait de *Ginkgo biloba*. La Presse Medicale 15:1455–1457
11. Sticher O, Hasler A, Meier B (1991) *Ginkgo biloba* – Eine Standortbestimmung. Dtsch Apoth Ztg 131:1827-35
12. Boralle N, Braquet P, Gottlieb OR (1988) *Ginkgo biloba*: a review of its chemical composition. In: Braquet P, ed. Ginkgolides – Chemistry, Biology Pharmacology and Clinical Perspectives. Vol. 1. Barcelona: J.R. Prous Science Publishers, pp 9–25
13. Schennen A (1988) Neue Inhaltsstoffe aus den Blättern von *Ginkgo biloba* L. sowie Präparation ^{14}C-markierter Ginkgo-Flavonoide. Marburg: University of Marburg, Thesis.
14. Hölzl J (1992) Inhaltsstoffe von *Ginkgo biloba*. Pharm unserer Zeit 21:215–223
15. Nakanishi K (1967) The ginkgolides. Pure Appl Chem 14:89–113
16. Okabe K, Yamada K, Yamamura S, Takada S (1967) Ginkgolides. J Chem Soc 2201–2206
17. Weinges K, Hepp M, Jaggy H (1987) Isolierung und Strukturaufklärung eines neuen Ginkgolides. Liebigs Ann Chem 6:521–526
18. Hosford D, Mencia-Huerta JM, Page C, Braquet P (1988) Natural antagonists of platelet-activating factor. Phytother Res 2:1–24
19. Weinges K, Bähr W (1969) Kondensierte Ringsysteme II. Bilobalid A, ein neues Sesquiterpen mit tert.-Butyl Gruppe aus den Blättern von *Ginkgo biloba* L. Liebigs Ann Chem 724:214–216
20. Nakanishi K, Habaguchi K, Nakadaira Y, Woods MC, Maruyama M, Major RT, Alauddin M, Patel AR, Weinges K, Bähr W (1971) Structure of bilobalide, a rare tert.-butyl containing sesquiterpenoid related to the C_{20}-ginkgolides. J Am Chem Soc 93:3544–3546
21. Beek TA van (1994) Unpublished material.
22. Beek TA van, Scheeren HA, Rantio T, Melger WC, Lelyveld GP (1991) Determination of ginkgolides and bilobalide in *Ginkgo biloba* leaves and phytopharmaceuticals. J Chromatogr 543:375–387
23. Beek TA van, Lelyveld GP (1992) Concentration of ginkgolides and bilobalide in *Ginkgo biloba leaves* in relation to the time of year. Planta Med 58:413–416
24. Hasler A, Meier B (1992) Determination of terpenes from *Ginkgo biloba* L. by capillary gas chromatography. Pharm Pharmacol Lett 2:187–190
25. Flesch V, Jacques M, Cosson L, Teng BP, Petiard V, Balz JP (1992) Relative importance of growth and light level on terpene content of *Ginkgo biloba*. Phytochemistry 31:1941–1945

26. Weinges K, Bähr W, Kloss P (1968) Natural phenolic compounds. X. Phenolic components of *Ginkgo biloba* leaves. Arzneimittelforsch 18:539–543
27. Geiger H (1979) 3'-O-Methylmyricetin-3-rhamnoglucoside, a new flavonoid from the autumnal leaf of *Ginkgo biloba* L. Z Naturforsch 34C:878–879
28. Briançon-Scheid F, Guth A, Anton R (1982) High-performance liquid chromatography of biflavones from *Ginkgo biloba* L. J Chromatogr 245:261–267
29. Briançon-Scheid F, Lobstein-Guth A, Anton R (1983) HPLC separation and quantitative determination of biflavones in leaves from *Ginkgo biloba*. Planta Med 49:204–207
30. Nasr C, Lobstein-Guth A, Haag-Berrurier M, Anton R (1987) Quercetin coumaroyl glucorhamnoside from *Ginkgo biloba*. Phytochemistry 26:2869–2870
31. Pietta P, Mauri P, Rava A (1988) Reversed-phase high-performance liquid chromatographic method for the analysis of biflavones in *Ginkgo biloba* L. extract. J Chromatogr 437:453–456
32. Victoire C, Haag-Berrurier M, Lobstein-Guth A, Balz JP, Anton R (1988) Isolation of flavonol glycosides from *Ginkgo biloba* leaves. Planta Med 54: 245–247
33. Lobstein-Guth A, Briançon-Scheid F, Victoire C, Haag-Berrurier M, Anton R (1988) Isolation of amentoflavone from *Ginkgo biloba*. Planta Med 54:555–556
34. Hasler AR (1990) Thesis. Flavonoide aus *Ginkgo biloba* L. und HPLC-Analytik von Flavonoiden in verschiedenen Arzneipflanzen.
35. Hasler A, Gross G-A, Meier B, Sticher O (1992) Complex flavonol glycosides from the leaves of *Ginkgo biloba*. Phytochemistry 31:1391–1394
36. Hasler A, Meier B, Sticher O (1990) *Ginkgo biloba*. Botanische, analytische und pharmakologische Aspekte. Schweiz Apoth Ztg 128:341–347
37. Sticher O (1992) *Ginkgo biloba* - Analytik und Zubereitungsformen. Pharm unserer Zeit 21:253–265
38. Sticher O (1993) Quality of *Ginkgo* preparations. Planta Med 59:2–11
39. Schilcher H (1988) *Ginkgo biloba* L. Untersuchungen zur Qualität, Wirkung, Wirksamkeit und Unbedenklichkeit. Z Phytother 9:119–127
40. Kircher HW (1970) β-Sitosterol in *Ginkgo biloba* leaves. Phytochemistry 9:1879
41. Plieninger H, Schwarz B, Jaggy H, Huber-Patz U, Rodewald H, Irngartinger H, Weinges K (1986) Naturstoffe aus Arzneipflanzen. XXIV. Isolierung, Strukturaufklärung und Synthese von (Z,Z)-4,4'-(1,4-Pentadien-1,5-diyl)diphenol, einen ungewöhnlichen Naturstoff aus den Blättern des Ginkgo-Baumes (*Ginkgo biloba* L.). Liebigs Ann Chem 1772–1778
42. Schennen A, Hölzl J (1986) 6-Hydroxykynurensäure, die erste N-haltige Verbindung aus den Blättern von *Ginkgo biloba*. Planta Med 52:235–236
43. Höllriegl H, Köhler H, Franz G (1986) High-molecular-weight polysaccharides of *Ginkgo biloba* leaves. Sci Pharm 54:321–330
44. Ibata K, Mizuno M, Takigawa T, Tanaka Y (1983) Long-chain betulaprenol-type polyprenols from the leaves of *Ginkgo biloba*. Biochem J 213:305–311
45. Gellerman JL, Schlenk H (1968) Methods for isolation and determination of anacardic acids. Anal Chem 40:739–743
46. Kraus J (1991) Water-soluble polysaccharides from *Ginkgo biloba* leaves. Phytochemistry 30:3017–3020
47. Huh H, Staba EJ, Singh J (1992) Supercritical fluid chromatographic analysis of polyprenols in *Ginkgo biloba* L. J Chromatogr 600:364–369
48. Fu-shun Y, Evans KA, Stevens LH, Beek TA van, Schoonhoven LM (1990) Deterrents extracted from the leaves of *Ginkgo biloba*: effects on feeding and contact chemoreceptors. Entomol Exp Appl 54:57–64
49. Steinegger E, Hänsel R (1992) Pharmakognosie. 5. Auflage. Berlin: Springer-Verlag, pp 586–588
50. Matsumoto T, Sei T (1987) Antifeedant activities of *Ginkgo biloba*. Agric Biol Chem 51:249–250

51. Verotta L, Peterlongo F (1993) Selective extraction of phenolic components from *Ginkgo biloba* extracts using supercritical carbon dioxide and off-line capillary gas chromatography/mass spectrometry. Phytochem Anal 4:178-182
52. Gülz P-G, Müller E, Schmitz K, Marner F-J, Güth S (1992) Chemical compostion and surface structures of epicuticular leaf waxes of *Ginkgo biloba, Magnolia grandiflora*, and *Liriodendron tulipifera*. Z Naturforsch 47C:516–526
53. Kimura H, Irie H, Ueda K, Uyeo S (1968) Constituents of the heartwood of *Ginkgo biloba*. V. Structure and absolute configuration of bilobanone. Yakugaku Zasshi 88:562–572
54. Irie H, Ohno K, Ito Y, Uyeo S (1975) Isolation and characterization of 10,11-dihydroatlantone and related compounds from *Ginkgo biloba* L. Chem Pharm Bull 23:1892–1894
55. Irie H, Kimura H, Otani N, Ueda K, Uyeo S (1967) The revised structure of bilobanone. Chem Commun 678–679
56. Del Tredici P (1989) *Ginkgo biloba*: Evolution and seed dispersal. In: Braquet P, ed. Ginkgolides – Chemistry, Biology, Pharmacology and Clinical Perspectives. Vol. 2. Barcelona: J.R. Prous Science Publishers, pp 1–13
57. Jensen U, Berthold H (1989) Legumin-like proteins in gymnosperms. Phytochemistry 28:1389–1394
58. Amato I (1993) Sniffing out the origins of ginkgo-stink. Science 261:1389
59. Morimoto H, Kawamatsu Y, Sugihara H (1968) Steric structure of the toxic substances from the fruit pulp of *Ginkgo biloba*. Chem Pharm Bull 16:2282–2286
60. Itokawa H, Totsuka N, Nakahara K, Takeya K, Lepoittevin JP, Asakawa Y (1987) Antitumor principles from *Ginkgo biloba* L. Chem Pharm Bull 35:3016–3020
61. Wada K, Ishigaki S, Ueda K, Sakata M, Haga M (1985) An antivitamin B_6, 4'-methoxypyridoxine, from the seed of *Ginkgo biloba* L. Chem Pharm Bull 33:3555–3557
62. Wada K, Ishigaki S, Ueda K, Take Y, Sasaki K, Sakata M, Haga M (1988) Studies on the constitution of edible and medicinal plants. I. Isolation and identification of 4-O-methylpyridoxine, toxic principle from seed of *Ginkgo biloba* L. Chem Pharm Bull 36:1779–1782
63. Lobstein A, Rietsch-Jako L, Haag-Berrurier M, Anton R (1991) Seasonal variations of the flavonoid content from *Ginkgo biloba* leaves. Planta Med 57:430–433
64. Steinke B, Müller B, Wagner H (1993) Biologische Standardisierunsmethode für Ginkgo-Extrakte. Planta Med 59:155–160
65. Hänsel R (1990) Analytische Differenzierung verschiedener Ginkgo-Extrakte. Ärztl Forsch 37:1–3
66. Jaggy H (1993) Die Inhaltsstoffe des *Ginkgo biloba*-Extraktes EGb 761. Hämostaseologie (Stuttgart) 13:7–10
67. Beek TA van, Veldhuizen A van, Lelyveld GP, Piron I (1993) Quantitation of bilobalide and ginkgolides A, B, C and J by means of NMR. Phytochem Anal 4:261–268
68. Ganzer BM (1990) Spezialextrakte aus Ginkgo-Pflanze – jeder ein Unikat. Pharm Ztg 135:2111
69. O'Reilly J (1993) *Ginkgo biloba* – cultivation, extraction and therapeutic use of the extract. In: van Beek TA, Breteler H, eds. Phytochemistry and Agriculture. Vol. 34. Oxford: Clarendon Press, pp 253–270
70. Braquet P (1987) The ginkgolides: potent platelet-activating factor antagonists isolated from *Ginkgo biloba* L.: chemistry, pharmacology and clinical applications. Drugs Future 12:643–699
71. Smith F, Stuart GA (1973) Chinese Medicinal Herbs, compiled by Li Shih-Chen, translated and researched. San Francisco (390–391). Cited from: Müller I (1992) Zur Einführung des *Ginkgo biloba* in die europäische Botanik und Pharmazie. Pharm unserer Zeit 21:201–205
72. Anonymous (1987) New compounds from old tree. Pharm J 283:309
73. Sowers WF, Weary PE, Collins OD, Cawley EP (1965) Ginkgo-tree dermatitis. Arch Dermatol 91:452–456
74. Weiß RF (1991) Lehrbuch der Phytotherapie, 7. Auflage. Stuttgart: Hippokrates Verlag, pp 238–239

75. Trunzler G (1989) Phytotherapeutische Möglichkeiten bei Herz- und arteriellen Gefäßerkrankungen. Z Phytother 10:147–156
76. Kleijnen J, Knipschild P (1992) Ginkgo biloba for cerebral insufficiency. Br J Clin Pharmacol 34:352–358
77. Kleijnen J, Knipschild P (1992) Ginkgo biloba. Lancet 1136–1139
78. Wichtl M (1992). Pflanzliche Geriatrika. Dtsch Apoth Ztg 132:1569–76
79. Amling R (1991) Phytotherapeutika in der Neurologie. Z Phytother 12:9–14
80. Krieglstein J, Oberpichler H (1989) Ginkgo biloba und Hirnleistungsstörungen. Pharm Ztg 134:2279–2289
81. Herrschaft H (1992) Zur klinischen Anwendung von Ginkgo biloba bei dementiellen Syndromen. Pharm unserer Zeit 21:266–275
82. Oberpichler-Schwenk H, Krieglstein J (1992) Pharmakologische Wirkungen von Ginkgo biloba-Extrakt und -Inhaltsstoffen. Pharm unserer Zeit 21:224–235
83. Oyama Y, Fuchs PA, Katayama N, Noda K (1994) Myricetin and quercetin, the flavonoid constituents of Ginkgo biloba extract, greatly reduce oxidative metabolism in both resting and Ca^{2+}-loaded brain neurons. Brain Res 635:125–129
84. Bruno C, Cuppini R, Sartini S, Cecchini T, Ambrogini P, Bombardelli E (1993) Regeneration of motor nerves in bilobalide-treated rats. Planta Med 59:302–307
85. Hofer RE, Christopherson TJ, Scheithauer BW, Milde JH, Lanier WL (1993) The effect of a platelet activating antagonist (BN 52021) on neurologic outcome and histopathology in a canine model of complete cerebral ischemia. Anesthesiology 79:347–353
86. Freire-Maia L, de Matos IM (1993) Heparin or a PAF antagonist (BN-52021) prevents the acute pulmonary edema induced by Tityus serrulatus scorpion venom in the rat. Toxicon 31:1207–1210
87. Wada K, Sakaki K, Miura K, Yagi M, Kubota Y, Matsumoto T, Haga M (1993) Isolation of bilobalide and ginkgolide A from Ginkgo biloba L. shorten the sleeping time induced in mice by anesthetics. Biol Pharm Bull 16:210–212
88. Various authors (1986) Special issue on GBE. Presse Med 15:1438–1604
89. Various authors (1991) Ginkgo biloba: Aktuelle Forschungsergebnisse 1990/1991. Münch Med Wschr 133:S1–S62
90. Braquet P, ed (1988) Ginkgolides – Chemistry, Biology, Pharmacology and Clinical Perspectives. Vol. 1. Barcelona: J.R. Prous Science Publishers
91. Braquet P, ed (1989) Ginkgolides – Chemistry, Biology, Pharmacology and Clinical Perspectives. Vol. 2. Barcelona: J.R. Prous Science Publishers
92. Kemper FH, Schmid-Schönbein H (1991) Rökan, Ginkgo biloba EGb 761. Vol. 1, Pharmakologie. Berlin: Springer-Verlag
93. DeFeudis FV (1991) Ginkgo biloba Extrakt EGb 761, Pharmacological Activities and Clinical Applications. Paris: Elsevier
94. Koch E, Chatterjee SS (1993) Experimentelle Grundlagen für die therapeutische Anwendung von Ginkgoextrakt EGb 761 bei der Behandlung vaskulärer Erkrankungen. Hämastaseologie (Stuttgart) 13:11–27
95. Anonymous (1989) Ginkgo biloba extract: over 5 million prescriptions a year. Lancet ii:1513–1514
96. Stein U (1990) Ginkgo biloba extracts. Lancet 335:475–476
97. Fünfgeld FW (1990) Ginkgo biloba extracts. Lancet 335:476
98. Schönhöfer PS (1990) Ginkgo biloba extracts. Lancet 335:788
99. Moebius UM, Becker-Brüser W, Schönhöfer PS (1989) Alarmtelegramm. A.V.I. Berlin: Arzneimittel-Verlags GmbH, pp 160, 181
100 Anonymous (1989) Ginkgo biloba - Wirksam und therapeutisch von Nutzen? Dtsch Apoth Ztg 129:440–442
101. Sprecher E (1990) Modedrogen. Z Phytother 11:103–112
102. Anonymous (1988) Ginkgo biloba im Blickpunkt. Placebo oder "Robin-Hood-Effekt"? Apoth Ztg 4 (nr.37):1–8
103. Anonymous (1988) Kommission E für Tebonin/Rökan. Arznei-Telegramm no. 5, pp 46–47

104. Anonymous (1989) Tebonin. Arnei-Telegramm no. 2, pp 26–27
105. Kimbel KH (1992) *Ginkgo biloba*. Lancet 340:1474
106. Held K, Schwabe U (1993) Durchblutungsförderende Mittel. In: Schwabe U, Paffrath D, eds. Arzneiverordnungs-Report '93. Aktuelle Daten, Kosten, Trends und Kommentare. Stuttgart: Gustav Fischer Verlag, pp 200–209
107. Subhan Z, Hindmarch I (1984) The psychopharmacological effects of *Ginkgo biloba* extract in normal healthy volunteers. Int J Clin Pharm Res 4:89–93
108. Schaffler K, Reeh PW (1985) Doppelblindstudie zur hypoxieprotektiven Wirkung eines standardisierten *Ginkgo biloba*-Präparates nach Mehrfachverabreichung an gesunden Probanden. Arzneimittelforsch 35:1283–1286
109. Künkel H (1993) EEG profile of three different extractions of *Ginkgo biloba*. Neuropsychobiology 27:40–45
110. Petkov VD, Kehayov R, Belcheva S, Konstantinova E, Petkov VV, Getova D, Markovska V (1993) Memory effects of standardized extracts of *Panax ginseng* (G115), *Ginkgo biloba* (GK501) and their combination Ginkcosan® (PHL-00701). Planta Med 59:106–114
111. Braquet P, Paubert-Braquet M, Koltai M, Bourgain R, Bussolino F, Hosford D (1989) Is there a case for PAF antagonists in the treatment of ischemic states? Trends Pharmacol Sci 10:23–30
112. Chung KF, Barnes PJ (1988) PAF antagonists. Their potential therapeutic role in asthma. Drugs 35:93–103
113. Braquet P, Esanu A, Buisine E, Hosford D, Broquet C, Koltai M (1991) Recent progress in ginkgolide research. Med Res Rev 11:295–355
114. Anonymous (1992) Monitor. Marketletter July 6, p 25
115. Braquet P, Etienne A, Touvay C, Bourgain RH, Lefort J, Vargaftig BB (1985) Involvement of platelet activating factor in respiratory anaphylaxis, demonstrated by PAF-acether inhibitor BN 52021. Lancet i:1501
116. Morley J, Page CP, Sanjar S (1985) PAF and airway hyperreactivity. Lancet ii:451
117. Chung KF, Dent G, McCusker M, Guinot Ph, Page CP, Barnes PJ (1987) Effect of a ginkgolide mixture (BN 52063) in antagonising skin and platelet responses to platelet activating factor in man. Lancet i:248–251
118. Guinot Ph, Summerhayes C, Berdah L, Ducher J, Revillaud RJ (1988) Treatment of adult systemic mastocytosis with a PAF-acether antagonist BN 52063. Lancet ii:114
119. Roberts NM, McCusker M, Chung KF, Barnes PJ (1988) Effect of a PAF antagonist, BN 52063, on PAF-induced bronchoconstriction in normal subjects. Br J Clin Pharmacol 26:65–72
120. Wilkens JH, Wilkens H, Uffmann J, Bövers J, Fabel H, Fröhlich JC (1990) Effects of a PAF-antagonist (BN 52063) on bronchoconstriction and platelet activation during exercise induced asthma. Br J Clin Pharmacol 29:85–91
121. Kemény L, Csató M, Braquet P, Dobozy A (1990) Effect of BN 52021, a platelet activating factor antagonist, on dithranol-induced inflammation. Br J Dermatol 112:539–544
122. Page CP (1990) The role of platelet activating factor in allergic respiratory disease. Br J Clin Pharmacol 30:99S–103S
123. Hsieh K-H (1991) Effects of PAF antagonist, BN 52021, on the PAF-, methacholine-, and allergen-induced bronchoconstriction in asthmatic children. Chest 99:877–882
124. Wiesenauer M (1991) Homöopathie für Ärzte. Stuttgart: Deutscher Apothcker Verlag, pp 3/77, 4/61
125. Hänsel R (1991) *Ginkgo biloba*: das Arzneimittelangebot aus pharmazeutischer Sicht. Ärztez Naturheilverfahren 32:295–303
126. Adawadkar PD, El Sohly MA (1981) Isolation, purification and antimicrobial activity of anacardic acids from *Ginkgo biloba* fruits. Fitoterapia 52:129–135
127. Itokawa H, Totsuka N, Nakahara K, Maezuru M, Takeya K, Kondo M, Inamatsu M, Morta H (1989) A quantitative structure-activity relationship for antitumor activity of long-chain phenols from *Ginkgo biloba* L. Chem Pharm Bull 37:1619–1621

128. Moreau JP, Eck CR, McCabe J, Skinner S (1986) Absorption, distribution and elimination of radiolabeled *Ginkgo biloba* leaf extract in the rat. Presse Med 15:1458–1461
129. Drieu K, Moreau JP, Eck CR, McCabe J, Skinner S (1986) Animal distribution and preliminary human kinetic studies of the flavonoid fraction of a standardized *Ginkgo biloba* extract (GBE 761). Stud Org Chem 23:351–359
130. Anonymous (1989) *Ginkgo biloba*-haltige Arzneimittel. Pharm Ztg 134:561
131. Dukes MNG (1988) Meyler's Side Effects of Drugs, 11th ed. Amsterdam: Elsevier, p 395
132. Fintelmann V, Menßen HG, Siegers CP (1989) Phytotherapie Manual. Stuttgart: Hippokrates Verlag, p 55
133. Anonymous (1994) Ginkgo-biloba-haltiger Trockenextrakt zu Infusion. Pharm Ztg 139:986–987
134. Anonymous (1994) Rückruf Tebonin p.i., Tebonin p.i. 175. Dtsch Apoth Ztg 134:1324–1326
135. Bonvoisin B, Guinot P (1989) Clinical studies of BN 52063 a specific PAF antagonist. In: Braquet P, ed. Ginkgolides – Chemistry, biology, pharmacology and clinical perspectives. Vol. 2. Barcelona: J.R. Prous Science Publishers, pp 845–854
136. Lepoittevin J-P, Benezra C, Asakawa Y (1989) Allergic contact dermatitis to *Ginkgo biloba* L.: relationship with urushiol. Arch Dermatol Res 281:227–230
137. Rote Liste 1994. Frankfurt/Main: Bundesverband der Pharmazeutischen Industrie e.V., 36001–36012
138. Becker LE, Skipworth GB (1975) Ginkgo-tree dermatitis, stomatitis, and proctitis. JAMA 231:1162–1163
139. Long R, Yin R, Zhen Y (1992) Partial purification and analysis of allergenicity, immunogenicity of *Ginkgo biloba* L. pollen. J West China Univ Med Sci 23:429–432
140. Vorberg G (1985) *Ginkgo biloba* extract (GBE) : a long-term study of chronical cerebral insufficiency in geriatric patients. Clin Trials J 22:149–157
141. Hirono I, Shibuya C, Shimizu M, Fushimi K, Mori H, Miwa T (1972) Carcinogenicity examination of some edible plants. GANN 63:383–386

Glycyrrhiza Glabra

R.F. Chandler

Botany

Licorice consists of the dried unpeeled roots and stolons of *Glycyrrhiza glabra* L., a member of the Leguminosae (Fabaceae) family [1]. It is commonly known as licorice, liquorice, glycyrrhiza, sweet wood, liquiritiae radix (English); Süssholz, Lakritzenwurzel (German); reglisse, bois doux (French); liquirizia (Italian); and regaliz (Spanish) [1–7].

The licorice of commerce is obtained from several varieties of *Glycyrrhiza glabra* L., including var. *typica* (Spanish and Italian licorice), var. *glandulifera* (Russian licorice) and var. *beta-violacea* (Persian licorice). *Glycyrrhiza uralensis* Fisch. (Chinese or Manchurian licorice) is also utilized [1,7,8], and other species have regionalized use and/or are under investigation [1,5,9].

Glycyrrhiza species are perennial herbs or subshrubs growing to a height of 2 m with horizontal underground stems (rhizomes or stolons). The plants have dark green leaflets and yellow, blue or violet flowers which resemble those of the garden pea. The roots are sweet-flavored [1–3,7,9]. It is the dried roots and rhizomes (collectively called "roots") which are used [2,7].

Typical Spanish licorice occurs in straight pieces from 14 to 20 cm or more in length and from 5 to 20 mm in diameter. If unpeeled, they have a dark, reddish brown cork and the rhizomes and stolons, which are more numerous than the roots, bear buds. The peeled drug has a yellow, fibrous exterior. The fracture is fibrous and the drug has a faint, characteristic odor and a sweet characteristic taste, almost free from bitterness [1]. Other varieties and species have similar, but usually less regular, features [1]. Macroscopical and microscopical descriptions can be found in several textbooks [1,4,5,10,11].

Chemistry

Licorice is one of the most extensively investigated medicinal and food plants. The most important constituent, and the one to which licorice owes its sweet taste and its main pharmacological actions, is the saponin glycoside, glycyrrhizin (synonyms are glycyrrhizic and glycyrrhizinic acids) [1,3,12]. It is present as the potassium and calcium salts in concentrations ranging from 1 to 24%, depending on the source and method of assay [2,3,13]. The usual range, however, is 6–14% (6–8%

for Spanish licorice and 10–14% for Russian licorice) [1,3]. Glycyrrhizin undergoes hydrolysis to yield two molecules of glucuronic acid and the pentacyclic triterpene aglycone, glycyrrhetinic (glycyrrhetic, glycyrretic) acid [12,14,15]. Other related triterpenoids are also present [1–4,8,12,14].

Other known constituents of licorice root include amines, amino acids, bitter principles (glycyramarin), coumarins (glycyrin, herniarin, licopyranocoumarin, licoarylcoumarin, liqcoumarin, umbelliferone, etc.), flavonoids and isoflavonoids (glicoricone, glisoflavone, isoliquiritigenin, isoliquiritin, licoflavonol, licoricidin, licoricone, liquiritigenin, liquiritin, etc.), chalcone and chalcone glycosides (isoliquiritigenin, isoliquiritin, isoliquiritoside, liquiritoside, neoisoliquiritin, rhamnoisoliquiritin, rhamnoliquiritin, etc.), gums, licofuranone, lignin, resins, starch, steroids (β-sitosterol, stigmasterol, 22,23-dihydrostigmasterol, etc.), stilbenes, sugars and related compounds (glucose, mannose, sucrose, mannitol), tannins, triterpenes (β-amyrin, glabrolide, 18-β-glycyrrhetinic acid, glycyrrhetol, isoglabrolide, licoric acid, liquirtic acid, etc.), volatile oil (consisting of many constituents but which includes acetylsalicylic acid, salicylic acid, and methylsalicylate), and a wax [1–3,8,9,13,16–19].

Glycyrrhizin content in confectionery and health products has been found to vary considerably [20–22]. The level of glycyrrhizin in 18 confectionery products was found to range between 0.26 and 7.9 mg/g, while its level in eight health products ranged between 0.30–47.1 mg/g of product [22]. The amount of glycyrrhizin in chewing tobacco ranged between 1.5–4.1 mg/g [22,23]. For approximations of the glycyrrhizin content of licorice-containing confectionery products, glycyrrhizin is considered to represent approximately 0.2% of the licorice [21,22]. Studies have demonstrated that the mean daily ingestion of glycyrrhizin for the UK, USA, Belgium and the Nordic countries to be 1, 3, 5, and 8 mg per day, respectively [21,22]. Other studies have shown that approximately 5% of Danish schoolchildren [24] and about 5% of New Zealand high school students [25] consume enough licorice to be at risk [21].

Pharmacology and Uses

In 1760, George Dunhill of Pontefract added sugar to the extract and licorice became a popular confection [26]. In addition to its use as a flavoring agent for foods, and confectionaries [1,2], licorice's virtues as a demulcent, an expectorant, and as an agent to treat stomach pains and mouth ulcers have been recognized for at least 4000 years [2–4,8,9,13,14,20,27–29]. It is noteworthy, however, that currently about 90% of the licorice imported into the U.S.A. is used to flavor tobacco products [21,27]. The remaining 10% is distributed equally between the food and pharmaceutical industries [21].

Pharmacological knowledge regarding glycyrrhizin, the main saponin of licorice, has expanded remarkably since Revers [18] reported that licorice extracts were clinically effective in treating gastric ulcers, but were associated with certain side effects.

As with many herbal medicines used for such an extended period of history, licorice has a long list of known and reputed uses and activities (Table 1) [2,6,9,14,29–31]. It is official in over 20 pharmacopoeias [6].

Licorice (*Gan Cao*) is one of the oldest and one of the most important herbs in Chinese medicine, either on its own or as a supporting herb [2,29,32–38]. Licorice is also reported to be a constituent of 73.5% of the Chinese herbal medicines available in Japan [39]. The traditional herbal remedies originally imported into Japan from China have evolved independently and are known as Kampo medicines [37]. Licorice is also used extensively in Ayurvedic medicine [35].

Structure-activity-relationship studies have shown that olean-12-en-3-β,30-diol has retained the antiallergic and antiulcerous activities without any inhibitory activity on the action of δ-4,5-α- and δ-4,5-β-reductases on δ-4,3-ketosteroids [40].

Table 1. Some known and reputed uses and activities of licorice and its derivatives*

I. **Therapeutic Uses**

  A. **Blood and Circulatory System:** Reputed uses of licorice include sweetening the blood (hypoglycemia), to treat fevers, "griefs of the liver", and for moderating the "shape of arteries". It has been shown to exhibit antiplatelet [41], antihypotensive [42], antihemolytic [43], and antihypercholesteremic activities [44].

  B. **Gastrointestinal Tract:** Licorice has been used as a demulcent, a "corrector" of cathartics, a laxative, to heal gastric, duodenal and oral ulcers, to moisten the mouth and quench thirst, to treat hoarseness, potentiate laxatives [2,3,16,28,45–51], and for dyspepsia [13].
  It has been shown in animal models that co-administered deglycyrrhinized licorice reduces acute gastric mucosal damage due to aspirin alone or in combination with taurodeoxycholic acid, prevents the potentiation of aspirin injury by bile acid, and does not greatly affect the aspirin absorption [51].

  C. **Respiratory Tract:** Licorice has been used for asthma, bronchitis, chest complaints, consumption, cough (antitussive), expectorant, "harshness of chest", and inflammation of lungs [2,9,42,52].

  D. **Urinary Tract:** Licorice has been used for "griefs" of kidney, nephritis, sores of bladder, strangury, infections [53] and as a diuretic [29].

  E. **Antiinfective Agent:** Glycyrrhizin and various derivatives have been shown to possess *in vitro* antibacterial activity against a number of bacteria, fungi and several unrelated DNA and RNA viruses, including herpes simplex [54–56], herpes genitalis and herpes zoster [57–59], hepatitis A virus [60] and HIV [17,20,55,61–65]. Additionally, the derivatives carbenoxolone and cicloxolone exhibit *in vivo* activity against the herpes virus in aphthous ulcers [66] and show promise in the treatment of herpes genitalis and herpes zoster [58,59]. Licochalcone A, a Chinese licorice derivative, has potent antimalarial activity *in vitro* in mice [70].
  Glycyrrhetinic acid and its salts exhibit potent antitumor promoter activity *in vitro* and in mice, and an inhibitory effect on the growth of several cancer lines [2,12,67,68]. A 1% aqueous extract of licorice fed to female mice resulted in significant protection against lung and forestomach tumorigenesis induced by oral benzo[a]pyrene or *N*-nitrosodiethylamine, which are known human carcinogens [69].

  F. **Immunological Agent:** Glycyrrhizin enhances antibody production, possibly through the production of interleukin 1 or through the induction of interferon [12,14,44]. It has been reported that a polysaccharide from *Glycyrrhiza uralensis* exhibits significant

Table 1. *(Continued)* Some known and reputed uses and activities of licorice and its derivatives[*]

	immunological activities [71]. Glycyrrhizin has been shown *in vitro* to augment the cell-surface expression of H-2 class I antigens as well as class I gene transcription on various cell lines [72].
G.	**Miscellaneous:** Other medicinal uses and activities of licorice include the following: to treat Addison's disease [3,5], as an antitoxic [2], to treat "griefs" of scabies, and to heal wounds [14]. It has been shown to exhibit positive effects in allergies [13,20,73], arthritis and rheumatism [13,74], and to exhibit anticariogenic [75,76], anti-inflammatory [12,18,44,74,76–79], antipyretic, cholagogue [44], antinauseant [80], antiseborrheic [13], anticonvulsive [2], antispasmodic [80], deodorant (leaf) [31], estrogenic [2,3,31,81], and antiestrogenic activities [29]. It is important to note that licorice has been reported to be an inhibitor of both monoamine oxidase [19] and xanthine oxidase [17].
II.	**Pharmaceutical Uses**
	Licorice has been employed in antismoking lozenges [28], mouthwashes and toothpaste [3], and as a filler, binder, flavor, flavor enhancer [3], sweetener, sweetening enhancer, and a vehicle for idoxuridine and bitter substances [82].
III.	**Other Reported Uses and Activities**
	Licorice is employed as a bakery, beverage, dairy, candy and meat flavor and color [2,3,8], a thickening agent [77,83], and a food antioxidant [12,84]. It is a common moisturizer and flavor for tobacco [14]. Licorice has also been employed in fire extinguishers, as a wetting, spreading and adhesive agent in insecticides, and an textile dye [85]. See also the section on chemistry regarding usage levels.

Adapted from reference [14] with supplementary data and references included. See also [2, 3, 9, 29, 31].

Pharmacokinetics

Anaerobic incubation of glycyrrhizin with human intestinal flora produces the aglycone, 18-β-glycyrrhetic acid, slowly at first but developing to about a 60% yield after 48 hours. About 25% of the active aglycone may be further metabolized, via a reversible epimerization, to the 3-α isomer, 3-epi-18-β-glycyrrhetic acid [86].

Five healthy human subjects each ingested an extract of *Glycyrrhiza* root containing 133 mg of glycyrrhizin. Their serum and urine were analyzed for glycyrrhizin and glycyrrhetinic acid using an enzyme immuno-antibody technique. Great individual differences in serum glycyrrhizin levels were found, but the peak serum concentration occurred in less than four hours. Serum levels rapidly decreased and glycyrrhizin could not be detected after 96 hours. Serum glycyrrhetinic acid, however, increased in concentration, reaching peak values 24 hours after administration of tne root extract. Glycyrrhetinic acid levels then gradually decreased but were still detectable in four cases at 72 hours and in two at 96 hours [15,87,88].

The serum levels of glycyrrhetinic acid in two patients who developed pseudoaldosteronism by using licorice-containing medications were very high (70–80 ng/ml), whereas their glycyrrhizin levels were very low. These data agree with the hypothesis that pseudoaldosteronism develops in association with glycyrrhetinic acid rather than glycyrrhizin [15,89].

The metabolites are probably excreted via the gastrointestinal route, as urinary glycyrrhizin and glycyrrhetinic acid accounted for only about 2% of the total administered extract [15,88].

The maximum plasma concentrations and AUCs for glycyrrhizin and glycyrrhetinic acid do not appear to be significantly influenced by the presence of food [36].

A recent study in humans examined the absorption and excretion of the constituents of the herbal remedy, Saiboku-To, which contains ten herbal extracts, including licorice. The researchers were unable to detect any glycyrrhizin or glycyrrhetinic acid in either the urine or blood but they failed to report their methodology. They indicate that further study is necessary to determine why fewer compounds were detected in the body than are known to be present and absorbed from single-constituent medicines [37].

Adverse Reaction Profile

General Animal Data

The syndrome, known as pseudoaldosteronism in humans, has also been seen in experimental animal species [90–93].

General Human Data

Licorice is generally regarded as safe for human consumption as a natural flavor and plant extract [2,7]. Adverse effects are common, however, when licorice is ingested in excess (more than 20 g/day) [13,94], with symptoms becoming apparent in less than a week when 100 g are consumed daily [61,95–102].

Symptoms are also seen, however, when only moderate amounts are consumed [7,8,94,103,104]. The clinical symptoms most commonly seen are lethargy, flaccid tetraparesis in almost all cases, with muscle pain in 32% and peripheral dysesthesia in the extremities, manifested mainly by numbness (27%). Cardiac arrhythmias and ECG abnormalities also occur secondary to the hypokalemia [13,101,105]. Laboratory findings included a mean serum potassium value of 1.98 mEq/l, a mean creatinine kinase of 5,385.7 IU/l, a mean blood aldosterone concentration of 2.92 ng/dl and a mean plasma renin activity of 0.17 ng/ml/h [105]. While rare, deaths have resulted from licorice ingestion [101,106].

Patients most frequently seen with licorice toxicity are those who ingest large amounts of licorice regularly, those who chew large amounts of tobacco, and those with pre-existing hypertension, renal or cardiac impairment [3,23,97,107,108]. Persons chewing licorice-flavored gum [103,109], eating licorice sweets [15,22,25,101,110], using licorice-flavored medications [105,110,111], utilizing certain licorice-containing laxatives [104,112], and glycyrrhizin-containing antacids [113] have also developed toxicity. Licorice toxicity is also common in eastern cultures [39,105,114].

Also reported to cause serious adverse reactions, particularly in ex-alcoholics, are the alcohol-free, licorice flavored French apertifs (pastis) [102,106,115–121]. Patients report with the usual licorice-induced symptoms ranging from hypokalemia and fatigue to hypertension, paresis, cardiac arrhythmias, and rhabdomyolysis. Death resulted from a prolonged cardiac arrest for a 32-year-old alcoholic patient [106]. These anise-based aperitifs contain 2.57–3.74 g/l of anethole (main constituent of aniseed oil) and 0.14–1.31 g/l of glycyrrhizin (from licorice root) [106,115]. Patients report drinking approximately 250 ml per day, the equivalent of up to 0.33 g of glycyrrhizin daily [106,115,117].

In a study done to provide a safety assessment of the glycyrrhizin content of licorice sweets, it was demonstrated that while most individuals can consume 400 mg of glycyrrhizin daily without adverse effects, some individuals will develop adverse effects following regular daily intake of as little as 100 mg of glycyrrhizin. Based on this information and using a safety factor of 10, it was estimated that 10 mg of glycyrrhizin (approximately 5 g of licorice candy) per day could be safely ingested on a regular basis [21]. On the other hand, the Dutch Nutrition Information Bureau has advised against a daily consumption of greater than 200 mg of glycyrrhizin [20]. This amount of glycyrrhizin is present in approximately 70 g of licorice offcuts, 46 g of Pontefract cakes or 220 g of licorice allsorts [22]. See also the section on chemistry for daily exposure data about licorice and glycyrrhizin.

The effects, similar to those from injections of large doses of deoxycorticosterone or ACTH, are thought to arise via a depressed renin-aldosterone-angiotensin system [14,95,122,123]. This leads to a set of symptoms and conditions, known as pseudo(hyper)aldosteronism, which includes headache, lethargy, quadriplegia, paraparesis, oedema, hypertension, hypertensive encephalopathy, electrolyte imbalance, myopathy, and possibly heart failure or cardiac arrest [13,23,61,98-100,124,125]. The symptoms are reversed by spironolactone administration [96,125]. Deglycyrrhizinized licorice is not usually associated with such effects [6,13,14].

Because of its ability to induce pseudoaldosteronism, licorice, its extracts and derivatives should be avoided by persons with cardiac problems, hypertension, cirrhosis, kidney complaints and those who are overweight, are ex-alcoholics, or are having difficult pregnancies [3]. Those patients taking antihypertensive, diuretic or cardiovascular medications should ingest licorice in moderation [13].

The mechanism underlying the pseudoaldosteronism is discussed in the section on Endocrine Reactions.

Allergic Reactions

Hypersensitivity reactions to glycyrrhiza-containing products appear to be rare and it is uncertain whether the allergic reaction is due to the licorice or to the other ingredients present [13,126–128]. For further discussion, see the section on Hepatic Reactions.

Autoimmune Reactions

There is one Japanese case report which associates Sjögren's syndrome, an autoimmune disease, with hypokalemic myopathy due to glycyrrhizin [129].

Cardiovascular Reactions

Excessive licorice ingestion can lead to severe hypertension,[39,107,112,120,130–133], cardiac arrhythmias [31,45,112,134–136], cardiomyopathy [132,135], and cardiac arrest [112,134]. Hypertensive retinopathy [130] and hypertensive encephalopathy have been reported [130,132]. Oedema occurs in about 20% of peptic ulcer patients being treated with licorice extracts [45].

Dermatological Reactions

Oedema of the face and limbs is the only reported visible effect from the ingestion of excess licorice [31,137].

Topical glycyrrhetinic acid (2%) potentiates the action of hydrocortisone in several inflammatory cutaneous disorders by inhibiting enzymatic metabolism to the inactive cortisone [138,139].

Discoloration of skin and serum after the ingestion of a particular licorice product manufactured during the summer of 1991 has been reported. It was suspected that the coloration was due to an unidentified pigment from licorice [140].

Endocrine Reactions

Ingestion of licorice has long been associated with increased sodium retention, increased potassium loss, suppression of the renin-angiotensin-aldosterone axis, and, more recently, with the increased urinary excretion of free hydrocortisone [3–7,13,14,44,94,122,139,141–144]. Glycyrrhetinic acid potentiates the activity of hydrocortisone in the skin [145], and glycyrrhetinic acid (but not glycyrrhizin) potentiates the action of hydrocortisone in human lung tissue. Licorice is believed to induce the state of pseudo(hyper)aldosteronism mainly through its aglycone, glycyrrhetinic acid [146].

Two hypotheses for the action of licorice have been proposed; binding of glycyrrhetinic acid to mineralocorticoid receptors, and blocking the action of 11-β-hydroxysteroid dehydrogenase. A recent paper suggests that both mechanisms are involved and confirms that the blocking of 11-β-hydroxysteroid dehydrogenase is only temporary and that afterwards the pseudoaldosteronism is directly related to the increased plasma concentration of the licorice metabolites and their binding to the mineralocorticoid receptors [147–149].

Normal physiological glucocorticoids are rapidly metabolized by 11-β-hydroxysteroid dehydrogenase to inactive products, thereby regulating glucocorticoid access to peripheral mineralocorticoid and glucocorticoid receptors in a site-specific manner [92,150].

By preventing the inactivation of hydrocortisone, licorice increases the glucocorticoid concentration in mineralocorticoid-responsive tissues. As a result, glucocorticoids occupy mineralocorticoid receptors and produce a mineralocorticoid response, as evidenced by increased sodium retention and hypertension [14,143,151].

It was believed that glycyrrhetinic acid caused the hypertension syndrome by binding directly to the renal mineralocorticoid receptor [125,150]. However, previous studies have shown that the hypertension was dependent on the presence of hydrocortisone or another ACTH-dependent steroid since the hypertension was reversed by dexamethasone [150,152], and absent in patients without intact adrenal glands [150].

Glycyrrhetinic acid inhibits 11-β-hydroxysteroid dehydrogenase, 3-β-hydroxysteroid dehydrogenase, 3-α-hydroxysteroid dehydrogenase, 5-β-reductase, and 5-α-reductase [14,78,90,91,143,151,153–155]. Consequently, it has been postulated that the inhibition of 5-β-reductase, 3-α-hydroxysteroid-dehydrogenase, and 11-β-hydroxysteroid dehydrogenase results in steroid-like action, anti-inflammatory action, and pseudoaldosteronism, respectively [91,122,150,155–157].

Other studies have indicated that glycyrrhetinic acid is a potent inhibitor of cytosolic 5-β-reductase and also inhibits 3-β-hydroxysteroid dehydrogenase, possibly by competitive inhibition, resulting in an accumulation of aldosterone and 5-α-dihydroaldosterone, both potent mineralocorticoids. In addition, glycyrrhetinic acid and, to a lesser extent, glycyrrhizin also inhibit hepatic δ-4,5-β-steroid reductase in vitro, an enzyme that reduces the A ring of steroids and thus inactivates both glucocorticoids and mineralocorticoids. Consequently, the inhibition of this enzyme results in an accumulation of both glucocorticoid and mineralocorticoid hormones [44,100]. Thus, more than one enzyme may be involved in the mechanism by which glycyrrhetinic acid causes mineralocorticoid actions in humans and experimental animals [44,90]. It has been demonstrated that the activity of 11-β-hydroxysteroid dehydrogenase returns to normal about two to four weeks after withdrawal of licorice, coinciding with the decrease in urinary glycyrrhizin levels. In contrast, the basal activity of the renin-angiotensin-aldosterone system remained suppressed for several months after licorice withdrawal. This prolonged suppression of the renin-angiotensin-aldosterone axis demonstrates the potential of licorice toxicity and emphasizes the need to consider licorice, and possibly other factors or drugs that affect 11-β-hydroxysteroid dehydrogenase activity, as a cause of low-renin hypertension [157,158].

It has been shown that 11-β-hydroxysteroid dehydrogenase and possibly other corticosteroid-metabolizing enzymes in the brain play a major role in the negative feedback control by corticosteroids of corticotrophin-releasing factor-41 release into hypophysial portal blood [92,93].

Several experiments have been reported indicating that 11-β-hydroxysteroid dehydrogenase, in mineralocorticoid target tissues, acts as a "protective" mechanism that prevents endogenous glucocorticoids from causing mineralocorticoid receptor-mediated effects on sodium and potassium [38,91,150,153,159]. Additional experiments have also indicated that a second distinct protective mechanism exists that prevents endogenous mineralocorticoids from eliciting excessive mineralocorticoid receptor-mediated sodium retention. This second protective mechanism may involve steroid-metabolizing enzymes other than 11-β-hydroxysteroid dehydrogenase. It is also possible that a third protective mechanism exists whereby renal 11-β-hydroxysteroid dehydrogenase prevents endogenous glucocorticoids from eliciting glucocorticoid receptor-mediated effects on sodium and potassium [91]. Furthermore, by converting active glucocorticoid to an inactive metabolite, 11-β-hydroxysteroid dehydrogenase has been shown to also be a powerful modulator of glucocorticoid hormone action [160].

It has been stated that glycyrrhetinic acid inhibits 15-hydroxyprostaglandin dehydrogenase and δ-13-prostaglandin reductase, two enzymes that are important in the metabolism of prostaglandins E and $F_{2\alpha}$ [13,143,161]. This hypothesis, however, has been rejected on the basis of recent experimental data which showed that glycyrrhetinic acid had no effect on 15-hydroxyprostaglandin dehydrogenase activity and, therefore, that it was unlikely that altered prostaglandin metabolism contributes to the salt-retaining or anti-inflammatory actions of licorice and its derivatives as postulated [143,151]. Glycyrrhizin inhibits the activity of phospholipase A_2 [161] and kinase P [162].

It has been observed that insulin-treated diabetic patients appear to be predisposed to hypokalemia, sodium retention, and suppression of both plasma aldosterone concentration and plasma renin activity. Urinary excretion of potassium, however, was not increased, indicating a different condition from pseudoaldosteronism [163].

Gastrointestinal Reactions

Data on gastrointestinal reactions, other than a mild laxative effect, have not been identified in the literature [1,2,4,30].

Hepatic Reactions

In the Japanese literature, two case reports have appeared about a hypersensitive hepatic reaction to Stronger-Neo-Minophagen C® (SNMC), a drug consisting of glycine, cysteine and glycyrrhizin which is used there for allergic diseases and chronic liver diseases [126,127]. Another report about allergic hepatitis comes from Spain [128]. It is, however, uncertain whether such reactions were due to the licorice or to the other ingredients present.

Considerable attention, especially in Japan, has recently been focused on the role of glycyrrhizin and glycyrrhetinic acid as a therapeutic agent in chronic hepatitis B, as an antihepatotoxic and for its therapeutic effects in hepatic injury. However, ambiguity remains because the benefits may be dependent on the lowering of serum transaminase levels [12,44,79,164–168].

Muscular Reactions

Hypokalemic myopathy is a well established iatrogenic disease from excessive licorice ingestion [105,136,169–175]. A recent review article reports on 116 cases of glycyrrhizin (licorice)-induced hypokalemic myopathy [124].

Patients usually present with lethargy, flaccid tetraparesis, and myalgia. Walking is impaired if not impossible. Rhabdomyolysis, secondary to licorice-induced hypokalemia has also occurred [113,136,175,176]. The diagnosis of rhabdomyolysis, the disintegration of the striated muscle fibers with excretion of myoglobin in the urine, is confirmed by the combination of extensively elevated CPK, high LDH, SGOT, and SGPT, with dark brown urine and elevated serum myoglobin concentrations [113,175]. In one reported case, myoglobinemia led to glomerulopathy and tubulopathy, but there was no clinical evidence of acute renal failure (ARF). It was proposed that the volume expansion caused by the steroid-like actions of licorice might have prevented the development of ARF [175]. Electromyographic studies indicate that the myopathy results from hypochloremia independent of associated hypokalemia [169].

A complete absence of myoadenylate deaminase (MADA) activity has been reported in humans. MADA is an important enzyme of the purine nucleotide cycle, the function of which is crucial during muscle exercise [136,177]. The absence of MADA activity has been associated with exertional myalgia and hypokalemia [136,178]. In one report, the MADA deficiency was not corrected in vitro by the addition of potassium, but completely returned following licorice withdrawal. The authors speculate that their observations suggest that, although the enzyme is highly dependent on potassium, MADA deficiency cannot simply be the result of hypokalemia, but may result from a direct toxic effect of glycyrrhizin or similar glycosides [136]. A similar effect is seen on cortisol oxidase [158].

Ocular Reactions

One instance of retinopathy resulting from licorice-induced hypertension has been reported [130].

Pulmonary Reactions

Acute pulmonary oedema has been reported in a 15-year-old boy following the intravenous administration of Stronger Neo-Minophagen C® (contains glycyrrhizin) and Chlor-Trimetron (chlorphentermine maleate). No pleural reaction was present. It was suggested that the pulmonary oedema was due to increased focal permeability as a result of injury to pulmonary endothelial cells. The authors conclude that both of these drugs should be considered as possible etiologic factors [179].

Renal Reactions

An early report documented acute renal failure due to rhabdomyolysis, which was a consequence of chronic licorice ingestion and, possibly, due to the administration of furosemide for the two days prior to presenting. Withdrawal of the licorice and renal dialysis brought about complete recovery [176].

In a subsequent case, myoglobinemia led to glomerulopathy and tubulopathy, but there was no clinical evidence of acute renal failure (ARF) [175]. It was proposed that the mineralocorticoid-like actions of glycyrrhizin cause sodium retention and volume expansion, and thereby prevent the decrease in the glomerular filtration rate and the development of ARF, in spite of evidence of tubular dysfunction [175,176]. Another case reported the development of reversible tubulopathy [180].

Most recently, a 72-year-old man developed acute renal failure following severe hypokalemic rhabdomyolysis, subsequent to chronic use of a glycyrrhizin-containing antacid [113]. This patient presented with several predisposing factors, complicating the implication of glycyrrhizin, but was stabilized via plasma exchange, hemodialysis, potassium supplementation, and modest use of a glycyrrhizin-containing preparation. These authors conclude that the mineralocorticoid-like actions explained above may be inadequate to protect all persons, especially elderly people with decreased renal function and severely dehydrated patients [113].

Drug Interactions

It has been reported that co-administered deglycyrrhizinated licorice not only increases the bioavailability of nitrofurantoin by over 50%, but simultaneously decreases the tendencies toward nausea and emesis [80].

The concurrent use of furosemide has been indicated as a contributing factor in the development of acute renal failure [113,176].

Topical glycyrrhetinic acid (2%) potentiates the action of hydrocortisone in several inflammatory cutaneous disorders by inhibiting enzymatic metabolism to the inactive cortisone [138,139].

Glycyrrhetinic acid (but not glycyrrhizin) potentiates the action of hydrocortisone in human lung tissue [146].

A study in healthy men has shown that oral administration of glycyrrhizin significantly increases the plasma concentration of intravenously administered prednisolone and influences its pharmacokinetics by inhibiting its metabolism, but not by affecting its distribution [181]. Similar results have been seen in rheumatoid arthritis and polyarteritis nodosa patients being treated with prednisolone [182].

Insulin may be synergistic with glycyrrhizin in causing electrolyte disturbances and suppression of renin and aldosterone [163].

Fertility, Pregnancy and Lactation

Glycyrrhizin and glycyrrhetinic acid have been shown to inhibit the conversion of androstenedione to testosterone in rat gonads, indicating that these compounds inhibit the activity of 17-β-hydroxysteroid dehydrogenase, and result in reduced testosterone production. While this could lead to unwanted symptoms in males, it has been used successfully to treat infertile women who have high serum concentrations of testosterone [183].

A rise in the concentration of progesterone and other steroids in the blood, due to competition by licorice for liver metabolism, has been observed. This may result in amenorrhea and hyperprolactemia with subsequent infertility in females [73].

Extracts of the aerial portion of licorice and a phenolic constituent (glycesterone) exert an estrogenic activity in experimental animals. Glycesterone has 1/533 the potency of estrone [2,3,8].

Glycyrrhetinic acid also stimulates the release of arginine vasopressin and oxytocin into portal blood of adrenal intact, but not adrenalectomized, rats [92].

Dominant lethal effect studies (dead fetuses as a consequence of male treatment) with ammoniated glycyrrhizin have shown a questionable statistically significant effect in the male rat but not in the male mouse [184], and an increased resorption rate in the mouse [185]. There were no significant effects in the rat treated with disodium glycyrrhizinate [186]. Ammoniated glycyrrhizin also failed to induce heritable chromosomal effects in male mice [184].

A teratogenicity study of ammoniated glycyrrhizin in the Sprague-Dawley rat gave a clear indication of a slight, though undesirable, action of ammoniated glycyrrhizin on the conceptus in the absence of any significant maternal toxicity, besides polydipsia [187].

An epidemiological study performed in Australia failed to show a relationship between the use of licorice-based cough mixtures and the occurrence of abnormal neonatal outcomes [188].

Glycyrrhizin may cause a rise in the concentration of progesterone and other steroids in the blood, due to competition with glycyrrhizin for liver metabolism. This may result in amenorrhea, decreased libido, and hyperprolactemia with subsequent infertility in females [73,189].

Mutagenicity and Carcinogenicity

Glycyrrhetinic acid and its salts are neither mutagenic nor cytotoxic. On the contrary, both the 18-α- and 18-β-isomers exhibit potent antitumor promoting activity in vitro and an inhibitory effect on the growth of several cancer lines [2,67,190,191]. Licorice has been used to treat and/or prevent some cancers [2,192].

Mutagenicity testing of ammoniated glycyrrhizin, used as a sweetener in foods and pharmaceutical preparations, was negative in *Salmonella typhimurium* G-46 and TA1530 and in *Saccharomyces cerevisae* D3. Tests for chromosome aberrations in anaphases of human WI-38 embryonic lung cells were also negative [193]. Mutagenic screening of licorice root with *Bacillus subtilis* rec-assay showed weakly positive activity [194], whereas screening with Ames strains TA98 and TA100 of *Salmonella typhimurium* were negative, actually exhibiting a cytotoxic effect [194,195]. Another study examining the mutagenicities of flavonoids and related compounds found that isoliquiritigenin showed mutagenicity to TA100, and only in the presence of the S9 liver homogenate. No mutagenicity was observed in the absence of S9 or with TA98 [196]. A recent study on the mutagenicity of raw pharmaceuticals used in Chinese traditional medicine utilizing the Ames test and strains TA98 and TA100 found *Glycyrrhiza uralensis* to be free of mutagenic activity, even in the presence of S9. Further, it did not cause any chromosomal aberrations [197].

References

1. Evans WC (1989) Trease and Evans' Pharmacognosy. 13th ed. London: Bailliere Tindall, pp.495–498
2. Leung AY (1980) Encyclopedia of Common Natural Ingredients Used in Food, Drugs, and Cosmetics. Glen Rock, NJ: Wiley Interscience, pp.220–223
3. Morton JF (1977) Major Medicinal Plants: Botany, Culture, and Uses. Springfield, IL: Thomas, pp.154–158
4. British Herbal Medicine Association (1983) British Herbal Pharmacopeia. Bournemouth, U.K.: Megaron Press, pp.104–105
5. Osol A, Farrar GE eds (1955) The Dispensatory of the United States of America. 25th ed. Philadelphia: Lippincott, pp.617–621
6. Reynolds JEF ed (1989) Martindale: The Extra Pharmacopoeia. 29th ed. London: Pharmaceutical Press, pp.1093–1094
7. Simon JE, Chadwick AF, Craker LE (1984) Herbs: An Indexed Bibliography, 1971–1980. Hamden, Connecticut: Shoe String Press, pp.159–161
8. Lutomski J (1983) Chemie und therapeutische Verwendung von Süssholz. Pharm Unserer Zeit 12:49–54
9. Grieve M (1974) A Modern Herbal. New York: Hafner, pp.487–492
10. Jackson BP, Snowdon DW (1990) Atlas of Microscopy of Medicinal Plants, Culinary Herbs and Spices. London: Belhaven Press, pp.144–145
11. Pharmaceutical Society of Great Britain (1934) The British Pharmaceutical Codex. London: The Pharmaceutical Press, pp.487–489
12. Hikino H, Kiso Y (1988) Natural products for liver diseases. In: Wagner H, Hikino H, Farnsworth NR eds. Economic and Medicinal Plant Research. Vol 2. London: Academic Press, pp.39–72
13. Der Marderosian AH, Liberti LE (1988) Natural Product Medicine. Philadelphia: George F Stickley, 317–321
14. Gibson MR (1978) *Glycyrrhiza* in old and new perspectives. Lloydia 41:348–354
15. Terasawa K, Bandoh M, Tosa H, Hirate J (1986) Disposition of glycyrrhetic acid and its glycosides in healthy subjects and patients with pseudoaldosteronism. J Pharmacobio–Dyn 9:95–100
16. Mitscher LA, Park YH, Clark D, Beal JL (1980) Antimicrobial agents from higher plants. Antimicrobial isoflavonoids and related substances from *Glycyrrhiza glabra* L. var. *typica*. J Nat Prod 43:259–269
17. Hatano T, Yasuhara T, Fukuda T, Noro T, Okuda T (1989) Phenolic constituents of licorice. II. Structures of licopyranocoumarin, licoarylcoumarin, and glisoflavone, and inhibitory effects of licorice phenolics on xanthine oxidase. Chem Pharm Bull 37:3005–3009
18. Revers FE (1946) Has licorice juice (*Succus liquiritiae*) a healing action on gastric ulcer? Ned Tijdsch Geneesk 90:135 *via* Shibata S (1977) Saponins with biological and pharmaco-

logical activity. In: Wagner H, Wolff P eds. New Natural Products and Plant Drugs with Pharmacological, Biological or Therapeutical Activity. Berlin: Springer-Verlag, pp.177–196
19. Hatano T, Fukuda T, Miyase T, Noro T, Okuda T (1991) Phenolic constituents of licorice. III. Structures of glicoricone and licofuranone, and inhibitory effects of licorice constituents on monoamine oxidase. Chem Pharm Bull 39:1238–1243
20. Nieman C (1989) Physiology and toxicology of liquorice. Glucose Informatie 9:173–192
21. Stormer FC, Reistad R, Alexander J (1993) Glycyrrhizic acid in liquorice - evaluation of health hazard. Food Chem Toxicol 31:303–312
22. Spinks EA, Fenwick GR (1990) The determination of glycyrrhizin in selected UK liquorice products. Food Add Contam 7:769–778
23. Bell JH (1980) Determination of glycyrrhizic acid in liquorice extracts and chewing tobaccos. Tobacco Science 24:126–129
24. Ibsen KK (1981) Liquorice consumption and its influence on blood pressure in Danish school-children. Dan Med Bull 28:124–126
25. Simpson FO, Currie IJ (1982) Licorice consumption among high school students. N Z Med J 95:31–33
26. Toner JM, Ramsey LE (1985) Liquorice can damage your health. Practitioner 229:858–859
27. Tyler VE (1987) The New Honest Herbal. Philadelphia: George F Stickley, pp.143–145
28. Nieman C (1957) Licorice. In: Nieman C, Mrak EM, Stewart GF eds. Advances in Food Research; Vol 7. New York: Academic Press, pp.339–381
29. Davis EA, Morris DJ (1991) Medicinal uses of licorice through the millenia: the good and plenty of it. Molecul Cell Endocrinol 78:1–6
30. Chandler RF (1985) Licorice, more than just a flavor. Can Pharm J 118:420–424
31. Duke JA (1985) CRC Handbook of Medicinal Herbs. Boca Raton, FL: CRC Press, pp.215–216, 519, 556
32. Huang KC (1993) The pharmacology of Chinese herbs. Boca Raton, FL: CRC Press, pp.27–178
33. Tierra M (1990) The way of herbs. New York: Pocket Books, pp.275–277
34. Bensky D, Gamble A (1993) Chinese herbal medicine materica medica. Seattle: Eastland Press, pp.323–325
35. Willard T (1991) The wild rose scientific herbal. Calgary: The Wild Rose College of Natural Healing, pp.206–210
36. Nishioka Y, Kyotani S, Miyamura M, Kusunose M (1992) Influence of time of administration of a Shosaiko-to extract granule on blood concentrations of its active constituents. Chem Pharm Bull 40:1335–1337
37. Homma M, Oka K, Niitsuma T, Itoh H (1993) Pharmacokinetic evaluation of traditional Chinese herbal remedies. Lancet 341:1595
38. Edwards CR (1991) Lessons from licorice. N Engl J Med 325:1242–1243
39. Itami N, Yamamoto K, Andoh T, Akutsu Y (1991) Herbal medicine can induce hypertension. Nephron 59:339–340
40. Takahashi K, Shibata S, Yano S, Harada M, Saito H, Tamura Y, Kumagai A (1980) Chemical modification of glycyrrhetinic acid in relation to the biological activities. Chem Pharm Bull 28:3449–3452
41. Tawata M, Aida K, Noguchi T, Ozaki Y, Kume S, Sasaki H, Chin M, Onaya T (1992) Anti-platelet action of isoliquiritigenin, an aldose reductase inhibitor in licorice. Eur J Pharmacol 212:87–92
42. Imagawa M, Kamei H, Arakawa K (1982) High renin low blood pressure and its treatment with calcium glycyrrhetinyl-glycinate. Jpn Heart J 23:201–209
43. Segal R, Milo-Goldzweig I, Kaplan G, Weisenberg E (1977) The protective action of glycyrrhizin against saponin toxicity. Biochem Pharmacol 26:643–645
44. Hikino H (1985) Recent research on oriental medicinal plants. In: Wagner H, Hikino H, Farnsworth NR eds. Economic and Medicinal Plant Research. Vol 1. London: Academic Press, pp.53–85

45. Lewis WH, Elvin-Lewis MPF (1977) Medical Botany: Plants Affecting Man's Health. New York: Wiley Interscience, pp.182, 215, 275
46. Barrowman JA, Pfeiffer CJ (1982) Carbenoxolone: A critical analysis of its clinical value in peptic ulcer. In: Pfeiffer CJ, ed. Drugs and Peptic Ulcer; Vol 1. Boca Raton. Florida: CRC Press, pp.123–132
47. Guslandi M (1980) Effect of anti-ulcer drugs on gastric mucous barrier and possible cyclic AMP involvement. Int J Clin Pharmacol Ther Toxicol 18:140–143
48. Sircus W (1972) Drugs in the treatment of peptic ulcer. Prescr J 12(Feb):1–10
49. Glick L (1982) Deglycyrrhizinated licorice for peptic ulcer. Lancet 2:817
50. Watanabe S, Chey WY, Lee KY, Chen YF, Chang T-M, Shiratori K, Takeuchi T (1984) Secretin is released by licorice extract in mammals. Gastroenterology 86:1293
51. Morgan RJ, Nelson LM, Russell RI, Docherty C (1983) The protective effect of deglycyrrhinized liquorice against aspirin and aspirin plus bile acid-induced gastric mucosal damage, and its influence on aspirin absorption in rats. J Pharm Pharmacol 35:605–607
52. Anderson DM, Smith WG (1961) The antitussive activity of glycyrrhetinic acid and its derivatives. J Pharm Pharmacol 13:396–404
53. Mooreville M, Fritz RW, Mulholland SG (1983) Enhancement of the bladder defense mechanism by an exogenous agent. J Urol 130:607–609
54. Pompei R, Pani A, Flore MA, Marcialis MA, Loddo B (1980) Antiviral activity of glycyrrhizic acid. Experientia 30:304
55. Hirabayashi K, Iwata S, Matsumoto H, Mori T, Shibata S, Baba M, Ito M, Shigeta S, Nakashima H, Yamamoto N (1991) Antiviral activities of glycyrrhizin and its modified compounds against human immunodeficiency virus type 1 (HIV-1) and *Herpes simplex* virus type 1 (HSV-1) *in vitro*. Chem Pharm Bull 39:112–115
56. Dargan DJ, Subak-Sharpe JH (1985) The effect of triterpenoid compounds on uninfected and herpes simplex virus-infected cells in culture. I. Effect on cell growth, virus particles and virus replication. J Gen Virol 66:1771–1784
57. Baba M, Shigeta S (1987) Antiviral activity of glycyrrhizin against varicella-zoster virus in vitro. Antiviral Research 7:99–107
58. Csonka GW, Tyrell DAJ 1984) Treatment of herpes genitalis with carbenoxolone and cicloxolone creams. Br J Ven Dis 60:178–181
59. Poswillo DE, Roberts GJ (1981) Topical carbenoxolone for orofacial herpes simplex infections. Lancet 2:142–144
60. Crance JM, Biziagos E, Passagot J, van Cuyck-Gandre H, Deloince R (1990) Inhibition of hepatitis A virus replication in vitro by antiviral compounds. J Med Virol 31:155–160
61. Vulto AG, Buurma H. Drugs used in non-orthodox medicine. In: Dukes MNG ed (1985) Side Effects of Drugs Annual 9. Amsterdam: Elsevier, pp.418–429
62. Mori K, Sakai H, Suzuki S, Sugal K, Akutsu Y, Ishikawa M, Seino Y, Ishida N, Uchida T, Kariyone S, Endo Y, Miura A (1989) Effects of glycyrrhizin (SNMC: Stronger Neo-Minophagen CR) in hemophilia patients with HIV infection. Tohoku J Exp Med 158:25–35
63. Hattori T, Ikematsu S, Koito A, Matsushita S, Maeda Y, Hada M, Fujimaki M, Takatsuki K (1989) Preliminary evidence for inhibitory effect of glycyrrhizin on HIV replication in patients with AIDS. Antiviral Research 11:255–262
64. Ito M, Sato A, Hirabayashi K, Tanabe F, Shigeta S, Baba M, De Clerq E, Nakashima H, Yamamoto N (1988) Mechanism of inhibitory effect of glycyrrhizin on replication of human immunodeficiency virus (HIV). Antiviral Research 10:289–298
65. Ito M, Nakashima H, Baba M, Pauwels R, De Clerq E, Shigeta S, Yamamoto N (1987) Inhibitory effect of glycyrrhizin on the in vitro infectivity and cytopathic activity of the human immunodeficiency virus [HIV (HTLV-III/LAV)]. Antiviral Research 7:127–137
66. Poswillo D, Partridge M (1984) Management of recurrent aphthous ulcers. Br Dent J 157:55–57
67. Kitagawa K, Nishino H, Iwashima A (1984) Inhibition of 12-O-tetradecanoylphorbol-13-acetate-stimulated 3-O-methyl-glucose transport in mouse Swiss 3T3 fibroblasts by glycyrrhetic acid. Cancer Lett 24:157–163

68. Nishino H, Yoshioka K, Iwashima A, Takizawa H, Konishi S, Okamoto H, Okabe H, Shibata S, Fujiki H, Sugimura T (1986) Glycyrrhetic acid inhibits tumor-promoting activity of teleocidin and 12-O-tetradecanoylphorbol-13-acetate in two-stage mouse skin carcinogenesis. Jpn J Cancer Res (Gann) 77:33–38
69. Wang ZY, Agarwal R, Khan WA, Muktar H (1992) Protection against benzo[a]pyrene- and N-nitrosodiethylamine-induced lung and forestomach tumorigenesis in A/J mice by water extracts of green tea and licorice. Carcinogenesis 13:1491–1494
70. Chen M et al. (1994) Licochalcone A, a new antimalarial agent, inhibits in vitro growth of the human malaria parasite *Plasmodium falciparum* and protects mice from *P. yoelii*. Antimicrob Agents Chemother 38:1470–1475; via Inpharma 1994 no.949:9
71. Shimizu N, Tomoda M, Takada K, Gonda R (1992) The core structure and immunological activities of glycyrrhizan UA, the main polysaccharide from the root of *Glycyrrhiza uralensis*. Chem Pharm Bull 40:2125–2128
72. Zhang YH, Yoshida T, Isobe K, Rahman SMJ, Nagase F, Ding L, Nakashima I (1990) Modulation by glycyrrhizin of the cell-surface expression of H-2 class I antigens on murine tumour cell lines and normal cell populations. Immunology 70:405–410
73. Vulto AG, Buurma H (1984) Drugs used in non-orthodox medicine. In: Dukes MNG ed. Meyler's Side Effects of Drugs, 10th ed. Amsterdam: Elsevier, pp.886–907
74. Capasso F, Mascolo N, Autore G, Duraccio MR (1983) Glycyrrhetinic acid, leucocytes and prostaglandins. J Pharm Pharmacol 35:332–335
75. Segal R, Pisanty S, Wormser R, Azaz E, Sela MN (1985) Anticariogenic activity of licorice and glycyrrhizine 1: Inhibition of in vitro plaque formation by *Streptococcus mutans*. J Pharm Sci 74:79–81
76. Deutchman M, Petrou ID, Mellberg JR (1989) Effect of fluoride and glycyrrhizin mouthrinses on artificial caries lesions in vivo. Caries Res 23:206–208
77. Kondo M, Minamino H, Okuyama G, Honda K, Nagasawa H, Otani Y (1985) Two glycyrrhizin isomers and their application to cosmetics. Cosmet Toilet 100:33–35
78. Amagaya S, Sugishita E, Ogihara Y, Ogawa S, Okada K, Aizawa T (1984) Comparative studies of the stereoisomers of glycyrrhetinic acid on anti-inflammatory activities. J Pharm Dyn 7:923–928
79. Shibayama Y (1989) Prevention of hepatotoxic responses to chemicals by glycyrrhizin in rats. Exp Molecul Path 51:48–55
80. Lahiri K, Raju DSN, Rao PR (1980) Influence of deglycyrrhizinated licorice on the bioavailability of nitrofurantoin. East Pharm, Scientific Section 23:191–193
81. Costello CH, Lynn EV (1950) Estrogenic substances from plants: I. *Glycyrrhiza*. J Am Pharm Assoc 39:177–180
82. Touitou E, Segal R, Pisanty S, Milo-Goldweig I (1988) Glycyrrhizin gel as vehicle for idoxuridine topical preparation: skin permeation behaviour. Drug Design Deliv 3:267–272
83. Azaz E, Segal KR (1980) Glycyrrhizin as gelling agent. Pharm Acta Helv 55:183–186
84. Maruzen Chemical Co Ltd (1984) Japanese patent no. 58,217,583 via Chem Abstr 100:119655r
85. Paksoy G (1985) Possibility of the use of *Glycyrrhiza glabra* L. as a textile dye. Doga Bilim Der, ser B, 9(2):135–148; via Chem Abstr 1986; 104:51971r
86. Hattori M, Sakamoto T, Kobashi K, Namba T (1983) Metabolism of glycyrrhizin by human intestinal flora. Planta Med 48:38–42
87. Ishida S, Sakiya Y, Ichikawa T, Taira Z, Awazu S (1990) Prediction of glycyrrhizin disposition in rat and man with liver failure by a physiologically based pharmacokinetic model. J Pharmacobio-Dyn 13:142–157
88. Bando M, Terasawa K, Kaneoka M, Yano S, Kato H, Hirate J, Isamu H (1985) Pharmacokinetics of glycyrrhetinic acid. Wakan Iyaku Gakkaishi 2(1):264–265, via Chem Abstr 1986; 104:28337e
89. Ulmann A, Menard J, Corvol P (1975) Binding of glycyrrhetinic acid to kidney mineralocorticoid receptors. Endocrinology 97:46–51

90. Latif SA, Conca TJ, Morris DJ (1990) The effects of the licorice derivative, glycyrrhetinic acid, on hepatic 3-alpha- and 3-beta-hydroxysteroid dehydrogenases and 5-alpha- and 5-beta-reductase pathways of metabolism of aldosterone in male rats. Steroids 55:52-58
91. Morris DJ, Souness GW (1992) Protective and specificity-conferring mechanisms of mineralocorticoid action. Am J Physiol 263 (Renal Fluid Electrolyte Physiol 32):F759–F768
92. Seckl JR, Dow RC, Low SC, Edwards CRW, Fink G (1993) The 11-beta-hydroxysteroid dehydrogenase inhibitor glycyrrhetinic acid affects corticosteroid feedback regulation of hypothalamic corticotrophin-releasing peptides in rats. J Endocrinol 136:471–477
93. Gomez-Sanchez EP, Gomez-Sanchez CE (1992) Central hypertensiogenic effects of glycyrrhizic acid and carbenoxolone. Am J Physiol 263 (Endocrinol Metab 26):E1125–1130
94. Vulto AG, De Smet PAGM (1988) Drugs used in non-orthodox medicine. In: Dukes MNG ed. Meyler's Side Effects of Drugs, 11th ed. Amsterdam: Elsevier, pp.999–1084
95. Epstein MT, Espiner EA, Donald RA, Hughes H (1977) Effect of eating liquorice on the renin-angiotensin-aldosterone axis in normal subjects. Br Med J 1:488–490
96. Stedwell RE, Allen KM, Binder LS (1992) Hypokalemic paralyses: A review of the etiologies, pathophysiology, presentation, and therapy. Am J Emerg Med 10:143–148
97. Blachley JD, Knochel JP (1980) Tobacco chewer's hypokalemia: licorice revisited. N Engl J Med 302:784–785
98. Haberer JP, Jouve P, Bedock B, Bazin PE (1984) Severe hypokalemia secondary to overindulgence in alcohol-free "pastis". Lancet i:575–576
99. Sundaram MBM, Swaminathan R (1981) Total body potassium depletion and severe myopathy due to chronic liquorice ingestion. Postgrad Med J 57:48–49
100. Morris DJ, Davis E, Latif SA (1990) Licorice, tobacco chewing, and hypertension. N Engl J Med 322:849–850
101. Nielsen I, Pedersen RS (1984) Life-threatening hypokalemia caused by liquorice ingestion. Lancet 1:1305
102. Achar KN, Abduo TJ, Menon NK (1989) Severe hypokalemic rhabdomyolysis due to ingestion of liquorice during Ramadan. Aust NZ J Med 19:365–367
103. Roseel M, Schoors D (1993) Chewing gum and hypokalaemia. Lancet 341:175
104. Cumming AMM, Boddy K, Brown JJ, Fraser R, Lever AF, Padfield PL, Robertson JIS (1980) Severe hypokalaemia with paralysis induced by small doses of liquorice. Postgrad Med J 56:526–529
105. Shintani S, Murase H, Tsukagoshi H, Shiigai T (1992) Glycyrrhizin (licorice) -induced hypokalemic myopathy. Eur Neurol 32:44–51
106. Beddock B, Janin-Mercier A, Jouve P, Lamaison D, Meyrieux J, Chipponi PN, Haberer JP (1985) Intoxication mortelle par le pastis sans alcool. Ann Franc Anesth Reanimat 4: 374–377
107. Westman EC, Guthrie GP Jr (1990) Licorice, tobacco chewing, and hypertension. N Engl J Med 322:850
108. Morris DJ, Davis E, Latif SA (1990) Licorice, tobacco chewing, and hypertension. N Engl J Med 322:849–850
109. Rosseel M, Schoors D (1993) Chewing gum and hypokalemia. Lancet 341:175
110. Holmes AM, Marrott PK, Young J, Prentice E (1970) Pseudohyperaldosteronism induced by habitual ingestion of liquorice. Postgrad Med J 46:625–629
111. Levesque H, Cailleux N, Poutrain JR, Noblet C, Moore N, Courtois H (1992) Pseudohyperaldosteronisme par surdosage chronique en pastilles "Pulmoll" marron. Therapie 47:439–440
112. Scali M, Pratesi C, Zennaro MC, Zampollo V, Armanini D (1990) Pseudohyperaldosteronism from liquorice-containing laxatives. J Endocrinol Invest 13:847–848
113. Chubachi A, Wakui H, Asakura K, Nishimura S, Nakamoto Y, Miura AB (1992) Acute renal failure following hypokalemic rhabdomyolysis due to chronic glycyrrhizic acid administration. Int Med 31:708–711

114. Ono T, Komatsu M, Inomata S, Inoue M, Tobori F, Yagisawa H, Mukojima T, Arakawa H, Inoue S, Masamune O (1984) A case of asymptomatic PBC accompanied by glycyrrhizin-induced pseudoaldosteronism. Jap J Gastroenterol 81:3023–3027
115. Cereda JM, Trono D, Schifferli J (1983) Liquorice intoxication caused by alcohol-free pastis. Lancet 1:1442
116. Trono D, Cereda JM, Favre L (1983) Pseudo-syndrome de Conn par intoxication au pastis sans alcool. Schweiz Med Wschr 113:1092–1095
117. Piette A-M, Bauer D, Chapman A (1984) Hypokaliemie majeure avec rhabdomyolyse secondaire a l'ingestion de pastis non alcoolise. Ann Med Interne 135:296–298
118. Brunin J-L, Bories P, Ampelas M, Mimran A, Michel H (1984) Pseudo-hyperaldosteronisme induit par le pastis sans alcool chez le cirrhotique alcoolique. Gastroenterol Clin Biol 8:711–714
119. Ferrari P, Trost BN (1990) Lakritzeninduzierter Pseudohyperaldosteronismus bei einer vormals alkoholsuchtigen Frau durch Genuss eines alkoholfreien Pastis-Ersatzgetränks. Schweiz Rsch Med (Praxis) 79:377–378
120. Toulon J, Bruyere G, Berthoux F, Moulin J (1983) Hypertension arterielle maligne provoquée par l'ingestion de "pastis sans alcool". Presse Med 12:1171–1172
121. Massari P, Bonmarchand G, Canet E, Droy JM (1983) Hypermineralocorticisme exogène, responsible d'une hypokaliemie grave. Complications de la consommation de pastis sans alcool. Presse Med 12:105
122. Stewart PM, Valentino R, Wallace AM, Burt D, Shackleton CHI, Edwards CRW (1987) Mineralocorticoid activity of liquorice: 11-beta-hydroxysteroid dehyrogenase deficiency comes of age. Lancet ii:821–825
123. Biglieri EG, Kater CE (1991) Steroid characteristics of mineralocorticoid adrenocortical hypertension. Clin Chem 37:1843–1848
124. Shintani S, Murase H, Tsukagoshi H, Shiigai T (1992) Glycyrrhizin (licorice)-induced hypokalemic myopathy. Eur Neurol 32:44–51
125. Armanini D, Karbowiak I, Funder JW (1983) Affinity of liquorice derivatives for mineralocorticoid and glucocorticoid receptors. Clin Endocrin 19:609–612
126. Akashi K, Shirahama M, Iwakiri R, Yoshimatsu H, Nagafuchi S, Hayashi J, Ishibashi H (1988) Drug-induced allergic hepatitis caused by glycyrrhizin, or extract of licorice root. Acta Hepatol Jap 29:1633–1637
127. Sugiyama T, Sugaya T, Chiba S, Suga M, Yabana T, Yachi A (1992) A case of drug-induced allergic hepatitis caused by glycyrrhizin. Jap J Gasterenterol 89:1450–1453
128. Estivill X, Puig ML, Santesmasses A, Cadafalch J, Nolla J (1983) Hipermineralcorticismo mixto: hepatopatica y acido glucirricinico. Med Clin Barcelona 81:325
129. Okada K, Kobayashi S, Tsunematsu T (1987) A case of Sjögren's syndrome associated with hypokalemic myopathy due to glycyrrhizin. J Jap Soc Int Med 76:744–745
130. Garnier-Fabre A, Chaine G, Paquet R, Robert N, Fischbein L, Robineau M (1987) Retinopathie hypertensive et oedeme papillaire. J Franç Ophthalmol 10:734–740
131. Beretta-Piccoli C, Salvade G, Crivelli PL, Weidmann P (1985) Body-sodium and blood volume in a patient with licorice-induced hypertension. J Hypertension 3:19–23
132. Van der Zwan A (1993) Hypertension encephalopathy after liquorice ingestion. Clin Neurol Neurosurg 95:35–37
133. Brandon S (1991) Liquorice and blood pressure. Lancet 337:557
134. Bocker D, Breithardt G (1991) Arrhythmieauslösung durch Lakritzabusus. Z Kardiol 80:389–391
135. Takabatake H, Hirai T, Shiotani K (1989) A case of glycyrrhizin-induced pseudoaldosteronism with congestive heart failure in hypertrophic cardiomyopathy. IRYO 43:1240–1241 and 1331–1335
136. Bannister B, Ginsburg R, Shneerson J (1977) Cardiac arrest due to liquorice-induced hypokalemia. Br Med J 2:738–739

136. Cardonna P, Gentiloni N, Servidei S, Perrone GA, Greco AV, Russo MA (1992) Acute myopathy associated with chronic licorice ingestion: Reversible loss of myodenylate deaminase activity. Ultrastructural Pathology 16:529–535
137. Mitchell J, Rook A (1979) Botanical Dermatology. Vancouver: Greengrass, p.404
138. Teelucksingh S, Mackie ADR, Burt D, McIntyre MA, Brett L, Edwards CRW (1990) Potentiation of hydrocortisone activity in skin by glycyrrhetinic acid. Lancet 335:1060–1063
139. MacKenzie MA, Hoefnagels WHL, Jansen RWMM, Benraad TJ, Kloppenborg PWC (1990) The influence of glycyrrhetinic acid on plasma cortisol and cortisone in healthy young volunteers. J Clin Endocrinol Metab 70:1637–1643
140. Anttila V-J, Makela JP, Soininen K, Helminen V, Tenhunen R (1993) Discoloration of skin and serum after sweet ingestion. Lancet 341:1476–1477
141. Frohne D, Pfander HJ (1984) A Colour Atlas of Poisonous Plants. Translated by NG Bisset. London: Wolfe Publishing, p.123
142. Monder C, Stewart PM, Lakshmi V, Valentino R, Burt D, Edwards CRW (1989) Licorice inhibits corticosteroid 11-beta-dehydrogenase of rat kidney and liver: *in vivo* and *in vitro* studies. Endocrinology 125:1046–1053
143. Baker ME, Fanestil DD (1991) Liquorice as a regulator of steroid and prostaglandin metabolism. Lancet 337:428–429
144. Elmadjian F, Hope JM, Pincus G (1956) The action of mono-ammonium glycyrrhizinate on adrenalectomized subjects and its synergism with hydrocortisone, J Clin Endocrinol Metab 16:338–349
145. Teelucksingh S, Mackie ADR, Burt D, McIntyre MA, Brett L, Edwards CRW (1990) Potentiation of hydrocortisone activity in skin by glycyrrhetinic acid. Lancet 335:1060–1063
146. Schleimer RP (1991) Potential regulation of inflammation in the lung by local metabolism of hydrocortisone. Am J Resp Cell Mol Biol 4:166–173
147. Pratesi C, Scali M, Zampollo V, Zennaro MC, De Lazzari P, Lewicka S, Vecsei P, Armanini D (1991) Effects of licorice on urinary metabolites of cortisol and cortisone. J Hypertension 9 (Suppl):S274–S275
148. Lonka L, Smith Pedersen R (1987) How liquorice works. Lancet 2:1206–1207
149. Hoefnagels WHL, Kloppenborg PWC (1987) How liquorice works. Lancet 2:1207
150. Walker BR, Edwards CRW (1991) 11-Beta-hydroxysteroid dehydrogenase and enzyme-mediated receptor protection: Life after licorice? Clin Endocrinol 35:281–289
151. Teelucksingh S, Benediktsson R, Lindsay RS, Burt D, Seckl JR, Edwards CRW, Nan CL, Kelly R (1991) Liquorice. Lancet 337:1549
152. Hoefnagels WHL, Kloppenborg PWC (1983) Antimineralocorticoid effects of dexamethasone in subjects treated with glycyrrhetinic acid. J Hypertension 1(Suppl 2):313–315
153. Edwards CRW, Stewart PM, Burt D, Brett L, McIntyre MA, Sutanto WS, Dekloet ER, Monder C (1988) Localization of 11β-hydroxysteroid dehydrogenase; tissue specific protector of the mineralocorticoid receptor. Lancet 2:986–989
154. Tamura Y, Nishikawa T. Yamada K, Yamamoto M, Kumagai A (1979) Effects of glycyrrhetic acid and its derivatives on 5α- and 5β-reductase in rat liver. Arzneim Forsch 29:647–649
155. Akao T, Terasawa T, Hiai S, Kobashi K (1992) Inhibitory effects of glycyrrhetic acid derivatives on 11β- and 3α-hydroxysteroid dehydrogenases of rat liver. Chem Pharm Bull 40:3021–3024
156. Oberfield SE, Levine RM, Carvey RM, Greig F, Ulick S, New MI (1983) Metabolic and blood pressure responses to hydrocortisone in the syndrome of apparent mineralocorticoid excess. J Clin Endocrinol Metab 56:332–339
157. Kageyama Y (1992) A case of pseudoaldosteronism induced by glycyrrhizin. Jap J Nephrol 34:99–102
158. Farese RV Jr, Biglieri EG, Shackleton CHL, Irony I, Gomez-Fontes R (1991) N Engl J Med 325:1223–1227

159. Stewart PM, Corrie JET, Shackleton CHL, Edwards CRW (1988) Syndrome of apparent mineralocorticoid excess: a defect in the cortisol-cortisone shuttle. J Clin Investigation 82:340–349
160. Whorwood CB, Sheppard MC, Stewart PM (1993) Licorice inhibits 11 beta-hydroxysteroid dehydrogenase messenger ribonucleic acid levels and potentiates glucocorticoid hormone action. Endocrinol 132:2287–2292
161. Shinada M, Azuma M, Kawai H, Sazaki K, Yoshida I, Yoshida T, Suzutani T, Sakuma T (1986) Enhancement of interferon-gamma production in glycyrrhizin-treated human peripheral lymphocytes in response to concanavakin A and to surface antigen of hepatitis B virus. Proc Soc Exp Biol Med 181:205–210
162. Ohtsuki K, Iahida N (1988) Inhibitory effect of glycyrrhizin on polypeptide phosphorylation by polypeptide-dependent protein kinase (kinase P) in vitro. Biochem Biophys Res Commun 157:597–604
163. Fujiwara Y, Kikkawa R, Nakata K, Kitamura E, Takama T, Shigeta Y (1983) Hypokalemia and sodium retention in patients with diabetes and chronic hepatitis receiving insulin and glycyrrhizin. Endocrinol Jap 20:243–249
164. Mizoguchi Y, Katoh H, Tsutsui H, Yamamoto S, Morisawa S (1985) Protection of liver cells from experimentally induced liver cell injury by glycyrrhizin. Gastroenterol Jap 20:99–103
165. Kiso Y, Tohkin M, Hikino H, Hattori M, Sakamoto T, Namba T (1984) Mechanism of antihepatotoxic activity of glycyrrhizin. Planta Med 50:298–302
166. Matsunami H, Lynch SV, Balderson GA, Strong RW (1993) Use of glycyrrhizin for recurrence of hepatitis B after liver transplantation. Am J Gastroenterol 88:152–153
167. Saito S, Sasaki Y, Kuroda K, Hayashi Y, Sumita S, Nagamura Y, Nishida K, Ishiguro I (1993) Preparation of glycyrrhetic acid beta-glycosides having beta(1→2)-linked disaccharides by the use of 2-O-trichloroacetyl-beta-D-pyranosyl chlorides and their cytoprotective effects on hepatic injury in vivo. Chem Pharm Bull 41:539–543
168. Nose M, Ito M, Kamimura K, Shimizu M, Ogihara Y (1993) A comparison of the antihepatotoxic activity between glycyrrhizin and glycyrrhetinic acid. Planta Med 60:136–139
169. Hayashi R, Maruyama T, Maruyama K, Yanagawa S, Tako K, Yanagisawa N (1992) Myotonic and repetitive discharges in hypokalemic myopathy associated with glycyrrhizin-induced hypochloremia. J Neurol Sci 107:74–77
170. Fujii S (1990) Glycyrrhizine-induced pseudoaldosteronism with hypokalemic myopathy and myoglobinuria: a case report and a review of the literature. Shinshu Med J 38:180–186
171. Sugimoto K, Shionoiri H, Inuoe K, Kaneko Y (1984) A case report of hypokalemic myopathy due to ingestion of large doses of "Jintan." J Jap Soc Int Med 73:66–70
172. Cibelli G, De Mari M, Pozio G, Lamberti P (1984) Hypokalemic myopathy associated with liquorice ingestion. Ital J Neurol Sci 5:463–466
173. Joseph R, Kelemen J (1984) Paraparesis due to licorice induced hypokalemia. NY State J Med 84:296
174. Corsi FM, Galgani S, Gasparini C, Giacanelli M, Piazza G (1983) Acute hypokalemic myopathy due to chronic licorice ingestion: report of a case. Ital J Neurol Sci 4:493–497
175. Heidemann HT, Kreuzfelder E (1983) Hypokalemic rhabdomyolysis with myoglobinuria due to licorice ingestion and diuretic treatment. Klin Wschr 61:303–305
176. Mourad G, Gallay P, Oules R, Mimran A, Mion C (1979) Hypokalemic myopathy with rhabdomyolysis and acute renal failure in the course of chronic liquorice ingestion. Kidney Int 15:452
177. Sabina RL, Swain JL, Olanow CW, Bradley WG, Fishbein WN, Di Mauro S, Holmes EW (1984) Myodenylate deaminase deficiency. Functional and metabolic abnormalities associated with the disruption of the purine nucleotide cycle. J Clin Invest 73:720–730
178. Engel AG, Potter CS, Rosevear JW (1964) Nucleotides and adenosine monophosphate deaminase activity of muscle in primary hypokalemic paralysis. Nature 202:670–672
179. Kuwatsuru R, Katayama H, Hirano A, Hiraiwa T, Miyano T (1991) Drug-induced acute pulmonary edema – sequential changes in CT images. Radiation Med 9:229–231

180. Delcroix C, Poncin E, Pourrat O, Thomas P, Allal J (1985) Tubulopathie proximale au cours d'une intoxication par le reglisse. Presse Med 14:2346–2347
181. Chen M-F, Shimada F, Kato H, Yano S, Kanaoka M (1991) Effect of oral administration of glycyrrhizin on the pharmacokinetics of prednisone. Endocrinol Jap 38:167–174
182. Ojima M, Itoh N, Satoh K, Fukuchi S (1987) The effects of glycyrrhizin preparations on patients with difficulty in release from steroids treatment. Minophagen Med Rev Suppl 17:120–125; via Chen M-F, Shimada F, Kato H, Yano S, Kanaoka M (1991) Effect of oral administration of glycyrrhizin on the pharmacokinetics of prednisone. Endocrinol Jap 38:167–174
183. Sakamoto K, Wakabayashi K (1988) Inhibitory effect of glycyrrhetinic acid on testosterone production in rat gonads. Endocrinol Jap 35:333–342
184. Sheu CW, Cain KT, Rushbrook CJ, Jorgenson TA, Generoso WM (1986) Tests for mutagenic effects of ammoniated glycyrrhizin, butylated hydroxytoluene, and gum arabic in rodent germ cells. Environ Mutagen 8:357–367
185. Jorgeson TA, Rushbrook CI (1977) Study of mutagenic effects of ammoniated glycyrrhizin (71-1) by dominant lethal test in rats. Government Report Announcement Index (U.S.) 78:84 via Mantovani A, Ricciardi C, Stazi AV, Macri C, Piccioni A, Badellino E, De Vincenzi M, Caiola S, Patriarca M (1988) Teratogenicity study of ammonium glycyrrhizinate in the Sprague-Dawley rat. Food Chem Toxicol 26:435–440
186. Itami T, Ema M, Kanoh S (1985) Effects of disodium glycyrrhizinate on pregnant rats and their offspring. J Food Hyg Soc, Japan 26:460 via Mantovani A, Ricciardi C, Stazi AV, Macri C, Piccioni A, Badellino E, De Vincenzi M, Caiola S, Patriarca M (1988) Teratogenicity study of ammonium glycyrrhizinate in the Sprague-Dawley rat. Food Chem Toxicol 26:435–440
187. Mantovani A, Ricciardi C, Stazi AV, Macri C, Piccioni A, Badellino E, De Vincenzi M, Caiola S, Patriarca M (1988) Teratogenicity study of ammonium glycyrrhizinate in the Sprague-Dawley rat. Food Chem Toxicol 26:435–440
188. Colley DP, Gibson GT (1982) Three common Australian cough mixtures; study of their use in pregnancy. Aust J Pharmac 63:213
189. Werner S, Brismar K, Olsson S (1979) Hyperprolactinemia and liquorice. Lancet 1:319
190. O'Brian CA, Ward NE, Vogel VG (1990) Inhibition of protein kinase C by the 12-O-tetradecanoylphorbol-13-acetate antagonist glycyrrhetic acid. Cancer Lett 49:9–12
191. Wang ZY, Agarwal R, Zhou ZC, Bickers DR, Mukhtar H (1991) Inhibition of mutagenicity in *Salmonella typhimurium* and skin tumor initiating and tumor promoting activities in SENCAR mice by glycyrrhetinic acid: comparison of 18-alpha- and 18-beta-stereoisomers. Carcinogenesis 12:187–192
192. Kobuke T, Inai K, Nambu S, Ohe K, Takemoto T, Matsuki K, Nishina H, Huang I-B, Tokuoka S (1985) Tumorigenicity study of sodium glycyrrhizinate administered orally to mice. Food Chem Toxicol 23:979–983
193. Green S (1977) Present and future uses of mutagenicity tests for assessment of the safety of food additives. J Environ Pathol Toxicol 1:49–54
194. Morimoto I, Watanabe F, Osawa T, Okitsu T (1982) Mutagenicity screening of crude drugs with *Bacillus subtilis* rec-assay and *Salmonella*/microsome reversion assay. Mutat Res 97:81–102
195. Yamamoto H, Mizutani T, Nomura H (1982) Studies on the mutagenicity of crude drug extracts, I. Yakugaku Zasshi 102:596–601
196. Nagao M, Morita N, Yahagi T, Shimizu M, Kuroyanagi M, Fukuoka M, Yoshihira M, Natori S, Fujino T, Sugimura T (1981) Mutagenicities of 61 flavonoids and 11 related compounds. Environment Mut 3:401–419
197. Yin X-J, Liu D-X, Wang H, Zhou Y (1991) A study on the mutagenicity of 102 raw pharmaceuticals used in Chinese traditional medicine. Mutat Res 260:73–82

Linum Usitatissimum

H.J. Woerdenbag, W. Van Uden and N. Pras

Botany

The Linaceae or flax family contains 500 species [1]. With approximately 250 species, the genus of *Linum* is the largest of this family [2]. Representatives, mostly herbs and shrubs, are found in the temperate and subtropical parts of the world, particularly in countries bordering the Mediterranean sea [3].

This monograph will principally focus on *Linum usitatissimum* L. (synonym *L. humile* Mill.), because it is a source of linseed, used in medicine. This species is of commercial importance, because it produces fibre from which linen is made and linseed oil, mainly used in the paint industry [2,4]. Vernacular names for *L. usitatissimum* are common flax, linen flax (E), Lein, Flachs (G), and lin (F). According to Penso's *Index Plantarum Medicinalium* [5], several other *Linum* species are or have been employed as medicinal plants in various parts of the world. They include *L. altaicum* Lab., *L. chamissonis* Schiede, *L. catharticum* L., *L. pallescens* Bge., *L. perenne* L., *L. strictum* L., and *L. usitatissimum* L. var. *vulgare* Boenn. (= *L. vulgare* Boenn.). In addition, recent data from some other *Linum* species, containing potentially toxic constituents, will be given attention in this monograph.

Chemistry

Linseed (flaxseed, Lini semen) is the dried ripe seed of *L. usitatissimum*. It contains 30–45% of fixed oil, which consists of triglycerides from mainly unsaturated fatty acids, and only small amounts of saturated fatty acids [2,6,7]. Analyses of linseed oil showed 36–50% linolenic acid, 23–24% linoleic acid, 10–18% oleic acid, together with 5–11% of the saturated acids myristic, palmitic and stearic acid [8]. In linseed oil, mono- and triglycerides, free sterols, sterol esters and hydrocarbons are also present. The following sterols have been found: Δ^5-avenasterol, campesterol, cholesterol, cycloartenol, daucosterol, 24-methylene cycloartenol, sitosterol and stigmasterol [9–11]. In addition, linseed contains nicotinamide, the lignan secoisolariciresinol diglucoside, and the phenylpropanoid glucosides linocinnamarin and linusitamarin [11].

Flaxseed contains ca. 25% of protein, characterized by the absence of the amino acids lysine and methionine [2,6]. In the epidermis of the seed 3–6% mucilage is present, which is composed of polysaccharides consisting of arabinose, galactose, rhamnose, xylose, galacturonic acid and mannuronic acid [8,12,13].

According to Martindale [14], crushed linseed (=coarsely powdered linseed) contains not less than 30% of fixed oil. Powdered linseed cake (=linseed meal), left after the extraction of oil, contains 6–8% of fixed oil.

In the seeds, leaves, stems, flowers and roots of *L. usitatissimum* four cyanogenic glucosides have been found: the monoglucosides linamarin and lotaustralin, and the diglucosides linustatin and neolinustatin. The monoglucosides occur in the vegetative parts of the plant, whereas the diglucosides are present in the seeds [15]. Their total concentration in linseed range between 0.1 and 1.5% [2,3,16]. Other cyanogenic *Linum* species include *L. alpinum, L. arboreum, L. campanulatum, L. catharticum, L. flavum, L. gallicum, L. grandiflorum, L. kingii, L. lewisii, L. marginale* and *L. maritimum* [6,7].

In the seeds of *L. usitatissimum*, tocopherol [17], the glutaminic acid derivative linatine, 0.7% of phosphatide, minerals and cadmium are also present [2].

In aerial parts of *L. usitatissimum*, the C-glycoflavones lucenin-1 and -2, orientin, iso-orientin, vicenin-1 and -2, vitexin and iso-vitexin occur [18–20]. In addition, anthocyanidins [21] and glycosides and esters of p-coumaric, caffeic, ferulic and sinapic acids [19] have been found.

Several *Linum* species contain podophyllotoxin-related lignans, mostly 5-methoxypodophyllotoxin, with cytotoxic activity [22,23]. They include *L. album, L. arboreum, L. campanulatum, L. capitatum, L. catharticum, L. elegans, L. flavum, L. pamphylicum, L. tauricum* and *L. thracicum* [24–28]. With 0.1–0.4% in dried aerial parts and up to 3.7% in the roots, *L. flavum* is the richest in 5-methoxypodophyllotoxin [27,28].

Pharmacology and Uses

Linseed, whole or crushed, is applied as a bulk laxative against chronic obstipation. The daily dose is 30–45 g and it should be taken with plenty of fluid (at least 150 ml per 15 g linseed). In controlled studies with healthy volunteers as well as with patients suffering from chronic obstipation, this has been proven to be an effective dose [29].

The laxative action is caused by the mucilage. If the crushed drug is used, the oil may contribute to this action. The theory is that the mucilage swells in the intestinal lumen, resulting in an increased volume, thereby stimulating the peristaltic movements of the large intestine. The oil, in addition, acts as a lubricant, facilitating the passage of the faeces through the bowels. In contrast to most other laxatives, a local irritating action by linseed on the intestinal wall is absent. After taking a dose of linseed, it takes at least 3 days before the laxative effect is obtained. The seeds should not be crushed too finely, as in that case swelling already occurs in the stomach. Persons with overweight should preferably use whole linseed: after ingestion the seeds will swell, but the oil will not be liberated, thereby limiting the caloric value for the user [2,29–32].

In the case of other fibers used as laxatives, microbial degradation products seem to be important for the action. Some authors propose the theory that fibers are just a good food for bacteria in the gut and that the increase of stool weight represents mainly an increase in bacterial mass [33,34]. However, data on the fermentability of linseed polysaccharides are lacking in humans.

In folk medicine, a decoct of linseed is used in the treatment of acute and chronic gastritis, because of its demulcent action on the mucosa. Crushed linseed has been used as a poultice (cataplasma lini) to apply warmth and moisture locally for the relief of superfacial or deep-seated inflammation [14,16].

In Ayurvedic medicine, the seeds, oil and flowers of *L. usitatissimum* are used. Linseed tea, a mucilaginous infusion, is used internally as a demulcent and expectorant to treat cold, cough, bronchial affection, irritation of the urinary tract, gonorrhoea, diarrhoea and dysentery. A poultice made from linseed meal is applied to sooth local inflammations and ulcers, boils and carbuncles. Such poultices dilatate the blood vessels locally and relax the tissue, thereby relieving the tension and pain. Linseed poultice is also used in bronchitis and has been recommended for gouty and rheumatic swellings. Seeds are valued as a laxative, but they are also said to have aphrodisiac properties. Roasted seeds act as an adstringent. The mucilage may be dropped into the eye in irritable conditions of the eyelid [3,35].

In homoeopathy, preparations of fresh aerial parts of *L. usitatissimum* are used to treat fever and irritable conditions of the urine bladder [36].

In veterinary practice, linseed infusion is used as a demulcent drink and linseed oil is employed as a purgative for horses and cattle [14]. Despite its laxative properties, linseed oil serves no longer for this purpose to man, because of its unpleasant taste. In human medicine, the oil is mainly applied externally, in liniments for eczema and psoriasis [3,8,13].

In addition, linseed oil may be used as a source of dietary linolenic acid [37]. This essential fatty acid is incorporated into cellular membranes, influencing the membrane strength, flexibility and permeability. In addition, it acts as a biological precursor of several hormone-like prostaglandins and leukotrienes. These substances have a positive influence on serum cholesterol levels, aggregation of red blood cells and smooth muscle performance [37]. Because of the presence of large amounts of unsaturated fatty acids, a possible antisclerotic action of linseed oil has been assumed [2,30,38].

Estrogenic activity has been observed in postmenopausal women taking a diet supplemented with 25 g linseed daily. After 6 weeks, significant differences in vaginal cytology were found and vaginal cell maturation was enhanced. Furthermore, serum concentrations of luteinising hormone (LH) and follicle stimulating hormone (FSH) were increased. It was concluded that taking foods containing phyto-estrogens may modulate the severity of the menopause, as this is an estrogen deficiency state [39]. It has been shown that secoisolariciresol diglucoside or it as aglycone is converted by the intestinal flora of animals to the metabolites enterodiol and enterolactone, which are structurally similar to diethylstilbestrol but without estrogenic activity. These metabolites have been postulated to possess antiestrogenic properties [11,40].

The lignans enterodiol and enterolactone are formed in the intestinal tract from humans, from precursors present in linseed. These lignans may both function as weak estrogenics or estrogen antagonists. The effect of ingestion of linseed powder has been evaluated on the menstrual cycle and serum hormone concentration in 18 normally cycling women, in a balanced randomized cross-over design. Longer luteal phase lengths were found after linseed ingestion, as well as increased progesterone / estradiol ratios, and fewer anovulatory cycles. Thus, there was a decreased tendency to ovarian dysfunction. Such dysfunction may be related to the later development of breast and other cancers [41].

In vitro, hydrolyzed linseed oil as well as linolenic acid inhibited the growth of methicillin-resistant strains of *Staphylococcus aureus*. It has been postulated that topical preparations containing these ingredients may find application in the eradication of staphylococcal carriers and could be useful for prophylaxis, especially in debilitated patients [42]. Linatine also possesses antibacterial properties [43,44].

Formerly, the fresh herb of *L. catharticum* (purging flax) had a limited use as a mild laxative and a diuretic. These properties were ascribed to the presence of linin [30,31,45]. The precise structure of linin is unclear as yet, but based on old phytochemical data concerning this compound [46] and data on 5-methoxypodophyllotoxin, originating from recent studies [22,26], linin is likely to be identical with 5-methoxypodophyllotoxin. A homoeopathic preparation of *L. catharticum* is used in diarrhoea [36].

Pharmacokinetics

The liberation of hydrocyanic acid from cyanogenic glucosides is mediated by the β-glucosidase linamarase (=linase). The pH optimum for this enzyme is 5.5–6.0. The amount of hydrocyanic acid that may be liberated depends on the grade of fineness of the seeds. Under optimal conditions, this is 2, 7 or 50 mg per 100 g of whole, crushed and milled seed, respectively. The reaction is completed only after 8 hours [29]. Although 50 mg hydrocyanic acid is sufficient to cause poisoning, the enzyme linamarase becomes rapidly deactivated in the acid gastric juice, resulting in less than 1% liberation of the theoretically available amount of hydrocyanic acid. Even under hypoacidic conditions in the stomach, only 8% is liberated [47]. The traces of hydrocyanic acid that are formed, are rapidly detoxified in the liver by the enzyme rhodanase, yielding the far less toxic thiocyanate [15,29,32]. Repeated doses of 150–300 g linseed, given to healthy volunteers as well as to obstipated patients, did not reveal any toxic effect [29]. After long-term use of linseed, a slight increase in blood and urine thiocyanate levels have been found in this study. These levels were comparable with those in heavy smokers and considered non-toxic [16].

In another study, the absorption of hydrocyanic acid after ingestion of linseed was investigated in 20 healthy volunteers and in 5 patients. The persons investigated took a single dose of 30 g or of 100 g of linseed, or they received throughout several weeks 15 g t.i.d. One volunteer took for comparison bitter almonds or potassium cyanide. Before, during and after the periods of ingestion, plasma levels of hydrocyanic acid and of thiocyanate were normal. During long-term trials urinary excretion of thiocyanate was monitored regularly. Intake of linseed even in extremely high dosages never caused significant rises of plasma thiocyanate levels. This, however, was the case after intake of bitter almonds or potassium cyanide. It was concluded that no intoxication by hydrocyanic acid can be caused by linseed.

Long-term intake of linseed, however, raised plasma levels of thiocyanate significantly; at the same time urinary excretion of thiocyanate increased [48].

The hydrocyanic acid intake resulting from 60 g ground linseed daily has been estimated in two male adults by 24 h urinary excretion of thiocyanate in 3 preceding days and on days 8–10. The mean increased sevenfold from the normal 32 μmol to 247 μmol, corresponding with a daily cyanide exposure of more than 0.25 mmol [49].

Adverse Reaction Profile

General Animal Data

In small animals, linseed oil should not be used as a laxative, as it produces extreme nausea. In large doses, the oil may cause superpurgation [3].

Linseed meal is valued as a protein supplement for livestock [3]. After feeding rats, chickens and turkeys with deoiled linseed meals, vitamin B6 deficiency symptoms have been observed in these animals, caused by the pyridoxine antagonist linatine. Also, growth inhibition of animals fed with linseed oil has been seen, based on a vitamin B6 deficiency [44,50]. An LD_{50} of 2 mg linatine, injected intraperitoneally to one-week-old chickens, was counteracted by the simultaneous injection of 1 mg pyridoxine [44].

Linseed meal has been reported to possess a goitrogenic effect on sheep and mice. Ewes on a diet containing linseed meal were found to produce lambs with acute goitre. The goitrogenic principle was identified as a thiocyanate. Hydrolysis of the cyanogenic glucosides in the rumen of sheep produces cyanide, which is detoxified in the liver to form thiocyanate [3].

The cyanogenic glucosides, present in all plant parts, have been held responsible for several cases of death among livestock, due to grazing on these plants and feeding with linseed meal [3]. In ewes and rats, linseed has been reported to cause hydrocyanic acid poisoning and goitre [50]. The mucilage of linseed has been found to cause beak necrosis in poultry [51].

General Human Data

Despite the presence of cyanogenic glucosides in linseed from which hydrocyanic acid may be liberated, no health risk due to poisoning seems to exist for humans. The traditional use of linseed as a laxative (10 g soaked overnight) is not associated with toxic effects. However, inquiries have shown that some Swedish users use ground linseed in doses op to 80 g daily. The grinding of the seeds might enhance the hazard of such excessive dosing by inducing hydrolysis of the glucosides to cyanohydrins and/or by making more glucosides accessible to intestinal glucosidases [49].

As already mentioned above, linamarase is rapidly deactivated by acid gastric juice. In elderly people, being a potentially large group of users of laxatives, achlorhydria is not uncommon, and has been found in one study in about 50% of elderly subjects without gastrointestinal problems [52]. However, the significance of achlorhydria on the potential increase in the liberation of hydrocyanic acid is still unclear.

Linseed may contain high cadmium contents. This heavy metal is taken up from the soil by the plant and accumulates in the seed. Levels ranging from 0.1–1.7 mg/kg seed have been found, depending on the degree of pollution of the soil on which the plants were cultivated [53]. Cadmium is already toxic for man and animals at low concentrations. Acute intoxications are often characterized by disturbance of the renal function and by hypertension [53]. By taking a daily dose of 45 g linseed per day for a longer period, the consumer may become exposed to higher amounts of cadmium than are considered tolerable. Therefore, the German health authorities have set the maximally tolerable level of cadmium in linseed at 0.3 mg/kg [54,55]. In addition, linseed may be considerably contaminated with bacteria, molds and pesticides [56,57].

Allergic Reactions

On the skin, flax plants may cause slight irritation [31]. In a study evaluating 79 uncommon food-antigen skin prick tests in 102 patients with the initial diagnosis of idiopathic anaphylaxis, linseed was shown to provoke anaphylaxis in several subjects [58].

Inhalation of powder of linseed may provoke allergic reactions, in the form of rhinitis and asthmatic attacks [2]. See also under Respiratory Reactions.

Gastrointestinal Reactions

Although long-term use of linseed as a laxative is considered to be safe, rebound obstipation may occur [29,47,56]. The use of linseed is contra-indicated in patients with any kind of ileus [16]. Due to the consumption of large amounts of bulky material, a considerable production of intestinal gas may occur, resulting in heavy flatulence [56].

In the literature, two cases of severe obstruction of the large intestine after taking linseed have been reported [56,59]. They were caused by clenched clumps of bulk material. The simultaneous consumption of too little fluid played a role here.

The Food and Drug Administration (FDA) in the United States of America has formulated the following warning for over-the-counter drugs containing water-soluble gums as active ingredients: "Taking this product without adequate fluid may cause it to swell and block your throat or esophagus and may cause choking. Do not take this product if you have difficulty in swallowing. If you experience chest pain, vomiting, or difficulty in swallowing or breathing after taking this product, seek immediate medical attention." [60].

Due to the high degree of unsaturation, linseed oil is susceptible to oxidation. Oxidized linseed oil irritates the stomach. Therefore, crushed linseed should not be stored for a longer period before use [30].

At a higher dose, *L. catharticum* may cause vomiting [31].

Metabolic Reactions

The concentration of the pyridoxine antagonist linatine in linseed is too low to cause vitamin B6 deficiency in humans, when normally used [2].

Respiratory Reactions

Several reports exist on the occupational hazards of flax, and ventilatory responses of normal subjects have been described after inhalation of flax dust. Steamed flax dust showed less impairment of the forced expirations than untreated flax, suggesting that autoclavation of the flax has a protective effect on long term airway effects [61]. The acute bronchostrictor response to flax dust was found to be increased by pre-harvest retting, suggesting an increased risk of byssinosis [62]. In a large retrospective study of ex-flax workers in Northern Ireland, an excess of respiratory symptoms was found compared to control subjects. In women, the reduction in lung function was confined to the younger subjects [63,64].

Drug Interactions

Disturbance of the absorption of calcium, magnesium, zinc, iron or phosphor is most probably irrelevant when taking linseed, but by using extremely bulky-rich food, a deficit of these minerals may occur [56]. The absorption of drugs, simultaneously taken with linseed, might become reduced [65], but there are no actual reports in the medical literature.

Fertility, Pregnancy and Lactation

No adverse reactions on fertility, pregnance or lactation caused by linseed have been recovered from the literature.

Mutagenicity and Carcinogenicity

For linseed no mutagenic or carcinogenic effects have been recovered from the literature. The podophyllotoxin-related lignans, as present in several *Linum* species, but not in *L. usitatissimum*, exhibit cytotoxic properties. For podophyllotoxin, mutagenic and carcinogenic properties have been described [66].

References

1. Frohne D, Jensen U (1979) Systematik des Pflanzenreichs. Stuttgart: Gustav Fischer Verlag, p 179
2. Steinegger E, Hänsel R (1988) Lehrbuch der Pharmakognosie und Phytopharmazie. 4. Auflage. Berlin: Springer-Verlag.
3. Anonymous (1962) The Wealth of India. Volume VI. New Delhi: Council of Scientific & Industrial Research, pp 119–140
4. Langer GM (1986) Leinöl für die Farbenherstellung. Farbe Lack 92: 1221–1223
5. Penso G (1983) Index Plantarum Medicinalium Totius Mundi Eorumque Synonymorum. Milan: Organizzazione Medico Farmaceutica, pp 574–575
6. Hegnauer R (1966) Chemotaxonomie der Pflanzen. Band 4. Basle: Birkhäuser Verlag, pp 393–401, 482
7. Hegnauer R (1989) Chemotaxonomie der Pflanzen. Band 8. Basle: Birkhäuser Verlag, pp 669–672
8. Evans WC (1989) Trease and Evans' Pharmacognosy, 13th edition. London: Ballière Tindall
9. Sukhija PS, Bhatia IS (1970) Lipids of taramira (*Eruca sativa*) & linseed (*Linum usitatissimun*) - tentative identification of various components & their fatty acid make-up. Ind J Biochem 7: 271–274
10. Middleditch BS, Knights BA (1971) Sterols of *Linum usitatissimum* seed. Phytochemistry 11: 1183
11. Luyengi L, Pezzuto JM, Waller DP, Beecher CWW, Fong HHS (1993) Linusitamarin, a new phenylpropanoid glucoside from *Linum usitatissimum*. J Nat Prod 56: 2012–2015
12. Davis EA, Derouet C, Herve du Penhoat C, Morvan C (1990) Isolation and NMR study of pectins from flax (*Linum usitatissimum*). Carbohydr Res 197: 205–215
13. Wagner H (1985) Pharmazeutische Biologie. 2. Drogen und ihre Inhaltstoffe, 3. Auflage. Stuttgart: Gustav Fischer Verlag, pp 283–284, 300
14. Reynolds JEF, Prasad AB, ed. (1982) Martindale The Extra Pharmacopeoia. 28th Edition. London: The Pharmaceutical Press, p 696
15. Nahrstedt A (1987) Flachs, Hornklee, Widderchen und Blausäure. Dtsch Apoth Ztg 127: 2385–2390
16. Willuhn G (1989) Leinsamen. In: Wichtl M, ed. Teedrogen. 2. Auflage. Stuttgart: Wissenschaftliche Verlagsgesellschaft mbH, pp 306–308
17. Marquard R (1990) Untersuchungen über den Einfluß von Sorte und Standort auf den Tocopherolgehalt verschiedener Pflanzenöle. Fat Sci Technol 92: 452–455
18. Ibrahim RK (1969) Chromatographic and spectrometric evidence for the occurrence of mixed O- and C-glycoflavones in flax (*Linum usitatissimum*) cotyledons. Biochem Biophys Acta 192: 549–552
19. Ibrahim RK, Shaw M (1970) Phenolic constituents of the oil flax (*Linum usitatissimum*). Phytochemistry 9: 1855–1858
20. Dubois J, Mabry TJ (1971) The C-glycosylflavonoids of flax, *Linum usitatissimum*. Phytochemistry 10: 2839–2840
21. Thakur ML, Ibrahim RK (1974) Biogenesis of flavonoids in flax seedlings. Z Pflanzenphysiol 71: 391–397
22. Van Uden W, Homan B, Woerdenbag HJ, Pras N, Malingré ThM, Wichers HJ, Harkes M (1992) Isolation, purification, and cytotoxicity of 5-methoxypodophyllotoxin, a lignan from a root culture of *Linum flavum*. J Nat Prod 55: 102–110
23. Van Uden W, Pras N, Woerdenbag HJ (1994) *Linum* species (flax): *in vivo* and *in vitro* accumulation of lignans and other metabolites. In: Bajaj YPS, ed. Biotechnology in Agriculture and Forestry, Volume 26. Medicinal and Aromatic Plants. Part VI. Berlin: Springer-Verlag, pp. 219–244
24. Weiss SG, Tin-Wa M, Perdue RE, Farnsworth NR (1975) Potential anticancer agents II: antitumor and cytotoxic lignans from *Linum album* (Linaceae). J Pharm Sci 64: 95–98

25. Berlin J Wray V, Mollenschott C, Sasse F (1986) Formation of β-peltatin-A-methylether and coniferin by root cultures of *Linum flavum*. J Nat Prod 49: 435–439
26. Broomhead AJ, Dewick PM (1990) Aryltetralin lignans from *Linum flavum* and *Linum capitatum*. Phytochemistry 29: 3839–3844
27. Wichers HJ, Harkes MP, Arroo RJ (1990) Occurrence of 5-methoxypodophyllotoxin in plants, cell cultures and regenerated plants of *Linum flavum*. Plant Cell Tiss Org Cult 23:93–100
28. Wichers HJ, Versluis-De Haan GG, Marsman JW, Harkes MP (1991) Podophyllotoxin related lignans in plants and cell cultures of *Linum flavum*. Phytochemistry 30: 3601–3604
29. Schilcher H, Schulz V, Nissler A (1986) Zur Wirksamkeit und Toxikologie von Semen Lini. Z Phytother 7: 113–117
30. Weiß RF (1991) Lehrbuch der Phytotherapie. 7. Auflage. Stuttgart: Hippokrates Verlag, pp 131–133
31. Madaus G (1938) Lehrbuch der Biologischen Heilmittel. Leipzig: Georg Thieme Verlag, pp 1765–1775
32. Härtling C (1969) Lein und Leinsamen, eine uralte Kulturpflanze, eine zu Unrecht umstrittene Droge. Dtsch Apoth Ztg 109: 1025–1028
33. Leng-Peschlow E. Pharmacological aspects of fiber. In: Csomós G, Kusche J, Meryn S, eds. Fibers. Berlin: Springer-Verlag, pp 69–88
34. Read NW. Fiber and colonic motility: relevance for constipation. In: Csomós G, Kusche J, Meryn S, eds. Fibers. Berlin: Springer-Verlag, pp 110–120
35. Kapoor LD (1990) Handbook of Ayurvedic Medicinal Plants. Boca Raton: CRC Press, p 217
36. Wiesenauer M (1989) Homöopathie für Apotheker und Ärzte. Stuttgart: Deutscher Apotheker Verlag, p 4/67
37. Hudson BJF (1987) Oilseeds as sources of essential fatty acids. Hum Nutr: Food Sci Nutr 41F: 1–13
38. Albrecht M, Klein M (1995) Oleum Lini: Portrait eines pflanzlichen Öls. Pharm Ztg 140: 572–576
39. Wilcox G, Wahlqvist ML, Burger HG, Medley G (1990) Oestrogenic effects of plant foods in postmenopausal women. Br Med J 301: 905–906
40. Setchell K, Alderkreutz H (1988) Mammalian lignans and phyto-oestrogens: recent studies on their formation, metabolism and biological role in health and disease. In: Rowland I, ed. Role of the gut flora in toxicity and cancer. London: Academic Press, pp. 315–345.
41. Phipps WR, Martini MC, Lampe JW, Slavin JL, Kurzer MS (1993) Effect of flax seed ingestion on the menstrual cycle. J Clin Endocrinol Metab 77: 1215–1219
42. McDonald MI, Graham I, Harvey KJ (1981) Antibacterial activity of hydrolysed linseed oil and linolenic acid against methicillin-resistant *Staphylococcus aureus*. Lancet 2: 1056
43. Windholz M, Budavari S, Stroumtsos LY, Fertig MN, eds. (1976) The Merck Index. 9th Edition. Rahway: Merck & Co, p 719
44. Klostermann HJ, Lamoureux GL, Parsons JL (1967) Isolation, characterization, and synthesis of linatine. A vitamin B6 antagonist from flax seed (*Linum usitatissimum*). Biochemistry 6: 170–177
45. Steinegger E, Hänsel R (1972) Lehrbuch der Pharmakognosie. 3. Auflage. Berlin: Springer-Verlag, p 103
46. Hills JS (1905) An investigation of *Linum catharticum*. Pharm J 18: 401–404, 436–438
47. Anonymous (1986) Leinsamen enthält kein Kaliumcyanid. Dtsch Apoth Ztg 126: 1794–1795
48. Schulz V, Löffler A, Gheorghiu T (1983) Resorption von Blausäure aus Leinsamen. Leber Magen Darm 13: 10–14
49. Rosling H (1993) Cyanide exposure from linseed. Lancet 341: 177
50. Mandokhot VM, Singh N (1983) Studies on linseed (*Linum usitatissimum*) as a protein source. 2. Evidence of toxicity and treatments to improve quality. J Food Sci Technol 20: 291–295

51. Mandokhot VM, Singh N (1979) Studies on linseed (*Linum usitatissimum*) as a protein source for poultry. I. Processes of demucilaging and dehulling of linseed and evaluation of processed materials by chemical analysis and with rats and chickens. J Food Sci Technol 16: 25–31
52. Prescott LF (1975) Pathological and physiological factors affecting drug absorption, distribution, elimination and response in man. In: Gillette JR, Mitchell JR, eds. Concepts in Biochemical Pharmacology. Part 3. New York: Springer Verlag, pp. 234–257
53. Marquard R, Böhm H, Friedt W (1990) Untersuchungen über Cadmiumgehalt in Leinsaat (*Linum usitatissimum* L.) Fat Sci Technol 92: 468–472
54. De Smet PAGM (1992) Toxicological outlook on the quality assurance of herbal remedies. In: De Smet PAGM, Keller K, Hänsel R, Chandler RF, eds. Adverse Effects of Herbal Drugs. Vol. 1. Heidelberg: Springer-Verlag, pp 1–72
55. Anonymous (1988) Zuviel Cadmium in Leinsamen. Dtsch Apoth Ztg 128: 145
56. Hardt M, Geisthövel W (1986) Schwerer Obstruktionsileus durch Leinsamenbezoar. Med Klin 81: 541–543
57. Anonymous (1987) Darmverschluß durch Leinsamen. Med Mo Pharm 10: 191
58. Stricker WE, Anorve-Lopez E, Reed CE (1986) Food skin testing in patients with idiopathic anaphylaxis. J All Clin Immunol 77: 516–519
59. Siem-Jorgensen P, Wamberg P (1984) Svaer obstipation efter 'fastekur'. Ugeskr Laeg 146: 195–196
60. Department of Health and Human Services, Food and Drug Administration (1993) Warning statements required for over-the-counter drugs containing water-soluble gums as active ingredients. Federal Register 58: 45194–45201
61. Jamison JP, Langlands JH, Lowry RC (1986) Ventilatory impairment from pre-harvest retted flax. Br J Industr Med 43: 809–813
62. Jamison JP, Langlands JH, Bodel CC (1985) Ventilatory responses of normal subjects to flax dust inhalation: the protective effect of autoclaving the flax. Br J Industr Med 42: 196–201
63. Elwood JH, Elwood PC, Campbell MJ, Stanford CF, Chivers A, Hey I, Brewster L, Sweetnam PM (1986) Respiratory disability in ex-flax workers Br J Industr Med 43: 300–306
64. Cotes JE (1986) Respiratory disability in ex-flax workers. Br J Industr Med 43: 845
65. Fintelmann V, Menßen HG, Siegers CP (1989) Phytotherapie Manual. Stuttgart: Hippokrates Verlag, p 90
66. Bowen IH, Cubbin IJ (1992) *Podophyllum* species. In: De Smet PAGM, Keller K, Hänsel R, Chandler RF, eds. Adverse Effects of Herbal Drugs. Vol. 2. Heidelberg: Springer-Verlag, pp. 263–273

Phoradendron Flavescens

P.A.G.M. De Smet

Botany

Phoradendron flavescens (Pursh.) Nutt. is a parasitic plant which has also been designated as *Viscum flavescens* Pursh., *Phoradendron serotinum* (Raf.) M.C. Johnst., and *Phoradendron tomentosum* (DC.) Engelm. ssp. *macrophyllum* (Cockerell) Wiens [1,2]. Its most recent Latin binomial is *Phoradendron leucarpum* (Raf.) Rev. & M.C. Johnst. (Viscaceae) [3]. The plant is the familiar mistletoe sold at Christmas in the United States. It is most commonly known as American mistletoe to distinguish it from the European mistletoe, *Viscum album*; other vernacular names are false mistletoe, birdlime and golden bough. The medicinal plant part is the leaf [4,5].

Chemistry

Samuelsson and co-workers obtained a small basic protein denoted as phoratoxin from the dried leaves and stems of *Phoradendron flavescens* grown on *Juglans hindsii*. This protein had similar chemical and pharmacological properties as the viscotoxins isolated from the European mistletoe, *Viscum album*, although phoratoxin had to be given in higher doses [6-8]. The substance was found to consist of 46 amino acids. Its amino acid sequence was elucidated [9], and the arrangement of the disulphide bonds in the molecule was reported [10].

Mellstrand [11] did not detect a chemical or toxicological difference between phoratoxin of *P.flavescens* grown on *Juglans hindsii* and phoratoxin obtained from the leaves of *P.flavescens* grown on *Populus fremontii*. Thunberg [12] later found that these phoratoxins do not have the same chemistry. She designated the phoratoxin of material grown on *Populus fremontii* as phoratoxin B, and determined its amino acid sequence. She showed that phoratoxin of *P.flavescens* grown on *Juglans hindsii* is apparently a mixture of at least two proteins. Further studies of the influence of the host plant on the composition of *P.flavescens* are certainly warranted. According to American Indians, only mistletoes grown on certain trees are poisonous [13], and it has been shown for other types of parasitic plants that they may extract toxic principles from their host plant. For instance, *Phrygilanthus celastroides*, *Dendrophtoe falcata* and *Amyema congener* extract polar cardiac glycosides from *Nerium oleander*, when grown on this plant species [14].

P.flavescens contains sterols, such as sitosterol and stigmasterol [15], as well as the pressor amine tyramine [16]. The leaves are reported to contain 3.9% of tannin [17]. Dossaji et al. [18] studied the flavonoids of air-dried leaf samples of *Phoradendron tomentosum* (DC.) Gray grown on different host trees (*Ulmus crassifolia, Prosopis glandulosa*, and *Celtis laevigata*). They found three apigenin C-glycosides (vitexin, schaftoside and isoschaftoside) as well as lesser amounts of apigenin and apigenin 4'-O-glucoside, and this pattern was uniform, irrespective of the host tree.

Up to now, the berries of the American mistletoe have not been submitted to a thorough phytochemical analysis.

Pharmacology and Uses

Hanzlik and French [19] showed that aqueous and alcoholic extracts of *Phoradendron flavescens* produced a marked tyramine-like action on the circulation of anesthetized dogs, when administered intravenously in doses of 0.2 ml/kg. Initially, there was a temporary fall of blood pressure, which could be prevented by atropine, and which was accompanied by an accelerated pulse rate. The initial fall was followed by a steep and sustained rise of blood pressure, with the pulse either slowing down or remaining accelerated. Circulatory effects were less marked after intramuscular or subcutaneous injection of 0.5 ml/kg, and gastric administration of 1 ml/kg did not elicit noteworthy effects in anesthetized dogs. In unanesthetized animals, however, a gastric dose of 1 ml/ kg produced an increase in pulse rate. In vitro testing of the mistletoe extracts showed a stimulant effect on smooth muscle in excised strips of intestine, bladder and uterus.

The effects of phoratoxin were studied by Rosell and Samuelsson [6]. Intravenous injection of 0.4 mg/kg decreased blood pressure, heart contractility and heart rate in anesthetized cats. Phoratoxin also produced vasoconstriction of the vessels in skeletal muscle, but only in higher doses than those required for reflex bradycardia and diminished contractile force.

Phoratoxin showed no antibacterial or antifungal activity and had no inhibiting effect on the enzymatic activity of trypsin or chymotrypsin [20].

In the past, American mistletoe was used for cholera, convulsions, hysteria, delirium, heart problems, and nervous debility. American Indians used it to cause abortion [4].

Pharmacokinetics

The pharmacokinetic behaviour of phoratoxin remains to be elucidated. Since this substance is a protein or a mixture of proteins, the question arises, whether it is able to resist digestive degradation following oral ingestion [21].

Adverse Reaction Profile

As was pointed out in the section on chemistry, it is still insufficiently known, to which extent the composition and toxicity of *Phoradendron flavescens* may depend on the host plant.

General Animal Data

The intraperitoneal LD_{50} of phoratoxin in mice was found to be 0.57 mg/kg body weight [8]. In anesthetized cats, the lethal intravenous dose of phoratoxin was about 1 mg/kg, which was ten times the lethal dose of viscotoxin [6].

See also the section on pharmacology and uses.

General Human Data

Both *Phoradendron* and *Viscum* species have been claimed in 19th century reports to produce poisoning. Reported symptoms were vomiting, purging, collapse, hallucinations, bounding pulse, stertorous respiration and dilated pupils [13]. On basis of these early reports, the berries of the American mistletoe are considered poisonous, and particularly children are said to have died from eating the berries [1,17,22,23].

Hall et al. [21] collected 14 cases, where one to three *Phoradendron* **berries** (11 cases) or one to two *Phoradendron* **leaves** (3 cases) had been ingested. Five individuals had emesis induced with syrup of ipecac, whereas nine were observed without intervention. No signs or symptoms other than ipecac-induced vomiting were noted [21]. However, persons drinking teas brewed from the American mistletoe are at risk of developing severe toxicity. In a fatal case, a 28-year-old female intentionally ingested an unknown quantity of a tea brewed from berries of the American mistletoe to bring on her period. She fell ill some 1-2 hours later, and suffered from vomiting, abdominal cramps and diarrhea over the next 8-10 hours. She was then transported to hospital and died there shortly after her arrival, apparently from cardiovascular collapse. When she came in the emergency room, she was in deep shock, with extreme paleness, profuse sweating, dilated pupils, mental confusion, moderate dehydration and subnormal temperature. Her blood pressure could not be obtained, and her pulse was barely perceptible. Many of her symptoms were those of acute digitalis poisoning, but no cardiac arrthythmias were noted [23]. In another case, the victim had drunk an unknown amount of tea prepared from unspecified plant parts of *Phoradendron* for use as a tonic. This patient also died, but no further details were presented [21].

Allergic Reactions

Repeated subcutaneous administration of phoratoxin to rabbits can result in antibody formation [20].

Fertility, Pregnancy and Lactation

Phoradendron flavescens is reputed to be abortifacient and has been used in the past for its oxytocic action. Intravenous administration of an alcoholic extract to a dog in oestrus and to a non-pregnant cat was found to increase uterine tonus and contractility [19].

Further data on the effects during pregnancy and lactation have not been recovered from the literature.

Mutagenicity and Carcinogenicity

No data have been recovered from the literature.

References

1. Osol A, Farrar GE (1955) The Dispensatory of the United States of America. 25th edn. Philadelphia: J.B. Lippincott Company, pp.1928–1929
2. Tyler VE (1987) The New Honest Herbal. A sensible guide to herbs and related remedies. 2nd edn. Philadelphia: George F. Stickley Company, pp.154–155
3. Reveal JL, Johnston MC (1989) A new combination in *Phoradendron* (Viscaceae). Taxon 38:107–108
4. Lust JB (1974) The Herb Book. New York: Bantam Books, p.278
5. Lampe KF, McCann MA (1985) AMA Handbook of Poisonous and Injurious Plants. Chicago: American Medical Association, pp.131–132
6. Rosell S, Samuelsson G (1966) Effects of mistletoe viscotoxin and phoratoxin on blood circulation. Toxicon 4:107–110
7. Samuelsson G, Ekblad M (1967) Isolation and properties of phoratoxin, a toxic protein from *Phoradendron serotinum* (Loranthaceae). Acta Chem Scand 21:849–856
8. Mellstrand ST, Samuelsson G (1973) Phoratoxin, a toxic protein from the mistletoe *Phoradendron tomentosum* subsp. *macrophyllum* (Loranthaceae). Improvements in the isolation procedure and further studies on the properties. Eur J Biochem 32:143–147
9. Mellstrand ST, Samuelsson G (1974) Phoratoxin, a toxic protein from the mistletoe *Phoradendron tomentosum* subsp. *macrophyllum* (Loranthaceae). The amino acid sequence. Acta Pharm Suec 11:347–360
10. Mellstrand ST, Samuelsson G (1974) Phoratoxin, a toxic protein from the mistletoe *Phoradendron tomentosum* subsp. *macrophyllum* (Loranthaceae). The disulfide bonds. Acta Pharm Suec 11:367–374
11. Mellstrand ST (1974) Phoratoxin, a toxic protein from the mistletoe *Phoradendron tomentosum* subsp. *macrophyllum* (Loranthaceae). Isolation of phoratoxin from *Phoradendron tomentosum* subsp. *macrophyllum* grown on *Populus fremontii*. Acta Pharm Suec 11:410–412
12. Thunberg E (1983) Phorotoxin B, a toxic protein from the mistletoe *Phoradendron tomentosum* subsp. *macrophyllum*. Acta Pharm Suec 20:115–122
13. Crawford AC (1911) The pressor action of an American mistletoe. JAMA 57:865–868
14. Boonsong C, Wright SE (1961) The cardiac glycosides in mistletoes growing on *Nerium oleander*. Austr J Chem 14:449–457
15. Orcutt DM, Calvin CL (1978) Comparison of the lipid composition of five species of mistletoe. Virginia Acad J Sci 29:75
16. Crawford AC, Watanabe WK (1914) Parahydroxyethylamine, a pressor compound in an American mistletoe. J Biol Chem 19: 303–304

17. Gill LS, Hawksworth FG (1961) The mistletoes – a literature review. Technical Bulletin no. 1242 of the United States Department of Agriculture. Washington: U.S. Government Printing Office, pp.24 and 40
18. Dossaji SF, Becker H, Exner J (1983) Flavone C-glycosides of *Phoradendron tomentosum* from different host trees. Phytochemistry 22:311–312
19. Hanzlik PJ, French WO (1924) The pharmacology of *Phoradendron flavescens* (American mistletoe). J Pharmacol Exp Ther 23:269–305
20. Mellstrand ST (1974) Phoratoxin, a toxic protein from the mistletoe *Phoradendron tomentosum* subsp. *macrophyllum* (Loranthaceae). Immunological properties and tests for proteinase inhibiting and antibiotic effects. Acta Pharm Suec 11:375–380
21. Hall AH, Spoerke DG, Rumack BH (1986) Assessing mistletoe toxicity. Ann Emerg Med 15:1320–1323
22. Haggerty RJ (1958) Christmas holiday poison hazards. New Engl J Med 259:1277–1278
23. Moore HW (1969) Mistletoe poisoning. A review of the available literature, and the report of a case of probable fatal poisoning. J South Carolina Med Assoc 59:269–271

Safrole – General Discussion

G. Abel

Botany

Safrole is found naturally as a constituent of numerous essential oils [1–3]. It is the principle constituent of oil of *Sassafras albidum* (Nutt.) Nees (up to 90%), oil of *Ocotea cymbarum* H.B.K., oil of *Cinnamomum micranthum* (Hayata) Hayata, and brown camphor oil from *Cinnamomum camphora* (L.) Sieb. (50–60%) [3,4].

Safrole is also reported as a minor component (< 1%) in a variety of other spices and essential oils, including nutmeg and mace (*Myristica fragrans* Houtt.), black pepper (*Piper nigrum* L.) and ginger (*Zingiber officinale* Roscoe) [1–4]. However, considering the age of these references, it may be that these results will not be confirmed, when an analysis is carried out with latest techniques, as was the case with star anise (*Illicium verum* Hooker). Star anise oil obtained from the Japanese tree (*Illicium anisatum* L.) contains considerable quantities of safrole (about 6%), but no safrole was detected in star anise oil obtained from the Chinese tree *Illicium verum* Hooker [5,6].

Chemistry

Safrole is chemically described as 4-allyl-1,2-methylenedioxybenzene and as 5-(2-propenyl)-1,3-benzodioxole.

Pharmacology and Uses

Safrole is used in perfumery and soaps and as a flavoring agent in pharmaceutical preparations. It was formerly used as a flavoring agent in soft drinks and root-beer [7,8].

Pharmacokinetics

Studies on safrole metabolism show that the compound gives rise to a large number of metabolites by two major pathways, oxidation of the methylenedioxy group with subsequent cleavage to form a catechol and oxidation of the allyl side chain.

In mouse and rat livers, safrole is hydroxylated at the 1'-position of the allyl side chain by microsomal P-450 enzymes [9]. In turn, the 1'-hydroxy metabolite is further metabolized by liver enzymes to three kinds of electrophilic metabolites: 1'-ester of sulfuric acid (1'-sulfoxy derivatives), 2',3'-epoxides, and 1'-oxo derivatives [10–15]. The epoxidation of safrole, as evidenced by the formation of the 2',3'-dihydrodiol, either in vivo or in rat liver cells in culture, has also been demonstrated [16–19].

Evidence for the metabolism of the 1'-hydroxy metabolites to reactive derivatives in vivo was provided by the formation of covalently bound adducts in liver DNA, RNA and protein [11,20–23]. Further characterization of the DNA adducts formed by the electrophilic esters of 1'-hydroxysafrole has been reported [24–26].

Benedetti et al. [27] examined the absorption and excretion of safrole in rats and humans. In rats fed safrole at levels varying from 0.6 to 750 mg/kg, low doses were rapidly eliminated while high doses produced a large decrease in the rate of safrole elimination. The major urinary metabolite was 4-allylcatechol, with smaller amounts of eugenol, 1'-hydroxysafrole, and 3'-hydroxysafrole also being detected (conjugated forms). In human volunteers given 0.17 and 1.66 mg of radiolabeled safrole, the compound was rapidly absorbed, and more than 90% of the test dose was eliminated within 24 hours. The major excretory product was 4-allylcatechol and small amounts of eugenol were also excreted; 1'-hydroxysafrole was not detected. However, as the dose levels were much lower than those given to rats, it is not known whether the apparent absence of this metabolite was due to a dose effect or to a species difference.

Adverse Reaction Profile

General Animal Data

The first toxicological study of safrole appears to be the work of Heffter [28]. He reported six experiments, the first one in a frog, the remaining five in four rabbits and a cat. In the frog, safrole induced narcosis with degradation of reflexes. Similar symptoms were observed in cats and rabbits, as well as death by paralysis of respiration. When the cat was given a subcutaneous injection of 1 ml safrole, its state of health was normal for the following two days. On the third day, the cat was given a second injection of 1 ml safrole. It vomited during the course of this day and died five days later. The subacute poisoning in general caused physical decline and after some time, death. Tissues from the animals were examined and fatty degeneration of liver and kidney was observed, primarily in the cat. The lethal dose for rabbits, as stated by Heffter, was approximately 1 g/kg via the stomach or subcutaneously and about 0.2 g/kg intravenously.

Acute LD_{50} values of 1.95 g/kg in rats and 2.35 g/kg in mice were reported [29,30]. The acute dermal LD_{50} value in rabbits exceeded 5 g/kg [31]. Four daily oral doses of 650 mg/kg given to rats produced macroscopic liver lesions, characterized by discoloration, enlargement and fatty infiltration [32]. After oral doses of 750 mg/kg administered to rats as a 25% solution in maize oil for 19 days, 9 of 10 animals died; with 500 mg/kg/day only 1 of 10 animals died after 46 days; and with 250 mg/kg/day no animal died within 34 days [30].

Studies in dogs showed extensive liver damage at 80 and 40 mg/kg, lesser damage at lower levels, but no tumors [33]. There was some evidence of adaptation to the stress of safrole ingestion [34].

Using partially hepatectomized rats, Gershbein [35] reported that the oral administration of safrole at 10 mg/kg for 10 days significantly stimulated hepatic regeneration.

General Human Data

The American Food and Drug Administration (FDA) has not permitted safrole to be used in foods since 1960 [4]. The Council of Europe listed safrole among toxicologically active flavoring substances for which it was considered necessary to set a limit for its occurrence in food. The limits for safrole were set as follows: < 1 mg/kg in beverages and food, 5 mg/kg in alcoholic beverages containing more than 25% of alcohol by volume, 15 mg/kg in food containing mace or nutmeg. The explanatory text contained the annotation that the toxicological limit should be lower but that the methods of analysis that were generally available did not permit a lower level of detection [36].

The EEC Guideline for Cosmetic Products and the derived German Cosmetics Regulation have laid down a permissible maximum concentration of safrole in ready-for-sale cosmetic products of 100 ppm safrole [1].

In 1981, safrole was listed as a carcinogen by the Environmental Protection Agency (EPA) [7]. The medicinal use of herbs with safrole as a major component in their volatile oil should be discouraged because of the carcinogenic potential of safrole. This is especially valid for those ways of administration in which safrole is systemic available, because safrole is less carcinogenic than its metabolites.

Central Nervous System Reactions

A 19-year-old man developed a schizophrenia-like psychosis after ingesting isosafrole, an analog of safrole, for approximately two weeks [37].

Hepatic Reactions

See the sections on general animal data, drug interactions, and mutagenicity and carcinogenicity.

Drug Interactions

Parke and Rahman [38] reported that safrole produced rat liver hypertrophy, and stimulated the activity of a number of hepatic drug metabolizing microsomal enzymes including biphenyl hydroxylase, nitro reductase, glucuronyl transferase and cytochrome P-450. These findings that administration of safrole resulted in induction of various microsomal enzymes are in agreement with several other investigations [39–46]. Friedman et al. [47] reported that safrole stimulated mouse aminopyrine demethylase activity while decreasing biphenyl-4-hydroxylase activity. Crampton and co-workers [48] studied the effect of prolonged feeding of 0.25% safrole on the liver weights and drug metabolizing system of female rats. After administration of safrole for 7 days the relative liver weight was increased and the activity of the drug metabolizing enzymes was markedly enhanced. This enzyme induction was shortlived, however, and continued administration of safrole led to inhibition of drug metabolizing activity. In spite of this, the liver remained enlarged and concentrations of NADPH-cytochrome C reductase, cytochrome B_5 and microsomal protein were markedly elevated. During the initial phase of enzyme induction no histochemical or morphological abnormalities were evident, but the loss of this inductive response was associated with histochemical and ultrastructural evidence of liver damage. Ligand-complex formation between cytochromes P-450 and P-448 and safrole was reported by Delaforge and co-workers [49] and by Fennell and Bridges [50].

Using rats, Homburger and co-workers [51] studied the effect of 1.0% safrole in diets deficient and supplemented with riboflavin, tocopherol, or casein. They reported that riboflavin and tocopherol supplements had little effect on hepatoma induction, but casein supplementation significantly stimulated hepatoma formation. The incidence of hepatocellular carcinomas in rats fed safrole was markedly increased by simultaneous administration of phenobarbital [52].

The evidence of drug interactions obtained so far is limited to animal studies. There are no data to prove or disprove that such effects are clinically relevant in human use.

Fertility, Pregnancy and Lactation

Transplacental and lactational carcinogenesis by safrole has been investigated by Vesselinovitch and co-workers [53]. Transplacental treatment did not induce liver tumors. Only male mice nursed during the preweaning period by mothers treated with safrole developed hepatocellular tumors; the vast majority of tumors were identified only after the offspring were 60 weeks old (see the section on mutagenicity and carcinogenicity below for details).

The binding of safrole and its proximate carcinogen, 1'-hydroxysafrole, to liver and kidney DNA was increased 2.3–3.5 fold in pregnant mice compared to nonpregnant mice [54]. The formation of DNA adducts in various maternal and fetal tissues after administration of safrole to pregnant mice was studied by Lu and co-workers [55]. In both maternal and fetal tissues, safrole exhibited preferential binding to liver DNA. The fetal adduct levels, however, were generally lower than the corresponding maternal adduct levels (42-fold) [55].

Possible teratogenic effects of safrole were studied in Swiss mice by treating groups of pregnant animals with multiple intragastric administrations at 0 to 200 mg/kg/day of safrole from day 6 to 14 of pregnancy. It was shown that safrole was toxic to fetuses and caused growth retardation, but no significant increase of malformations was observed [56].

Treatment of male mice with safrole did not lead to an increase in the incidence of abnormally shaped sperm heads [57].

Mutagenicity and Carcinogenicity

Safrole has been studied extensively in numerous mutagenicity assays, and has been used often for evaluation of test systems. Attempts to demonstrate the mutagenicity of safrole in bacteria have been largely unsuccessful. Although certain investigators have reported safrole to be mutagenic in the *Salmonella*/microsome assay [58,59], it has generally been found inactive in this assay [60–73]. Negative results were also obtained in tests using *Escherichia coli* WP2 uvrA [66]. In tests using a mouse-liver postmitochondrial fraction, Green and Savage [58] showed that safrole was mutagenic to *Salmonella typhimurium* strains TA 1530 and TA 1532, but not to strains TA 1531 and TA 1964. Concentrations tested ranged from 50 to 500 µg/plate. These authors also obtained positive results for safrole in a host-mediated assay using male mice and *Salmonella typhimurium* strains TA 1950 and TA 1952 [58].

In contrast, 1'-acetoxysafrole, the 2',3'-oxides of safrole, 1'-hydroxysafrole, 1'-acetoxysafrole and 1'-oxosafrole were reported to be directly mutagenic for *Salmonella typhimurium* strains TA 1535 and TA 100. No significant mutagenicity was detected in this assay with safrole, isosafrole, 1'-hydroxysafrole, 3'-hydroxyisosafrole, 3'-acetoxyisosafrole, or 1'-oxosafrole [52]. The mutagenic activities of the 2',3'-oxides of safrole were confirmed by Swanson and co-workers [64].

A variety of yeast assay systems were used that detect several types of genetic events as gene mutations [74–81], recombinogenic effects [82–86], mitotic aneuploidy [81,87,88] and repair activity [89]. There was a wide variation in the methods used in these tests. Contradictory results were reported: results were predominantly negative, but weakly positive or positive results were obtained in part after modifying a routine test. Growing cells were generally more sensitive than were stationary phase cells.

In DNA repair assays, safrole induced significant UDS (unscheduled DNA synthesis). This result was only apparent in scintillation counting assays [90–94], but not in autoradiographic/hepatocyte assays [95–98]. One possible explanation for the discrepancy between the autoradiographic and scintillation UDS results is the latter's theoretically greater sensitivity due to the great number of cells sampled ($2–5 \times 10^7$ versus 50) and the statistical reliability of scintillation counting [99]. The most effective dose was 10^{-2} to 10^{-3} M. However, the genotoxicity of safrole was relatively weak compared to the activity of 2-acetylaminofluorene. Isosafrole was negative [94]. The structure-dependent genotoxic activity of naturally occurring flavors, structurally related to safrole, revealed in this study [94] is consistent with their known tumorigenicities in rodents and their DNA binding as revealed by the sensitive ^{32}P-post-labelling assay [91,100]. The highest quantities and most persistent adducts were found after treatment of mice with safrole, estragole and methyleugenol.

Data concerning gene mutation assays in mammalian cells were reported on a variety of cell lines, such as mouse lymphoma L5178Y cells (mainly the TK$^{+/-}$ system), Chinese hamster V79 cells (HGPRT locus), Chinese hamster ovary cells, and human lymphoblastoid cell lines. The most common procedure for metabolic activation was the use of a rat liver S9 mix from either Aroclor or phenobarbitone/naphtoflavone induced animals. The final concentrations of liver S9 varied considerably from laboratory to laboratory. Sometimes uninduced rat liver S9 was used or activation was performed, for example, with various primary cell cultures (rat hepatocytes, Syrian hamster embryo cells, chick embryo hepatocytes).

The majority of the laboratories failed to detect safrole as a mammalian cell mutagen. Only two laboratories obtained acceptable positive results in the presence of S9, but the magnitude of response was small [101,102]. Other laboratories obtained negative or equivocal results [103–111]. Evidence for the mutagenicity at the ouabain resistance locus, HGPRT locus, or the TK locus without S9 was reported, but was not convincing (reported active concentration range: 1-625 μg/ml) [102,112,113]. When the data for safrole that were considered positive by several laboratories were rigorously examined using suitable statistical tests, the results reported by some of these labs were found to be incorrect [114].

Measurement of DNA single-strand breaks by alkaline elution in rat hepatocytes gave positive results for safrole [115,116]. In Chinese hamster ovary cells, Lakhaniski and Hendrickx [117] reported a strong dose-related response for the induction of DNA single-strand breaks by alkaline sucrose sedimentation, however, in a very narrow range of concentrations: 10^{-3} M to 3.4x 10^{-3} M. Douglas and co-workers [118] revealed negative results in this assay, testing concentrations from 5x 10^{-5} M to 2x 10^{-3} M. Safrole has been studied for the induction of chromosomal aberrations mainly in Chinese hamster cells with and without metabolic activation and it is generally found inactive [119–122]. In rat liver cells, safrole did not induce structural aberrations either [123,124]. Jain [109] reported that safrole is clastogenic in V79 Chinese hamster cells, but judging from the published data this statement seems questionable, because dose-dependency was not evident, only a few breaks were scored and the effect was not reproduced. This is also true for the weak positive effect reported by Palitti [121] with Chinese hamster ovary cells in the absence of S9. Ishidate [125] revealed an induction of structural chromosome aberrations with metabolic activation (S9) in Chinese hamster lung fibroblast cells.

When albino rats were injected with different doses of safrole (0.6 to 1.0 ml/kg body weight, i.p., for 96 h), the chromosome preparations of bone-marrow cells revealed numerical and structural chromosome aberrations [126]. The relevance of this paper seems questionable, however, as the results were not confirmed and evaluation criteria were not clearly defined. In vitro, safrole induced neither polyploidy nor aneuploidy [119,124,125,127].

As described for structural chromosome aberrations, the results for safrole in the SCE (sister chromatid exchange) assay are negative [109,118,122,124,128–130]. Two tests with Chinese hamster cells are reported as positive, but the effect was not dose-dependent and the SCE-rate was increased less than a factor of two [120,131]. Darroudi and Natarajan [132] studied drug metabolites: exponentially growing Chinese hamster ovary cells were incubated with plasma from rats that contained active metabolites of the test chemicals. In this assay, safrole was marginally positive, enhancing the spontaneous SCE-rate by a factor of about two. Safrole was negative by in vivo SCE-tests in male CBA/J mice; SCE-frequencies were determined in the bone marrow and liver cells [133].

In *Drosophila* safrole gave reproducible effects in the wing and eye mosaic assay [134]. The clone size produced by safrole was generally small, pointing to an induction late during larval development. Safrole was tested for mutagenicity in the sex-linked recessive-lethal (SLRL) mutation assay after being fed to *Drosophila melanogaster* adult males and larvae and was found to be non-mutagenic [135,136]. Safrole did not show mutagenic activity in the unstable zeste-white somatic eye color system [137].

The micronucleus test is an *in vivo* cytogenetic screen based on the observation that cells with chromosome breaks and/or exchanges often have had aberrations in the distribution of chromatin during cell division. After division, the daughter cells displayed chromatin as distinct micronuclei in the cytoplasm. The cell population tested consists of the erythrocytes of the bone marrow of mice. The existing studies revealed consistent negative results for safrole [138–140].

Pienta [141] found a positive effect of safrole in the transformation of Syrian hamster embryo cells; the lowest transforming dose was indicated as 0.001 µg/ml. Styles [142] also reported a positive result for safrole in the BHK-21 cell transformation test, using growth in semisolid agar as the endpoint. Safrole increased the transformation frequency over the control values by a factor of 10 at the LD$_{50}$ dose (20 µg/ml). In 1985, a summary report on the performance of cell transformation assays was published by McGregor and Ashby [143]. Safrole was reported to induce morphological transformation of Syrian hamster embryo cells [144,145], of C3H/10 T 1/2 CL8 mouse embryo fibroblasts [146,147], and of Balb/c-3T3 cells only under conditions of rat-liver cell-mediated exogenous metabolic activation [148]. Safrole was assayed for its capacity to enhance the adenovirus (SA7) transformation of Syrian hamster embryo (SHE) cells and produced negative results [149]. Additionally, safrole did not induce cell transformation (cell invasive growth in agar) in Chinese hamster ovary cells [150]. There is evidence that the initiation of carcinogenesis may result from the mutational activation of a cellular proto-oncogene. Recently, reactive derivatives of safrole, e.g., 1'-acetoxysafrole, were reported to modify the human c-Ha-ras-1 proto-oncogene in vitro. The modifications are specific point-mutations and these are responsible for activating the proto-oncogene [151].

In the nineteensixties, it was first reported that safrole caused liver tumors in rats fed the substance at high dietary dose levels (1%) for 150 to 360 days [51]. At the 0.1% level safrole had no effect. These findings were confirmed by Long and co-workers [152]. Animals fed 0.5% safrole developed malignant liver tumors in high incidence (14/50 animals), whereas lower levels (0.1%) induced benign tumors in lower incidence (statistically not significant). At lower dosages (0.05% and 0.01%, respectively) there was no increase in tumor production. Other research groups also reported that safrole is a very weak carcinogen when fed to adult male or female rats or male mice. Dietary concentrations of up to 0.5-1.0% for one year or more were required to induce appreciable incidences of liver tumors [30,153–155].

However, total doses of only a few milligrams of safrole injected subcutaneously to male mice during infancy will induce high incidences of hepatocellular carcinomas after a year or more, with no hepatomas developing in treated females [156]. Similarly, Lipsky and co-workers [157] reported that only 16 weeks of safrole treatment (0.4%) is needed in young male BALB/c mice (6–8 weeks old) to produce initiated hepatocytes that have sufficiently developed to progress to hepatocellular carcinomas without further carcinogenic stimulation. When mice exposed to safrole for 16 weeks were allowed to live 36 more weeks on a control diet, 15% developed grossly visible neoplasms. This increased to 50% in mice allowed to live for 52 weeks on the control diet subsequent to the safrole exposure. However, safrole did not produce a pulmonary tumor response in strain A mice. In this study, groups of 15 male and 15 female mice were given total doses of 0.9 and 4.5 g/kg body weight (12 i.p. injections). All surviving mice were killed at 24 weeks [158].

Transplacental and lactational carcinogenesis has been reported by Vesselinovitch and co-workers [53,159]. Groups of pregnant or lactating mice were treated with doses of 120 mg/kg body weight which were administered by gastric intubation at 2-day intervals. The pregnant mice were given four doses, starting on day 12 of gestation, and the first of the 12 doses during lactation was administered on the day of delivery. Starting at 28 days of age offspring of untreated mothers were given 120 mg safrole per kg body weight twice weekly for 90 weeks. Two additional groups of offspring were given combined treatments; one was exposed during gestation and via the mother's milk and the other was exposed pre- and postnatally and for 90 weeks after weaning. The mice exposed to safrole or its metabolites prenatally and/or via the mother's milk had a high survival rate (at least 90%) at 92 weeks, but those subjected to direct intubation beginning at the time of weaning (with or without prenatal treatment) had lower rates of survival (about 50% for males and 30% for females). The vast majority of tumors (97%) were identified only after the offspring were 60 weeks old.

Transplacental treatment with safrole did not induce liver tumors. However, renal epithelial tumors occurred in females that were exposed transplacentally. Although the incidence of these tumors was low (7%), they were not seen in controls, in females exposed via the milk and/or during weaning, or in males.

Only male mice nursed during the preweaning period by mothers treated with safrole developed hepatocellular tumors (34%). A similar incidence of liver tumors was observed in male mice exposed during gestation and via the milk (32%). No neoplastic activity was observed following in utero or adult exposure of male mice to safrole. The greater sensitivity of newborn mice compared with adults to safrole carcinogenesis may, besides other facts, be attributable also to the greater proportion of DNA adducts that persist in the target organ. Thus, high levels of DNA adducts were detected with safrole when injected in newborn male mice. Most of these adducts were still present at 43 days [100]. This is in marked contrast to the situation in adult female mice, where 80% of the adducts initially formed after administration of safrole and 1'-hydroxysafrole are lost from the DNA within the first week of treatment [160].

Safrole was not carcinogenic in prenatal or infant females. In contrast, direct administration of safrole, beginning at the time of weaning and continuing throughout the experiment, resulted in a significantly high incidence of hepatocellular tumors in females (48%), but not in males (8%). Of the liver tumors found in females, 86% were hepatocellular carcinomas and there was a high incidence (42%) of pulmonary metastases.

The results indicate strong modifying effects of sex and of age on the liver carcinogenicity of safrole. Some earlier studies have indicated that adult female mice are more susceptible than males to the carcinogenic effects of orally administered safrole and its metabolites [52,161]. However, the reverse seems to be true for infant mice and for rats [12,53,156,162].

1'-Hydroxysafrole is a more potent carcinogen than the parent compound safrole [153,163,164]. Detailed studies have provided strong evidence that the hepatocarcinogenicity in mice of 1'-hydroxysafrole requires conversion to 1'-sulfo-oxysafrole by sulfotransferase activity in hepatic cytosol and the reaction of this highly electrophilic ester with DNA [11,12]. Thus, concurrent administration of the hepatic sulfotransferase inhibitor, pentachlorophenol, strongly inhibited hepatic sulfotransferase activity for 1'-hydroxysafrole in vitro, as well as the formation of DNA-adducts and hepatic tumors after administration of 1'-hydroxysafrole to mice [160,165].

Recently, a weak initiating and, additionally, a promoting activity of 1'-hydroxysafrole for the formation of enzyme-altered foci and tumors in rat liver was reported [166]. The intubation of a single dose of N,N-diethylnitrosamine into partially hepatectomized rats, followed by long-term (10 months) dietary administration of 1'-hydroxysafrole (0.10% and 0.25%, respectively), resulted in a strong synergistic effect on the induction of hepatic tumors. Thus, whereas treatment with N,N-diethylnitrosamine alone or with 0.1% 1'-hydroxysafrole alone did not result in the development of any gross hepatic tumors by ten months, their sequential administration resulted in a 67% incidence of liver-tumor-bearing rats. Concurrent administration of the hepatic sulfotransferase inhibitor, pentachlorophenol, almost completely inhibited the initiating and promoting activities of 1'-hydroxysafrole [166].

Neoplasms of the forestomach developed in mice ingesting dihydrosafrole. The maximal tolerated doses of dihydrosafrole, safrole, and isosafrole were given by continuous oral administration, starting at the age of 7 days, to both sexes of two hybrid strains of mice. Hyperplasia and carcinomas of the forestomach were significantly increased in female mice of both strains and in male mice of one of the strains ingesting dihydrosafrole. On the contrary, neoplasms of the forestomach were not increased in mice receiving safrole or isosafrole [167].

References

1. Fiedler HP (1981) Safrole: A Literature Survey. Drugs made Germ 24:163–166
2. Gildemeister E, Hoffmann F (1966) Safrol. In: Treibs W (ed) Die ätherischen Öle, Band IIId. 4. Auflage. Berlin:Akademie-Verlag

3. Hoppe HA (1975) Drogenkunde. Band 1. Angiospermen. 8. Auflage. Berlin: Walter de Gruyter
4. Opdyke DLJ (1974) Monographs on fragrance raw materials: Safrole. Fd Cosmet Toxicol 12:983–986
5. Kämpf R, Steinegger E (1974) Dünnschicht- und gaschromatographische Untersuchungen an Oleum anisi und Oleum anisi stellati. Pharm Acta Helv 49:87–93
6. Seger V, Miething H, Hänsel R (1987) Pharm Ztg 132:2747–2748
7. Windholz M (ed) (1983) The Merck Index. 10th Edition. Rahway, NJ: Merck & Co.
8. Anonymous (1976) Safrole, Isosafrole and Dihydrosafrole. IARC Monogr Eval Carcinog Risk Chem Man 10:231–244
9. Swanson AB, Miller EC, Miller JA (1981) The side-chain epoxidation and hydroxylation of the hepatocarcinogens safrole and estragole and some related compounds by rat and mouse liver microsomes. Biochim Biophys Acta 673:504–516
10. Oswald EO, Fishbein L, Corbett BJ, Walker MP (1971) Identification of tertiary amino methylenedioxy-propiophenones as urinary metabolites of safrole in the rat and guinea pig. Biochim Biophys Acta 230:237–247
11. Wislocki PG, Borchert P, Miller JA, Miller EC (1976) The metabolic activation of the carcinogen 1'-hydroxysafrole in vivo and in vitro and the electrophilic reactivities of possible ultimate carcinogens. Cancer Res 36:1686–1695
12. Miller JA, Swanson AB, Miller EC (1979) The metabolic activation of safrole and related naturally occurring alkenylbenzenes in relation to carcinogenesis by these agents. Proc Int Symp Princess Takamatsu Cancer Res Fund 9th: 111–125
13. Peele JD, Oswald EO (1978) Metabolism of the proximate carcinogen 1'-hydroxysafrole and the isomer 3'-hydroxyisosafrole. Bull Environ Contam Toxicol 19:396–402
14. Fennell TR, Miller JA, Miller EC (1984) Characterization of the biliary and urinary glutathione and N-acetylcysteine metabolites of the hepatic carcinogen 1'-hydroxysafrole and its 1'-oxo metabolite in rats and mice. Cancer Res 44:3231–3240
15. Miller EC, Miller JA, Boberg EW, Delclos KB, Lai CC, Fennell TR, Wisemann RW, Liem A (1985) Sulfuric acid esters as ultimate electrophilic and carcinogenic metabolites of some alkenylbenzenes and aromatic amines in mouse liver. Carcinog Compr Surv 10:93-108
16. Stillwell WG, Carman MJ, Bell L, Horning MG (1974) The metabolism of safrole and 2',3'-epoxysafrole in the rat and guinea pig. Drug Metab Dispos 2:489–498
17. Delaforge M, Janiaud P, Chessebeuf M, Padieu P, Maume BF (1976) Possible occurrence of the epoxid-diol metabolic pathway for hepatocarcinogenic safrole in cultured rat liver cells, as compared with whole animal: a metabolic study by mass spectrometry. Adv Mass Spectr Biochem Med 2:65–89
18. Delaforge M, Janiaud P, Maume BF, Padieu P (1978) Direct evidence of epoxide metabolic pathway for natural allylbenzene compounds in adult rat liver cell culture. Recent Dev Mass Spectr Biochem Med 1:521–539
19. Delaforge M, Janiaud P, Levi P, Morizot JP (1980) Biotransformation of allylbenzene analogues in vivo and in vitro through the epoxide-diol pathway. Xenobiotica 10:737–744
20. Phillips DH, Hanawalt PC, Miller JA, Miller EC (1981) The in vivo formation and repair of DNA adducts from 1'-hydroxysafrole. J Supramol Struct Cell Biochem 16:83–90
21. Levy GN, Weber WW (1988) High-Performance Liquid Chromatographic Analysis of ^{32}P-Postlabeled DNA-Aromatic Carcinogen Adducts. Anal Biochem 174:381–392
22. Phillips DH (1990) Further evidence that eugenol does not bind to DNA in vivo. Mutat Res 245:23–26
23. Reddy MV, Randerath K (1990) A comparison of DNA adduct formation in white blood cells and internal organs of mice exposed to benzo(a)pyrene, dibenzo(c,g)carbazole, safrole and cigarette smoke condensate. Mutat Res 241:37–48
24. Phillips DH, Miller JA, Miller EC, Adams B (1981) N^2 atom of guanine and N^6 atom of adenine residues as sites for covalent binding of metabolically activated 1'-hydroxysafrole to mouse liver DNA in vivo. Cancer Res 41:2664–2671

25. Miller JA, Miller EC (1983) The metabolic activation and nucleic acid adducts of naturally-occurring carcinogens: recent results with ethylcarbamate and the spice flavors safrole and estragole. Br J Cancer 48:1–15
26. Wiseman RW, Fennell TR, Miller JA, Miller EC (1985) Further characterization of the DNA adducts formed by electrophilic esters of the hepatocarcinogens 1'-hydroxysafrole and 1'-hydroxyestragole in vitro and in mouse liver in vivo, including new adducts at C-8 and N-7 of guanine residues. Cancer Res 45:3096–3105
27. Benedetti MS, Malnoe A, Broillet AL (1977) Absorption, metabolism and excretion of safrole in the rat and man. Toxicology 7:69–83
28. Heffter A (1894–1895) Zur Pharmakologie der Safrolgruppe. Arch Exp Pathol Pharmacol 35:342–374
29. Jenner PM, Hagan EC, Taylor JM, Cook EL, Fitzhugh OG (1964) Food Flavourings and Compounds of Related Structure. I. Acute Oral Toxicity. Fd Cosmet Toxicol 2:327–343
30. Hagan EC, Jenner PM, Jones WI, Fitzhugh OG, Long EL, Brouwer JG, Webb WK (1965) Toxic properties of compounds related to safrole. Toxicol Appl Pharmacol 7:18–24
31. Moreno OM (1972) Report to RIFM, 31. May
32. Taylor JM, Jenner PM, Jones WI (1964) A comparison of toxicity of some allyl, propenyl and propyl compounds in the rat. Toxicol Appl Pharmacol 6:378–387
33. Hagan EC, Hansen WH, Fitzhugh OG, Jenner PM, Jones WI, Taylor JM, Long EL, Nelson AA, Brouwer JB (1967) Food Flavourings and Compounds of Related Structure. II. Subacute and Chronic Toxicity. Fd Cosmet Toxicol 5:141–157
34. Weinberg MS, Sternberg SS (1966) Effect of chronic safrole administration on hepatic enzymes and functional activity in dogs. Toxicol Appl Pharmacol 8:363–380
35. Gershbein LL (1977) Regeneration of rat liver in the presence of essential oils and their components. Fd Cosmet Toxicol 15:173–182
36. Anonymous (1981) Flavouring substances and natural sources of flavourings. Council of Europe, Partial Agreement in the Social and Public Health Field. Strasbourg
37. Keitner GI, Sabaawi M, Haier RJ (1984) Isosafrole and schizophrenia-like psychosis. Am J Psychiatry 141:997–998
38. Parke DV, Rahman H (1970) The induction of hepatic microsomal enzymes by safrole. Biochem J 119:53–54 p
39. Parke DV, Rahman H (1971) Induction of a new hepatic microsomal haemoprotein by safrole and isosafrole. Biochem J 123:9–10 p
40. Lotlikar PD, Wasserman MB (1972) Effects of safrole and isosafrole pretreatment on N- and Ring-hydroxylation of 2-acetamidofluorene by rat and hamster. Biochem J 129:937–943
41. Lake BG, Parke DV (1972) Induction of aryl hydrocarbon hydroxylase in various tissues of the rat by methylenedioxyphenyl compounds. Biochem J 130:86 p
42. McPherson FJ, Bridges JW, Parke DV (1976) The effects of benzopyrene and safrole on biphenyl 2-hydroxylase and other drug metabolizing enzymes. Biochem J 154:773–780
43. Parke DV, Gray TJB (1978) A comparative study of the enzymic and morphological changes of livers of rats fed butylated hydroxytoluene, safrole, ponceau MX or 2-acetamidofluorene. Falk Symp 25:335–353
44. Batt AM, Martin N, Siest G (1981) Induction of group-1 and group-2 UDP-glucuronosyl-transferase in microsomes from the livers of C57 B1/6 mice. Toxicol Lett 9:355–360
45. Cook JC, Hodgson E (1983) Induction of cytochrome P-450 by methylenedioxyphenyl compounds: importance of the methylene carbon. Toxicol Appl Pharmacol 68:131–139
46. Ioannides C, Lum PY, Parke DV (1984) Cytochrome P–448 and the activation of toxic chemicals and carcinogens. Xenobiotica 14:119–137
47. Friedmann MA, Arnold E, Bishop Y, Epstein SS (1971) Additive and synergistic inhibition of mammalian microsomal enzyme functions by piperonyl butoxide, safrole and other methylenedioxyphenyl derivatives. Experientia 27:1052–1054
48. Crampton RF, Gray TJB, Grasso P, Parke DV (1977) Long-term studies on chemically induced liver enlargement in the rat: II. Transient induction of microsomal enzymes leading

to liver damage and nodular hyperplasia produced by safrole and Ponceau MX. Toxicology 7:307–326
49. Delaforge M, Ioannides C, Parke DV (1985) Ligand-complex formation between cytochromes P-450 and P-448 and methylenedioxyphenyl compounds. Xenobiotica 15:333–342
50. Fennell TR, Bridges JW (1979) Structure-activity relationship for "Safrole-type" cytochrome P-450 induction. Biochem Soc Trans 7:1104–1106
51. Homburger F, Kelley T, Friedler G, Russfield AB (1961) Toxic and possible carcinogenic effects of 4-allyl-1,2-methylenedioxybenzene (safrole) in rats on deficient diets. Med Exp 4:1–11
52. Wislocki PG, Miller EC, Miller JA, McCoy EC, Rosenkranz HS (1977) Carcinogenic and mutagenic activities of safrole, 1'-hydroxysafrole, and some known or possible metabolites. Cancer Res 37:1883–1891
53. Vesselinovitch SD, Rao KVN, Mihailovich N (1979) Transplacental and lactational carcinogenesis by safrole. Cancer Res 39:4378–4380
54. Lu LJW, Disher RM, Randerath K (1986) Differences in the covalent binding of benzo(a)pyrene, safrole,1'-hydroxysafrole, and 4-aminobiphenyl to DNA of pregnant and non-pregnant mice. Cancer Lett 31:43–52
55. Lu LJW, Disher RM, Reddy MV, Randerath K (1986) ^{32}P-Postlabeling assay in mice of transplacental DNA damage induced by the environmental carcinogens safrole, 4-aminobiphenyl, and benzo(a)pyrene. Cancer Res 46:3046–3054
56. Moro MG, Ognio E, Rossi L, Ferreri-Santi L, Santi L (1985) Tossicita prenatale indotta da safrolo in animali di laboratorio. Rivista di Tossicologia Sperimentale e Clinica 15:91–97
57. Topham JC (1981) Evaluation of some chemicals by the sperm morphology assay. Prog Mutat Res 1:718–720. Amsterdam: Elsevier Science Publishers-Geneva: World Health Organisation
58. Green NR, Savage JR (1978) Screening of safrole, eugenol, their ninhydrin positive metabolites and selected secondary amines for potential mutagenicity. Mutat Res 57:115–121
59. Anderson D, Styles JA (1978) An evaluation of 6 short-term tests for detecting organic chemical carcinogens. Appendix 2. The bacterial mutation test. Br J Cancer 37:924–930
60. McCann J, Ames BN (1976) Detection of carcinogens as mutagens in the *Salmonella* /microsome test: Assay of 300 chemicals: Discussion. Proc Natl Acad Sci USA 73:950–954
61. Dorange JL, Delaforge M, Janiaud P, Padieu P (1977) Pouvoir mutagene de metabolites de la voie epoxyde-diol du safrol et d'analogues. Etude sur *Salmonella typhimurium*. C R Seances Soc Biol Fil 171:1041–1048
62. Rosenkranz HS, Poirier LA (1979) Evaluation of the mutagenicity and DNA modifying activity of carcinogens and noncarcinogens in microbial systems. J Natl Cancer Inst 62:873–892
63. Simmon VF (1979) In vitro mutagenicity assays of chemical carcinogens and related compounds with *Salmonella typhimurium*. J Natl Cancer Inst 62:893–899
64. Swanson AB, Chambliss DD, Blomquist JC, Miller EC, Miller JA (1979) The mutagenicities of safrole, estragole, trans-anethole, and some of their known or possible metabolites for *Salmonella typhimurium*. Mutat Res 60:143–153
65. Gocke E, King MT, Eckhardt K, Wild D (1981) Mutagenicity of cosmetic ingredients licensed by the European communities. Mutat Res 90:91–109
66. Sekizawa J, Shibamoto T (1982) Genotoxicity of safrole-related chemicals in microbial test systems. Mutat Res 101:127–140
67. To LP, Hunt TP, Andersen ME (1982) Mutagenicity of trans-anethole, estragole, eugenol, and safrole in the Ames *Salmonella typhimurium* assay. Bull Environ Contam Toxicol 28:647–654
68. Baker RSU, Bonin AM (1985) Tests with the *Salmonella* plate-incorporation assay. Prog Mutat Res 5:177–180. Amsterdam: Elsevier Science Publishers - Geneva: World Health Organisation

69. Liber H (1985) Mutation tests with *Salmonella* using 8-azaguanine resistance as the genetic marker. Prog Mutat Res 5:213–216. Amsterdam: Elsevier Science Publishers – Geneva: World Health Organisation
70. Matsushima T, Muramatsu M, Haresaku M (1985) Mutation test on *Salmonella typhimurium* by the preincubation method. Prog Mutat Res 5:181–186. Amsterdam: Elsevier Science Publishers – Geneva: World Health Organisation
71. Rexroat MA, Probst GS (1985) Mutation tests with *Salmonella* using the plate–incorporation assay. Prog Mutat Res 5:201–212. Amsterdam: Elsevier Science Publishers – Geneva: World Health Organisation
72. Venitt St, Baker R, Liber H, Matsushima T, Probst G, Zeiger E (1985) Summary report on the performance of the bacterial mutation assays. Prog Mutat Res 5:11–23. Amsterdam: Elsevier Science Publishers – Geneva: World Health Organisation
73. Zeiger E, Haworth St (1985) Tests with a preincubation modification of the *Salmonella*/microsome assay. Prog Mutat Res 5:187–199. Amsterdam: Elsevier Science Publishers – Geneva: World Health Organisation
74. Loprieno N (1981) Screening of coded carcinogenic/noncarcinogenic chemicals by a forward-mutation system with the yeast *Schizosaccharomyces pombe*. Prog Mutat Res 1:424–433. Amsterdam: Elsevier Science Publishers – Geneva: World Health Organisation
75. Mehta RD, von Borstel RC (1981) Mutagenic activity of 42 encoded compounds in the haploid yeast reversion assay, strain XV185–14C. Prog Mutat Res 1:414–423. Amsterdam: Elsevier Science Publishers – Geneva: World Health Organisation
76. Arni P (1985) Induction of various genetic effects in the yeast *Saccharomyces cerevisiae* strain D7. Prog Mutat Res 5:217–224. Amsterdam: Elsevier Science Publishers – Geneva: World Health Organisation
77. Brooks TM, Gonzales LP, Calvert R, Parry JM (1985) The induction of mitotic gene conversion in the yeast *Saccharomyces cerevisiae* strain JD1. Prog Mutat Res 5:225–228. Amsterdam: Elsevier Science Publishers – Geneva: World Health Organisation
78. Harrington TR, Nestmann ER (1985) Tests for mutagenic activity in growing cells of the yeast *Saccharomyces cerevisiae* strain XV185–14C. Prog Mutat Res 5:257–260. Amsterdam Elsevier Science Publishers – Geneva: World Health Organisation
79. Inge-Vechtomov SG, Pavlov YI, Noskov VN, Repnevskaya MV, Karpova TS, Khromov-Borisov NN, Chekuolene J, Chitavichus D (1985) Tests for genetic activity in the yeast *Saccharomyces cerevisiae*: study of forward and reverse mutation, mitotic recombination and illegitimate mating induction. Prog Mutat Res 5: 243–255. Amsterdam: Elsevier Science Publishers – Geneva: World Health Organisation
80. Mehta RD, von Borstel RC (1985) Tests for genetic activity in the yeast *Saccharomyces cerevisiae* using strains D7–144, XV185–14C and RM52. Prog Mutat Res 5:271–284. Amsterdam: Elsevier Science Publishers – Geneva: World Health Organisation
81. Parry JM, Eckhardt F (1985) The induction of mitotic aneuploidy, point mutation and mitotic crossing-over in the yeast *Saccharomyces cerevisiae* strains D61-M and D6. Prog Mutat Res 5:285–295. Amsterdam: Elsevier Science Publishers – Geneva: World Health Organisation
82. Simmon VF (1979) In vitro assays for recombinogenic activity of chemical carcinogens and related compounds with *Saccharomyces cerevisiae* D3. J Natl Cancer Inst 62:901–910
83. Jagannath DR, Vultaggio DM, Brusick DJ (1981) Genetic activity of 42 coded compounds in the mitotic gene conversion assay using *Saccharomyces cerevisiae* strain D4. Prog Mutat Res 1:457–467. Amsterdam: Elsevier Science Publishers – Geneva: World Health Organisation
84. Sharp DC, Parry JM (1981) Induction of mitotic gene conversion by 41 coded compounds using the yeast culture JD1. Prog Mutat Res 1:491–501. Amsterdam: Elsevier Science Publishers – Geneva: World Health Organisation
85. Zimmermann FK, Scheel I (1981) Induction of mitotic gene conversion in strain D7 of *Saccharomyces cerevisiae* by 42 coded chemicals. Prog Mutat Res 1:481–490. Amsterdam: Elsevier Science Publishers – Geneva: World Health Organisation

86. Schiestl RH, Chan WS, Gietz RD, Mehta RD, Hastings PJ (1989) Safrole, eugenol and methyleugenol induce intrachromosomal recombination in yeast. Mutat Res 224:427–436
87. Parry JM, Sharp DC (1981) Induction of mitotic aneuploidy in the yeast strain D6 by 42 coded compounds. Prog Mutat Res 1:468–480. Amsterdam: Elsevier Science Publishers – Geneva: World Health Organisation
88. Zimmermann FK, Heinisch J, Scheel I (1985) Tests for the induction of mitotic aneuploidy in the yeast *Saccharomyces cerevisiae* strain D61.M. Prog Mutat Res 5:235–242. Amsterdam: Elsevier Science Publishers – Geneva: World Health Organisation
89. Sharp DC, Parry JM (1981) Use of repair-deficient strains of yeast to assay the activity of 40 coded compounds. Prog Mutat Res 1:502–516. Amsterdam: Elsevier Science Publishers – Geneva: World Health Organisation
90. Martin CN, Campbell J (1985) Tests for the induction of unscheduled DNA repair synthesis in HeLa cells. Prog Mutat Res 5:375–379. Amsterdam: Elsevier Science Publishers – Geneva: World Health Organisation
91. Barrett RH (1985) Assays for unscheduled DNA synthesis in HeLa S3 cells. Prog Mutat Res 5:347–352. Amsterdam: Elsevier Science Publishers – Geneva: World Health Organisation
92. Glauert HP, Kennan WS, Sattler GL, Pitot HC (1985) Assays to measure the induction of unscheduled DNA synthesis in cultured hepatocytes. Prog Mutat Res 5:371–373. Amsterdam: Elsevier Science Publishers – Geneva: World Health Organisation
93. Althaus FR, Lawrence SD, Sattler GL, Longfellow DG, Pitot HC (1982) Chemical quantification of unscheduled DNA synthesis in cultured hepatocytes as an assay for the rapid screening of potential chemical carcinogens. Cancer Res 42:3010–3015
94. Howes AJ, Chan VSW, Caldwell J (1990) Structure-specifity of the genotoxicity of some naturally occurring alkenylbenzenes determined by the unscheduled DNA synthesis assay in rat hepatocytes. Fd Chem Toxicol 28: 537–542
95. Probst GS, Hill LE (1985) Tests for the induction of DNA- repair synthesis in primary cultures of adult rat hepatocytes. Prog Mutat Res 5:381–386. Amsterdam: Elsevier Science Publishers – Geneva: World Health Organisation
96. Williams GM, Tong C, Brat SV (1985) Tests with the rat hepatocyte primary culture/DNA repair test. Prog Mutat Res 5:341–345. Amsterdam: Elsevier Science Publishers – Geneva: World Health Organisation
97. Klaunig JE, Goldblatt PJ, Hinton DE, Lipsky MM, Trump BF (1984) Carcinogen induced unscheduled DNA synthesis in mouse hepatocytes. Toxicol Pathol 12:119–125
98. Mirsalis JC, Tyson CK, Butterworth BE (1982) Detection of genotoxic carcinogens in the in vivo – in vitro hepatocyte DNA repair assay. Environ Mutagen 4:553–562
99. Williams GM, Barrett R, Bradley M, Douglas G, Glauert H, Lakhanisky T, Martin C, Probst G (1985) Summary report on the performance of the assays for DNA damage. Prog Mutat Res 5:59–67. Amsterdam: Elsevier Science Publishers – Geneva: World Health Organisation
100. Phillips DH, Reddy MV, Randerath K (1984) ^{32}P-Postlabelling analysis of DNA adducts formed in the livers of animals treated with safrole, estragole and other naturally-occurring alkenylbenzenes. II. Newborn male B6C3F1 mice. Carcinog 5:1623–1628
101. Amacher DE, Turner GN (1985) Tests for gene mutational activity in the L5178Y/TK assay system. Prog Mutat Res 5:487–496. Amsterdam: Elsevier Science Publishers – Geneva: World Health Organisation
102. Styles JA, Clay P, Cross MF (1985) Assays for the induction of gene mutations at the thymidine kinase and the Na$^+$/K$^+$ ATPase loci in two different mouse lymphoma cells in culture. Prog Mutat Res 5:587–596. Amsterdam: Elsevier Science Publishers – Geneva: World Health Organisation
103. Fox M, Delow GF (1985) Tests for mutagenic activity at the HGPRT locus in Chinese hamster V79 cells in culture. Prog Mutat Res 5:517–523. Amsterdam: Elsevier Science Publishers – Geneva: World Health Organisation
104. Knaap AGAC, Langebroek PB (1985) Assays for the induction of gene mutations at the thymidine kinase locus and the hypoxanthine guanine phosphoribosyltransferase locus in

L5178Y mouse lymphoma cells in culture. Prog Mutat Res 5:531–536. Amsterdam: Elsevier Science Publishers – Geneva: World Health Organisation
105. Kuroki T, Munakata K (1985) Assays for the induction of mutations to ouabain resistance in V79 Chinese hamster cells in culture with cell- or microsome-mediated metabolic activation. Prog Mutat Res 5:543–545. Amsterdam: Elsevier Science Publishers – Geneva: World Health Organisation
106. Lee CG, Webber TD (1985) The induction of gene mutations in the mouse lymphoma L5178Y/TK$^{+/-}$ assay and the Chinese hamster V79/HGPRT assay. Prog Mutat Res 5:547–554. Amsterdam: Elsevier Science Publishers – Geneva: World Health Organisation
107. Oberly TJ, Bewsey BJ, Probst GS (1985) Tests for the induction of forward mutation at the thymidine kinase locus of L5178Y mouse lymphoma cells in culture. Prog Mutat Res 5:569–582. Amsterdam: Elsevier Science Publishers – Geneva: World Health Organisation
108. Zdzienicka MZ, Simons JWIM (1985) Assays for the induction of mutations to 6-thioguanine and ouabain resistance in Chinese hamster ovary (CHO) cells in culture. Prog Mutat Res 5:583–586. Amsterdam: Elsevier Science Publishers – Geneva: World Health Organisation
109. Jain AK (1989) 6-Thioguanine (6TG) resistant mutation, chromosomal aberrations and sister chromatid exchanges (SCE's) in V79 cells. I. Induced by safrole. Cytologia 54:145–148
110. Elmore E, Korytynski EA, Smith MP (1985) Tests with the Chinese hamster V79 inhibition of metabolic cooperation assay. Prog Mutat Res 5:597–612. Amsterdam: Elsevier Science Publishers – Geneva: World Health Organisation
111. Umeda M, Noda K, Tanaka K (1985) Assays for inhibition of metabolic cooperation by a microassay method. Prog Mutat Res 5:619–622. Amsterdam: Elsevier Science Publishers – Geneva: World Health Organisation
112. Garner RC, Campbell J (1985) Tests for the induction of mutations to ouabain or 6-thioguanine resistance in mouse lymphoma L5178Y cells. Prog Mutat Res 5:525–529. Amsterdam: Elsevier Science Publishers – Geneva: World Health Organisation
113. Kuroda Y, Yokoiyama A, Kada T (1985) Assays for the induction of mutations to 6-thioguanine resistance in Chinese hamster V79 cells in culture. Prog Mutat Res 5:537–542. Amsterdam: Elsevier Science Publishers – Geneva: World Health Organisation
114. Garner RC, Amacher D, Caspary W, Crespi C, De Low G, Knaap A, Kuroda Y, Kuroki T, Lee C, Myrh B, Oberly T, Styles J, Zdzienicka M (1985) Summary report on the performance of gene mutation assays in mammalian cells in culture. Prog Mutat Res 5:85–94. Amsterdam: Elsevier Science Publishers – Geneva: World Health Organisation
115. Sina JF, Bean CL, Dysart GR, Taylor VI, Bradley MO (1983) Evaluation of the alkaline elution rat/hepatocyte assay as a predictor of carcinogenic/mutagenic potential. Mutat Res 113:357–391
116. Bradley MO (1985) Measurement of DNA single-strand breaks by alkaline elution in rat hepatocytes. Prog Mutat Res 5:353–357. Amsterdam: Elsevier Science Publishers – Geneva: World Health Organisation
117. Lakhanisky Th, Hendrickx B (1985) Induction of DNA single-strand breaks in CHO cells in culture. Prog Mutat Res 5:367–370. Amsterdam: Elsevier Science Publishers – Geneva: World Health Organisation
118. Douglas GR, Blakey DH, Liu-Lee VW, Bell RDL, Bayley JM (1985) Alkaline sucrose sedimentation, sister-chromatid exchange and micronucleus assays in CHO cells. Prog Mutat Res 5:359–366. Amsterdam: Elsevier Science Publishers – Geneva: World Health Organisation
119. Danford N (1985) Tests for chromosome aberrations and aneuploidy in the Chinese hamster fibroblast cell line CH1-L. Prog Mutat Res 5:397–411. Amsterdam: Elsevier Science Publishers – Geneva: World Health Organisation
120. Gulati DK, Sabharwal PS, Shelby MD (1985) Tests for the induction of chromosomal aberrations and sister chromatid exchanges in cultured Chinese hamster ovary (CHO) cells. Prog Mutat Res 5:413–426. Amsterdam: Elsevier Science Publishers – Geneva: World Health Organisation

121. Palitti F, Fiore M, De Salvia R, Tanzarella C, Ricordy R, Forster R, Mosesso P, Astolfi S, Loprieno N (1985) Tests for the induction of chromosomal aberrations in Chinese hamster ovary (CHO) cells in culture. Prog Mutat Res 5:443–450. Amsterdam: Elsevier Science Publishers – Geneva: World Health Organisation
122. Natarajan AT, van Kesteren-van Leeuwen AC (1981) Mutagenic activity of 20 coded compounds in chromosome aberrations/sister chromatid exchanges assay using Chinese hamster ovary (CHO) cells. Prog Mutat Res 1:551–559. Amsterdam: Elsevier Science Publishers – Geneva: World Health Organisation
123. Dean BJ (1981) Activity of 27 coded compounds in the RL_1 chromosome assay. Prog Mutat Res 1:570–579. Amsterdam: Elsevier Science Publishers – Geneva: World Health Organisation
124. Priston RAJ, Dean BJ (1985) Tests for the induction of chromosome aberrations, polyploidy and sister-chromatid exchanges in rat liver (RL_4) cells. Prog Mutat Res 5:387–395. Amsterdam: Elsevier Science Publishers – Geneva: World Health Organisation
125. Ishidate M, Sofuni T (1985) The in vitro chromosomal aberration test using Chinese hamster lung (CHL) fibroblast cells in culture. Prog Mutat Res 5:427–432. Amsterdam: Elsevier Science Publishers – Geneva: World Health Organisation
126. Sharma GP, Sobti RC, Sahi K (1982) Effects of some natural carcinogens on hemopoietic tissue of Rattus norvegicus. Nucleus (Calcutta) 25:142–147
127. Parry EM (1985) Tests for effects on mitosis and the mitotic spindle in Chinese hamster primary liver cells (CHL-L) in culture. Prog Mutat Res 5:479–485. Amsterdam: Elsevier Science Publishers – Geneva: World Health Organisation
128. Lane AM, Phillips BJ, Anderson D (1985) Tests for the induction of sister chromatid exchanges in Chinese hamster ovary (CHO) cells in culture. Prog Mutat Res 5:451–455. Amsterdam: Elsevier Science Publishers – Geneva: World Health Organisation
129. Obe G, Hille A, Jonas R, Schmidt S, Tenhaus U (1985) Tests for the induction of sister-chromatid exchanges in human peripheral lymphocytes in culture. Prog Mutat Res 5:439–442. Amsterdam: Elsevier Science Publishers – Geneva: World Health Organisation
130. Evans EL, Mitchell AD (1981) Effects of 20 coded chemicals on sister chromatid exchange frequencies in cultured Chinese hamster cells. Prog Mutat Res 1:538–550. Amsterdam: Elsevier Science Publishers – Geneva: World Health Organisation
131. Van Went GF (1985) Test for sister-chromatid exchange in Chinese hamster V79 cells in culture. Prog Mutat Res 5:469–477. Amsterdam: Elsevier Science Publishers – Geneva: World Health Organisation
132. Darroudi F, Natarajan AT (1985) Cytostatic drug acticity in plasma, a bioassay for detecting mutagenicity of directly and indirectly acting chemicals, an evaluation of 20 chemicals. Mutat Res 143:263–269
133. Paika IJ, Beauchesne MT, Randall M, Schreck RR, Latt SA (1981) In vivo SCE analysis of 20 coded compounds. Prog Mutat Res 1:673–681. Amsterdam: Elsevier Science Publishers – Geneva: World Health Organisation
134. Würgler FE, Graf U, Frei H (1985) Somatic mutation and recombination test in wings of *Drosophila melanogaster*. Prog Mutat Res 5:325–340. Amsterdam: Elsevier Science Publishers – Geneva: World Health Organisation
135. Valencia R, Houtchens K (1981) Mutagenic activity of 10 coded compounds in the *Drosophila* sex-linked recessive lethal test. Prog Mutat Res 1:651–659. Amsterdam: Elsevier Science Publishers – Geneva: World Health Organisation
136. Zimmering S, Mason JM, Valencia R (1989) Chemical Mutagenesis Testing in *Drosophila* VII. Results of 22 Coded Compounds Tested in Larval Feeding Experiments. Environ Mol Mutagen 14:245–251
137. Fujikawa K, Ryo H, Kondo S (1985) The *Drosophila* reversion assay using the unstable zeste-white somatic eye color system. Prog Mutat Res 5:319–324. Amsterdam: Elsevier Science Publishers – Geneva: World Health Organisation

138. Tsuchimoto T, Matter BE (1981) Activity of coded compounds in the micronucleus test. Prog Mutat Res 1:705–711. Amsterdam: Elsevier Science Publishers – Geneva: World Health Organisation
139. Salamone F, Heddle JA, Katz M (1981) Mutagenic activity of 41 compounds in the in vivo micronucleus assay. Prog Mutat Res 1:686–697. Amsterdam: Elsevier Science Publishers – Geneva: World Health Organisation
140. Kirkhart B (1981) Micronucleus test on 21 compounds. Prog Mutat Res 1:698–704. Amsterdam: Elsevier Science Publishers – Geneva: World Health Organisation
141. Pienta RJ (1980) Transformation of Syrian hamster embryo cells by diverse chemicals and correlation with their reported carcinogenic and mutagenic activities. Chem Mutagens 6:175–202
142. Styles JA (1981) Activity of 42 coded compounds in the BHK-21 cell transformation test. Prog Mutat Res 1:638–646. Amsterdam: Elsevier Science Publishers – Geneva: World Health Organisation
143. McGregor D, Ashby J (1985) Summary report on the performance of the cell transformation assays. Prog Mutat Res 5:103–115. Amsterdam: Elsevier Science Publishers – Geneva: World Health Organisation
144. Barrett JC, Lamb PW (1985) Tests with the Syrian hamster embryo cell transformation assay. Prog Mutat Res 5:623–628. Amsterdam: Elsevier Science Publishers – Geneva: World Health Organisation
145. Sanner T, Rivedal E (1985) Tests with the Syrian hamster embryo (SHE) cell transformation assay. Prog Mutat Res 5:665–671. Amsterdam: Elsevier Science Publishers – Geneva: World Health Organisation
146. Nesnow S, Curtis G, Garland H (1985) Tests with the C3H/10T 1/2 clone 8 morphological transformation bioassay. Prog Mutat Res 5:659–664. Amsterdam: Elsevier Science Publishers – Geneva: World Health Organisation
147. Lawrence N, McGregor DB (1985) Assay for the induction of morphological transformation in C3H/10T 1/2 cells in culture with and without S9-mediated metabolic activation. Prog Mutat Res 5:651–658. Amsterdam: Elsevier Science Publishers – Geneva: World Health Organisation
148. Matthews EJ, DelBalzo T, Rundell JO (1985) Assays for morphological transformation and mutation to ouabain resistance of Balb/c-3T3 cells in culture. Prog Mutat Res 5:639–650. Amsterdam: Elsevier Science Publishers – Geneva: World Health Organisation
149. Hatch GG, Anderson TM (1985) Assay for enhanced viral transformation of primary Syrian hamster embryo (SHE) cells. Prog Mutat Res 5:629–638. Amsterdam: Elsevier Science Publishers – Geneva: World Health Organisation
150. Zdzienicka MZ, de Kok AJ, Simons JWIM (1985) Assays for the induction of cell transformation in Chinese hamster ovary (CHO) cells and in Syrian hamster embryo (SHE) cells. Prog Mutat Res 5:685–688. Amsterdam: Elsevier Science Publishers – Geneva: World Health Organisation
151. Ireland CM, Cooper CS, Marshall CJ, Hebert E, Phillips DH (1988) Activating mutations in human c-Ha ras 1 gene induced by reactive derivatives of safrole and the glutamic pyrolysis product, Glu-P-3. Mutagenesis 3:429–435
152. Long EL, Nelson AA, Fitzhugh OG, Hansen WH (1963) Liver tumors produced in rats by feeding safrole. Arch Pathol 75:595–604
153. Borchert P, Miller JA, Miller EC, Shires TK (1973) 1'-Hydroxysafrole, a proximate carcinogenic metabolite of safrole in the rat and mouse. Cancer Res 33:590–600
154. Lipsky MM, Hinton DE, Klaunig JE, Trump BF (1981) Biology of hepatocellular neoplasia in the mouse. I. Histogenesis of safrole-induced hepatocellular carcinomas. J Natl Cancer Inst 67:365–376
155. Lipsky MM, Hinton DE, Klaunig JE, Trump BF (1981) Biology of hepatocellular neoplasia in the mouse. II. Sequential enzyme histochemical analysis of BALB/c mouse liver during safrole-induced carcinogenesis. J Natl Cancer Inst 67:377–392

156. Epstein SS, Fujii K, Andrea J, Mantel N (1970) Carcinogenicity testing of selected food additives by parenteral administration to infant swiss mice. Toxicol Appl Pharmacol 16:321–334
157. Lipsky MM, Tanner DC, Hinton DE, Trump BF (1984) Reversibility, persistence, and progression of safrole-induced mouse liver lesions following cessation of exposure. Mouse Liver Neoplasia Corp 11:161–177
158. Stoner GD, Shimkin MB, Kniazeff AJ, Weisburger JH, Weisburger EK, Gori GB (1973) Test for the carcinogenicity of food additives and chemotherapeutic agents by the pulmonary tumor response in strain A mice. Cancer Res 33:3069–3085
159. Vesselinovitch SD (1983) Perinatal hepatocarcinogens. Biol Res Pregnancy Perinatal 4:22–25
160. Randerath K, Haglund RE, Phillips DH, Reddy MV (1984) ^{32}P-Postlabeling analysis of DNA adducts formed in the livers of animals treated with safrole, estragole and other naturally-occurring alkenylbenzenes. I. Adult female CD-1 mice. Carcinog 5:1613–1622
161. Innes JRM, Ulland BM, Valerio MG, Petrucelli L, Fishbein L, Hart ER, Pallotta AJ, Bates RR, Falk HL, Gart JJ, Klein M, Mitchell I, Peters J (1969) Bioassay of pesticides and industrial chemicals for tumorigenicity in mice: a preliminary note. J Natl Cancer Inst 42:1101–1114
162. Homburger F, Kelley T, Baker TR, Russfield AB (1962) Sex effect on hepatic pathology from deficient diet and safrole in rats. Arch Pathol 73:118–125
163. Drinkwater NR, Miller EC, Miller JA, Pitot HC (1976) Hepatocarcinogenicity of estragole (1-allyl-4-methoxybenzene) and 1'-hydroxyestragole in the mouse and mutagenicity of 1'-acetoxyestragole in bacteria. J Natl Cancer Inst 57:1323–1331
164. Miller EC, Swanson AB, Phillips DH, Fletcher TL, Liem A, Miller JA (1983) Structure-activity studies of the carcinogenicities in the mouse and rat of some naturally occurring and synthetic alkenylbenzene derivatives related to safrole and estragole. Cancer Res 43:1124–1134
165. Boberg EW, Miller EC, Miller JA, Poland A, Liem A (1983) Strong evidence from studies with brachymorphic mice and pentachlorophenol that 1'-sulfooxysafrole is the major ultimate electrophilic and carcinogenic metabolite of 1'-hydroxysafrole in mouse liver. Cancer Res 43:5163–5173
166. Boberg EW, Liem A, Miller EC, Miller JA (1987) Inhibition by pentachlorophenol of the initiating and promoting activities of 1'-hydroxysafrole for the formation of enzyme-altered foci and tumors in rat liver. Carcinog 8:531–539
167. Reuber MD (1979) Neoplasms of the forestomach in mice ingesting dihydrosafrole. Digestion 19:42–47

Safrole – *Sassafras Albidum*

G. Abel

Botany

Sassafras albidum (Nutt.) Nees (syn. *Sassafras officinale* Nees et Eberm.; *Sassafras variifolium* (Salisb.) Kuntze) belongs to the Lauraceae. Vernacular names include sassafras, saxifrax, ague tree, cinnamon wood, saloop (E.); Fenchelholz (G.); and Bois de Sassafras (F.) [1,2]. Sassafras is native to North America and China [3]. The root with or without bark and the volatile oil are used medicinally [1,2,4]. Because of their sassafras–like odor, which is presumably due to the content of safrole, the following herbal drugs are also called "sassafras": *Atherosperma moschatum* Labill. (Australian sassafras), *Mespilodaphne sassafras* Meister (Brazilian sassafras), and *Doryphora sassafras* Endl. (New Caledonian sassafras). Brazilian sassafras oil is obtained from *Ocotea pretiosa* (Nees.) Mez. [4].

Chemistry

Sassafras root contains about 2 % volatile oil, tannins and sassafrid (a decomposition product of tannic acid), resin, wax, and mucilage [2,4]. The essential oil contains about 80 % safrole as the main component; minor components are α-pinene, phellandrene, camphor, eugenol, and sesquiterpenes [2,4]. Sassafras root bark oil was examined by GC-MS first by Sehti and co-workers [5]. Solvent extraction of 150 g of the powdered plant yielded two fractions of oily residues, namely 439 mg of oil A and 4.87 mg of oil B. In both fractions, nineteen components were identified; eleven out of these nineteen sassafras constituents were reported for the first time. Safrole was the major volatile constituent (about 90%) in oil A, while oil B contained 5-methoxyeugenol (30%), asarone (18%), piperonylacrolein (11%), coniferaldehyde (7%), safrole (6%), and camphor (5%). The remaining constituents were present in trace quantities (< 1%). 1'-Hydroxysafrole was not detected. The presence of safrole as the major component in sassafras oil, analysed by GC-MS, was confirmed by Noggle and co-workers [6,7]. These authors also reported smaller quantities of camphor and eugenol, and additionally of a dimethoxyallyl- and a trimethoxyallylbenzene.

Sassafras root bark contains aporphine and tetrahydrobenzylisoquinoline alkaloids. The following alkaloids were identified in the alkaloidal fraction from 500 g of root bark: boldine (ca. 10 mg), isoboldine (ca. 2 mg), norboldine (ca. 25 mg), cinnamolaurine (ca. 6 mg), norcinnamolaurine (ca. 4 mg), and reticuline (ca. 20 mg) [8].

Höke and Hänsel [9] isolated from a methylene chloride extract of sassafras root (wood) the lignans D-(+)-sesamine (3.4%) and desmethoxyashantin (2.5%), as well as β-sitosterol (0.33%), piperonylacrolein (0.28%), and (+)-2,3-dihydroxy-1-(3,4-methylendioxyphenyl)-propane (0.47%).

Dried sassafras leaves were found to contain 1.40–1.96 mg safrole per g [10]. Citral and D-phellandrene were also identified as components of the essential oil of the leaves [2].

The oil of *Ocotea cymbarum* H.B.K. (Brazilian sassafras oil) was reported to contain 90–93% safrole and about 5% sesquiterpenes; camphor and phellandrene were not detected [11].

Pharmacology and Uses

Sassafras root and oil of sassafras have been used as aromatic, flavoring agents and as a sudorific [1].

Liver regeneration increased over a 10-day period in partially hepatectomized rats that were given subcutaneous injections of sassafras oil daily for the first 7 days at high levels (50 mg/rat/day). The liver increment (the amount of tissue regenerated) also increased significantly when the diet of partially hepatectomized rats was supplemented with 7.0% or 1.5% sassafras bark tea for a period of 10 days [12].

Segelman et al. [13] reported that, in "preliminary pharmacological experiments", certain aqueous and alcoholic extracts of sassafras root bark were "capable of eliciting a variety of pharmacological responses in mice, including ataxia, ptosis, hypersensitivity to touch, central nervous system depression, and hyperthermia" [13]. Unfortunately, no data or detailed information were ever presented.

Oil of sassafras and safrole have been investigated for antifungal properties against eight strains with known pathogenicity for humans; no activity was discovered [14]. The related *Sassafras randaiense* (Hayata) Rehder, however, was found to exhibit antimicrobial activity against a number of microorganisms. These included *Staphylococcus aureus*, *Mycobacterium smegmatis*, *Saccharomyces cerevisiae*, and *Trichophyton mentagrophytes*. This antimicrobial activity was due to the presence of the neolignans, magnolol and isomagnolol [15].

Sassafras oil may be used as starting material in the synthesis of ecstacy (3,4-methylene-dioxymethamphetamine = MDMA). Noggle and co-workers [6,7] proved that treatment of sassafras oil with hydrobromic acid followed by bromide displacement with methylamine gives MDMA as the major amine product.

Adverse Reaction Profile

General Animal Data

The acute LD_{50} of sassafras oil in rats was reported to be 1.90 g/kg (1.52–2.37 g/kg); the acute dermal LD_{50} in rabbits exceeded 5 g/kg [16].

General Human Data

The FDA does not permit sassafras to be used in foods [17]. In 1974, the Council of Europe included sassafras in its list of natural flavoring substances that are deemed to contain a toxicologically unacceptable component [18]. Sassafras has been banned in at least one EC member state, according to a recent CPMP annual report [19]. The medicinal use of sassafras should be discouraged because of the carcinogenic potential of safrole. This is especially valid for those ways of administration in which safrole is systemic available, because the metabolites are more carcinogenic than safrole itself.

In the Netherlands, several brands of oil of sassafras are sold to be used in so-called aromatherapy. Although packages usually do not specify the application, accompanying leaflets recommend, inter alia, the internal use of maximally 12 drops per day which could lead to a daily intake of approximately 0.2 g of safrole [20].

The earliest source cited in the literature described a case of poisoning following the ingestion of a teaspoonful of oil of sassafras [21–23]. The young man, who took the oil by error began to vomit shortly afterwards, and later suffered from hallucinations and intermittent unconsciousness. Treated with emetics, he responded rapidly, regained consciousness and recovered within a short time [21]. Unfortunately, Craig [24] mistakenly reported the death of this patient, whose short illness is noted by Allbright [21]. This incorrect statement may have caused an inaccurate basis for the estimation of the toxicity of sassafras oil.

Recently, a second case of sassafras oil ingestion resulted in minor symptoms, which resolved with only supportive care [25]. A 47-year-old female inadvertently ingested one teaspoonful of oil of sassafras. She vomited spontaneously, and developed tachycardia and tremors. These symptoms were ameliorated by administration of activated charcoal. The woman was discharged the following day from the emergency department with normal liver and kidney function [25].

A case report by Kläsi and Roth [26] described the symptoms following ingestion of several swallows of a putative Macassar Oil. In view of the confusion of the compound ingested – the patient himself reported it as labeled "Eglisauerwasser" – and the vagueness of the analytical data, no definite conclusions as to the toxicity of sassafras or safrole can be drawn from this case.

Craig [24] reported five cases of poisoning among children (1 year 2 months to 2 years 6 months) following ingestion of undetermined amounts of oil of sassafras. He described that all the patients vomited, all but one showed signs of shock, three of the five showed vertigo, two became stuporous and one was aphasic. Miosis and respiratory symptoms were not apparent in the five cases discussed in this paper. In one case, the use of emetics was successfully tried and Craig stated this may well have averted serious symptoms.

The consumption of sassafras tea in amounts up to 10 cups a day was recently associated with a case of perspiration and hot flashes in an elderly woman [27]. Since there is no explanation available as to how sassafras tea could elicit such effects, the causal relationship remains uncertain. The woman was reported as obese (body weight of 112.5 kg), which is a well-known cause of excessive perspiration.

Dermatological Reactions

Mitchell and Rook [3] claim that oil of sassafras is said to produce dermatitis in hypersensitive individuals. However, the reference cited does not support this statement [28].

Fertility, Pregnancy and Lactation

Human data on the ingestion of sassafras or sassafras oil preparations during pregnancy or lactation were not found in the literature, nor data with regard to a teratogenic potential.

For animal data, see the corresponding section in the general discussion of safrole elsewhere in this volume.

Mutagenicity and Carcinogenicity

Data on the mutagenicity of sassafras root or sassafras oil have not been recovered from the literature. The following two studies on carcinogenicity have been reported.

An ethanolic extract of *Sassafras albidum* (root bark) was reported to be tumorigenic in rats [29]. Subcutaneous injections were given to NIH black rats once a week up to 72 weeks and produced tumors in a mean time of 59 weeks for males (11/15) and 65 weeks for females (9/15). These tumors showed the characteristics of malignant mesenchymal tumors similar to those of human malignant fibrous histiocytoma. The authors claimed that they used a safrole-free extract, but no data were reported to support this claim. The relevance of this study seems unclear because of the lack of sufficient information.

Natural oil of sassafras (Southern, NFX) was fed to animals (species not indicated!) in the dry diet at 390 and 1170 ppm for up to 2 years [30]. At 22 months, no liver tumors were detected. At 24 months, however, cellular changes in the liver compatible with carcinoma were observed. These liver findings were considered by the authors to be indicative of a weak carcinogen, requiring prolonged insult to a biological system before manifesting cellular changes. These conclusions were not supported by convincing data, however, and the significance of this paper remains unclear.

See also the section on mutagenicity and carcinogenicity in the general discussion of safrole elsewhere in this volume.

References

1. Windholz M (ed) (1983) The Merck Index. 10th Edition. Rahway, NJ: Merck & Co.
2. List PH, Hörhammer L (1979) Hagers Handbuch der Pharmazeutischen Praxis. Vollständige (vierte) Neuausgabe. Sechster Band. Chemikalien und Drogen (R,S) Berlin: Springer-Verlag

3. Mitchell J, Rook A (1979) Botanical dermatology. Plants and plant products injurious to the skin. Greengrass: Vancouver, p. 377
4. Hoppe HA (1975) Drogenkunde. Band 1. Angiospermen. 8. Auflage. Berlin: Walter de Gruyter
5. Sehti ML, Rao GS, Chowdhury BK, Morton JF, Kapadia GJ (1976) Identification of volatile constituents of *Sassafras albidum* root oil. Phytochemistry 15:1773–1775
6. Noggle FT, Clark CR, De Ruiter J (1991) Gas chromatographic and mass spectrometric analysis of samples from a clandestine laboratory involved in the synthesis of ecstacy from sassafras oil. J Chromatogr Sci 29:168–173
7. Noggle FT, Clark CR, De Ruiter J (1991) Gas chromatographic and mass spectrometric analysis of N-Methyl-1-aryl-2-propanamines synthesized from the substituted allylbenzenes present in sassafras oil. J Chromatogr Sci 29:267–271
8. Chowdhury BK, Sehti ML, Lloyd HA, Kapadia GJ (1976) Aporphine and tetrahydrobenzylisoquinoline alkaloids in *Sassafras albidum*. Phytochemistry 15:1803–1804
9. Höke M, Hänsel R (1972) Eine Neuuntersuchung des Lignum Sassafras. Arch Pharm 305:33–39
10. Sultatos LG (1986) Occurrence of the carcinogen safrole in the food additive file. Fed Proc 45:343
11. Gemballa G (1958) Scientia Pharmaceutica pp.8–14
12. Gershbein LL (1977) Regeneration of rat liver in the presence of essential oils and their components. Fd Cosmet Toxicol 15:173–181
13. Segelman AB, Segelman FP, Karliner J, Sofia RD (1976) Sassafras and Herb Tea. Potential Health Hazards. JAMA 236:477
14. Chaumont JP, Bardey I (1989) In-Vitro Antifungal Activity of Seven Essential Oils. Fitoterapia 60:263–266
15. El-Feraly FS, Cheatham SF, Breedlove RL (1983) Antimicrobial neolignans of *Sassafras randaiense* roots. J Nat Prod 46:493–498
16. Moreno OM (1976) Report to RIFM, 7 September; cited in 11
17. Opdyke DLJ, Letizia C (1982) Monographs on fragrance raw materials: Sassafras Oil. Fd Cosmet Toxicol 20:825–826
18. Anonymous (1974) Natural Flavouring Substances. Their Sources, and Added Artificial Flavouring Substances. Council of Europe, Partial Agreement in the Social and Public Health Field. List N(2), no. 424. Strasbourg
19. Anonymus (1993) Report on the operation of the Committee for Proprietary Medicinal Products in 1991 and 1992. Brussels: Commission of the European Communities, p. 49
20. De Smet PAGM (1994) Een alternatieve olie met een luchtje. Pharm Weekbl 129:258
21. Allbright M (1888) A case of poisoning by oil of sassafras. Cincinnati Lancet and Clinic 21:631–632
22. Jacobs MB (1958) Toxicity of Safrole. Am Perfum Aromat 71:57–58
23. Leidy WPh (1958) Safrole – a critical bibliographical review of available literature on the physiological effects of safrole. Am Perfum Aromat 71:61–63
24. Craig JO (1953) Poisoning by the volatile oils in childhood. Arch Dis Child 29:475–483
25. Grande GA, Dannewitz SR (1987) Symptomatic Sassafras Oil Ingestion. Vet Hum Toxicol 29:147
26. Kläsi J, Roth O (1915) Über einen Fall von Safrolvergiftung. Monatsschr Psych Neurol 38:235–250
27. Haines Jr JD (1991) Sassafras tea and diaphoresis. Postgraduate Medicine 90, no.4, 75–76
28. Tulipan L (1938) Cosmetic irritants. Arch Dermatol Syph 38:906–917
29. Kapadia GJ, Chung EB, Ghosh B, Shukla YN, Basak SP, Morton JF, Pradhan SN (1978) Carcinogenicity of some folk medicinal herbs in rats. J Natl Cancer Inst 60:683–686
30. Abbott DD, Packman EW, Wagner BM, Harrisson JWE (1961) Chronic oral toxicity of oil of sassafras and safrole. Pharmacologist 3:62

# *Spirulina* Species

P.A.G.M. De Smet

Botany

Spirulina is a genus of blue-green algae belonging to the family of Oscillatoriaceae. The two species which are most commonly utilized are *Spirulina platensis* and *Spirulina maxima* [1,2]. In India, *Spirulina fusiformis* is also regarded as a source plant [3].

Chemistry

Spirulina is rich in crude protein: *S.platensis* and *S.maxima* can yield as much as 56–77% and 60–77% of the dry weight, respectively [1]. The actual level depends on the medium in which the algae are cultivated; in one study, the protein content of *S.platensis* declined from 55–60% to 35–40%, when an alternative source of nitrogen was used [4]. In comparison to standard alimentary proteins, such as those of eggs and milk, the amino acid spectrum of *Spirulina* protein tends to be deficient in the essential sulphur-containing amino acid methionine [1,4,5]. The high level of protein in *Spirulina* species is accompanied by a high concentration of nucleic acids; reported values are 4.2% in *S.platensis* and 4.5% in *S.maxima* [2].

S.platensis yields 10–20% of carbohydrates and 9–14% of lipids, whereas *S.maxima* contains 8–16% of carbohydrates and 4–15% of lipids. In both species, total lipids consist for 70–80% of free fatty acids. The presence of γ-linolenic acid has been reported but in one study one of the three isolates of *Spirulina* that were examined had a predominance of α-linolenic acid. This makes it uncertain that γ-linolenic acid is present in all isolates [1].

The most abundant pigment is chlorophyll *a*, which is the only chlorophyll present. It accounts for 0.8–1.5% of the dry weight in *S.platensis* and *S.maxima*. The major carotenoids, which represent approximately 0.2–0.4% of the dry weight, are mixoxanthophyll and β-carotene [1]. As β-carotene alone makes up more than 0.1% of the dry weight [2], *Spirulina* products contain almost enough of this provitamin A to meet the recommended dietary allowance for adults. Promotional sources sometimes emphasize that *Spirulina* also provides various other vitamins and minerals, but almost all of these constituents occur in much lower concentrations than those needed for nutritional purposes (Table 1). The only apparent exception is vitamin B_{12} but recent research has shown that more than 80% of what

Table 1. Comparison of the United States recommended dietary allowances (RDA) for vitamins and minerals [6,7] with the amounts in a Dutch commercial product providing 2.4 g of *Spirulina* per day [8]

Nutrient	Recommended dietary allowance (RDA) values for adults	Daily amount supplied by Dutch product
Vitamins		
Provitamin A (β-carotene)	4800–6000 µg	4080 µg
Vitamin B_1 (thiamin)	1000–1500 µg	120 µg
Vitamin B_2 (riboflavin)	1200–1700 µg	96 µg
Provitamin B_3 (niacin)	13–19 mg	283 µg
Vitamin B_5 (pantothenate)	4000–7000 µg[*]	27 µg
Vitamin B_6 (pyridoxine)	1600–2000 µg	7 µg
Vitamin B_{11} (folic acid)	180–200 µg	1 µg
Vitamin B_{12} (cyanocobalamin)	2 µg	5 µg
Vitamin C (ascorbic acid)	60 mg	–
Vitamin D (cholecalciferol)	5–10 µg	–
Vitamin E (α-tocopherol)	8–10 mg	460 µg
Vitamin K (phytomenadione)	60–80 µg	–
Minerals		
Calcium	800–1200 mg	2.5–3.2 mg
Phosphorus	800–1200 mg	18–21 mg
Magnesium	280–350 mg	3.4–4.6 mg
Iron	10–15 mg	1.1–1.4 mg
Zinc	12–15 mg	65–94 µg
Iodine	150 µg	–
Selenium	55–70 µg	1 µg
Copper	1500–3000 µg[*]	3 µg
Manganese	2000–5000 µg[*]	43–60 µg
Chromium	50–200 µg[*]	–
Molybdenum	75–250 µg[*]	–

[*] This is not a recommended dietary allowance but a suggested safe and adequate daily intake for adults

registers as vitamin B_{12} in the microbiological assay consists in reality of B_{12} analogues. These analogues give a cobalamin-like growth response in the microbiological assay but they have no affinity for binding to intrinsic factor, when measured by a differential radioassay [9–11].

Pharmacology and Uses

Experimental studies of *Spirulina* have primarily focused on its potential as an alternative source of nutritional protein. Feeding experiments in animals have shown that although *Spirulina* is inferior to animal proteins, such as lactalbumin and casein, it ranks among the best vegetable sources of protein. Reports about the experimental feeding of humans with *Spirulina* still are so few and incomplete, however, that they do not yet provide sufficient reliable information about the possibility of utilizing spirulina as a major source of protein for human consumption [1,2].

In the health food circuit, *Spirulina* is promoted for a variety of purposes. Among other things, it is advocated as a nutritional supplement for busy people and vegetarians [8], even though most of the vitamins and minerals in *Spirulina* occur in quantities that are too low for such purposes (Table 1). *Spirulina* is also promoted as an energizing and restoring preparation for sportsmen and convalescing patients, as a natural aid to losing weight, and as an internally or externally applied beauty product [8,12]. The reputation of *Spirulina* as a weight-losing agent is based on unproven theories, such as the claim that its constituent phenylalanine affects the appetite center in the brain [5,12]. The American Food and Drug Administration has ruled that there is no convincing evidence for the effectiveness of this amino acid as a weight control product [13].

Schwartz et al. [14] reported that an oral preparation from *Spirulina* and *Dunaliella* prevented the tumor development in hamster buccal pouch following the topical application of 7,12-dimethylbenz[a]anthracene (DMBA). They also found that local injection of the *Spirulina/Dunaliella* preparation into DMBA-induced carcinomas of hamster buccal pouch resulted in tumor regression in part of the animals [15].

Adverse Reaction Profile

Johnson and Shubert [16] cautioned against the regular use of large doses of *Spirulina*, after they had found high concentrations of mercury (9.1–24.4 µg/g) and lead (1.3–6.7 µg/g) in commercial or cultured samples. However, their findings were later challenged by Slotton and co-workers [17], because Johnson and Shubert used a flawed analytical technology: the high levels attributed to mercury were due to iron interference and it is likely that this also resulted in high lead values. When Slotton et al. [17] examined 33 samples of *Spirulina* by more specific methods, they found acceptable low levels of mercury (up to 0.65 ppm) and lead (up to 6.5 ppm).

General Animal Data

Various feeding experiments in different animal species (such as mice, rats, pigs, chicken, and calves) have shown that *Spirulina* is non-toxic and promotes growth as well as other types of more conventional feeds, when their protein requirement was supplied totally or in part by substitution of this alga [1,2]. For instance, no changes of toxicological significance were observed in rats after the administration of *Spirulina* in single oral doses up to 800 mg/kg body weight [18], after subchronic dietary administration of 10–30% for 12–13 weeks [18–20], after chronic feeding with 20% in the diet for 6 months [21], and in long-term feeding trials that lasted 18 months [1].

In a study by Mitchell et al. [22], *Spirulina maxima* adversely affected the utilization of vitamin E (reduced plasma and liver levels of α-tocoferol) when fed to male rats at a level as low as 2.7%; plasma levels of retinol were also decreased, whereas liver retinoid levels were increased.

General Human Data

As a vegetarian or macrobiotic diet entails the risk of vitamin B_{12} deficiency, its reported presence in *Spirulina* has made this alga appear as an attractive non-animal source of the vitamin for those adhering to a vegetarian or macrobiotic life style [11]. However, as was already pointed out in the section on chemistry, most of what registers as vitamin B_{12} in a microbiological assay consists in reality of B_{12} analogues. Two of these analogues behaved in the laboratory as agents blocking vitamin B_{12} metabolism, and concern has arisen that such vitamin B_{12} antagonists could actually be harmful to humans [9,10]. In a recent study, the inclusion of *Spirulina* in the diet of macrobiotically fed children with vitamin B_{12} deficiency resulted in further deterioration of their hematological status, even though rises in the plasma levels of "vitamin B_{12}" suggested a good absorption [23].

Dermatological Reactions

In an acute dermal toxicity test, single doses up to 2 g/kg body weight were applied for 24 hours to the clipped skin of rats without producing local signs of reddishness or oedema [18].

There are no reports about skin eruptions in persons harvesting and handling *Spirulina* algae [18]. The literature has not yielded any data either about the induction of skin reactions by ingestion of a *Spirulina* product. Perhaps it should be noted, however, that another chlorophyll-containing alga, *Chlorella*, has been associated with an outbreak of photosensitive reactions in Japan, where this alga is a popular health food. The outbreak was attributed to certain factors in the manufacturing process, because *Chlorella* did not appear to be toxic per se. Pheophorbide-a, a degradation product of chlorophyll, was identified as a major etiologic agent [24].

Haematological Reactions

See the section on general human data.

Metabolic Reactions

Spirulina species have a nucleic acid content of more than 4% (see the section on chemistry). As uric acid is produced in the metabolism of these purines, the question arises, whether *Spirulina* may cause gout [1]. In one study, five undernourished adults were fed by gastric tube for some days with *Spirulina* at concentrations sufficient to provide up to 50% of their protein requirement. This resulted in a slight increase in the serum level, but not in the urinary level of uric acid [1,2].

According to Slotton et al. [17], the possibility of uric acid deposition in kidneys or joints may be avoided by limiting *Spirulina* consumption to a maximum of 50 g per day. Typical daily intakes are much less than this recommended maximum. Moreover, the uricosuric agents that are nowadays available for the treatment of hyperuricemia are so effective that they have greatly reduced the need of restricting purine intake by patients with gout [25].

Respiratory Reactions

During pulverization of dried algae using grinders, minute dust particles may enter the nostrils of personnel and may cause respiratory reactions (nasal discharge, wheezing, cough and expectoration). These reactions can easily be prevented by wearing a mask over the nose [18].

Fertility, Pregnancy and Lactation

Chamorro and co-workers tested dietary levels up to 30% of *Spirulina* in pregnant hamsters through days 7–11, 1–11 and 1–14 of gestation [26], in pregnant mice through days 7–13, 1–13 and 1–19 [27], and in pregnant rats through days 7–14, 1–14 and 1–21 [28] without evoking signs of embryotoxic or fetotoxic effects. Kapoor and Mehta [29] reported that dietary feeding of 48% of *S.platensis* to pregnant rats was without negative effects on dam's weight gain, litter size and litter weight.

Chamorro et al. [30] also gave *Spirulina* at dietary levels up to 30% to three successive generations of rats without observing adverse effects on fertility, gestation, viability and lactation. Negative results were also found in a toxicological multigeneration study in mice [1].

Chamorro et al. [31] also reported that short-term feeding (5 days) and prolonged-term feeding (5 days per week for 10 weeks) of *S.maxima* to male CD-1 mice at dietary levels up to 30% did not decrease fertility. Pregnancies resulting from mating with untreated females were normal in terms of pregnancy rates, numbers of corpora lutea and implants, pre-implantation and postimplantation losses. It was therefore concluded that, at the tested dose levels, spirulina did not cause dominant lethal mutations in the germinal cells of male mice. Similar negative results have been obtained in rats [32].

Mutagenicity and Carcinogenicity

Negative results were observed in mutagenicity tests with *Salmonella typhimurium* and *Schizosaccharomyces pombe* performed on urines of animals fed *Spirulina* for 4 months [1].

Specific data about the carcinogenicity of *Spirulina* have not been recovered from the literature.

References

1. Ciferri O (1983) *Spirulina*, the edible microorganism. Microbiol Rev 47:551–578
2. Ciferri O, Tiboni O (1985) The biochemistry and industrial potential of *Spirulina*. Ann Rev Microbiol 39:503–526
3. Annapurna VV, Deosthale YG, Bamji MS (1991) Spirulina as a source of vitamin A. Plant Foods Hum Nutr 41:125–134
4. Saxena PN, Ahmad MR, Shyam R, Misra PS (1982) Chemical composition of sewage-grown *Spirulina platensis*. Experientia 38:1438
5. Tyler VE (1993) The Honest Herbal. A sensible guide to the use of herbs and related remedies. 3rd edn. New York: Pharmaceutical Products Press, pp.299–301
6. Reynolds JEF, red. (1993) Martindale The Extra Pharmacopoeia. 30th edn. London: The Pharmaceutical Press, pp.1033–1064
7. McEvoy GK, red. (1994) AHFS Drug Information 94. Bethesda: American Society of Hospital Pharmacists, p.2389
8. Anonymous (undated) Een boekje open over Marcus Rohrer Spirulina. Tilburg: Spirulina Import
9. Herbert V, Drivas G (1982) *Spirulina* and vitamin B_{12}. JAMA 248:3096–3097
10. Herbert V (1987) The 1986 Herman Award Lecture. Nutrition science as a continually unfolding story: the folate and vitamin B-12 paradigm. Am J Clin Nutr 46:387–402
11. Van den Berg H, Dagnelie PC, Van Staveren WA (1988) Vitamin B_{12} and seaweed. Lancet 1:242–243
12. Popovich NG (1982) Spirulina. Am Pharm NS22:288–290
13. Kessler DA (1991) Weight control products for over-the-counter human use; certain active ingredients. Federal Register 56:37792–37799
14. Schwartz J, Shklar G, Reid S, Trickler D (1988) Prevention of experimental oral cancer by extracts of Spirulina-Dunaliella algae. Nutr Cancer 11:127–134
15. Schwartz J, Shklar G (1987) Regression of experimental hamster cancer by beta carotene and algae extracts. J Oral Maxillofac Surg 45:510–515
16. Johnson PE, Shubert LE (1986) Accumulation of mercury and other elements by *Spirulina* (Cyanophyceae). Nutr Rep Int 34: 1063–1070
17. Slotton DG, Goldman CR, Franke A (1989) Commercially grown *Spirulina* found to contain low levels of mercury and lead. Nutr Rep Int 40:1165–1172
18. Krishnakumari MK, Ramesh HP, Venkataraman LV (1981) Food safety evaluation: acute oral and dermal effects of the algae *Scenedesmus acutus* and *Spirulina platensis* on albino rats. J Food Protect 44:934–935
19. Chamorro GA, Herrera G, Salazar M, Salazar S, Ulloa V (1988) Subchronic toxicity study in rats fed *Spirulina*. J Pharm Belg 43:29–36
20. Chamorro GA, Herrera G, Salazar M, Salazar S, Ulloa V (1988) Short-term toxicity study of *Spirulina* in F^{3b} generation rats. J Toxicol Clin Exp 8:163–167
21. Yoshino Y, Hirai Y, Takakashi H, Yamamoto N, Yamazaki N (1980) The chronic intoxication test on Spirulina product fed to Wistar-strain rats. Jpn J Nutr 38:221–225
22. Mitchell GV, Grundel E, Jenkins M, Blakely SR (1990) Effects of graded dietary levels of *Spirulina maxima* on vitamins A and E in male rats. J Nutr 120:1235–1240
23. Dagnelie PC, Van Staveren WA, Van den Berg H (1991) Vitamin B-12 from algae appears not to be bioavailable. Am J Clin Nutr 53:695–697,988
24. Jitsukawa K, Suizu R, Hidano A (1984) Chlorella photosensitization. New phytophotodermatosis. Int J Dermatol 23:263–268

25. Den Oudsten SA, Meima GR (1990) Voeding bij arthritis urica (jicht). In: Carbasius Weber EC, Post GB, Swager TW, ed. Informatorium voor Voeding en Dietetiek. Band 3: Dieetleer (vervolg) Gezondheidszorg. Houten: Bohn Stafleu Van Loghum, pp. XIII–1 to XIII–4
26. Chamorro G, Salazar S, Salazar M, Pages N (1987) Evaluation teratologique de la spiruline chez le hamster. Belg J Food Chem Biotechnol 42:188–191
27. Chamorro G, Salazar M (1990) Estudio teratogenico de *Spirulina* en raton. Arch Latinoam Nutr 40:86–94
28. Chamorro G, Salazar M, Salazar S (1989) Estudio teratogenico de *Spirulina* en rata. Arch Latinoam Nutr 39:641–649
29. Kapoor R, Mehta U (1993) Effect of supplementation of blue green alga (*Spirulina*) on outcome of pregnancy in rats. Plant Foods Hum Nutr 43:29–35
30. Chamorro G, Salazar M, Izquierdo E, Salazar S, Ulloa V (1985) Multi-generation study on reproduction and lactation in rats fed with *Spirulina*. Arch Hydrobiol Beih 20:165–171
31. Chamorro GA, Salazar M (1989) Dominant lethal assay of *Spirulina maxima* in male CD-1 mice after short-term and prolonged-term feeding. J Food Protect 52:125–127
32. Salazar M, Chamorro G (1990) Study of lethal dominant of *Spirulina maxima* in male rats. Sci Aliments 10:713–718

Teucrium Chamaedrys

P.A.G.M. De Smet

Botany

Teucrium chamaedrys L. (= *Teucrium officinale* Lam. = *Chamaedrys officinalis* Moench.) belongs to the Lamiaceae. Vernacular names are common germander, wall germander (E); Gamander, Edelgamander (D); germandrée petit-chêne, germandrée chamaedrys (F) [1–3]. The plant part which is used medicinally is the flowering herb [3,4].

Chemistry

The aerial parts of *T.chamaedrys* contain various neo-clerodane diterpenoids; the exact composition seems to vary with the country of collection (Table 1). Teucrin A appears to be the predominant diterpenoid in Spanish material (1.5 mg/g) and in Italian material (0.3 mg/g) [12].

Grzybek [14,15] investigated the above-ground parts of Polish material and reported the presence of flavonoids (diosmine and isoquercetin), choline, tannins, chlorogenic acid, stigmasterol and β-sitosterol, β-amyrin and ursolic acid. β-Sitosterol was also found in aerial parts of Spanish origin [9,10]. Gross et al. [16] isolated a phenylpropanoid glycoside named teucrioside from a commercially available herb sample.

Harborne et al. [17] studied the flavonoid composition of the leafy stem of *T.chamaedrys* and isolated cirsiliol (principal flavonoid) and cirsimaritin as free flavone aglycones, together with flavone glycosides of luteolin, apigenin, hypolaetin and isoscutellarein.

The herb contains 0.07% of essential oil [2]. Chialva et al. [18] recovered 31 different compounds from the essential oil, with caryophyllene (20.7%) and humulene (14.2%) as the major constituents; headspace analysis of the finely ground herb yielded 18 substances, with α-pinene (22.5%) as principal component.

Table 1. Diterpenoid composition of aerial parts of *Teucrium chamaedrys* plants of different geographical origin

Diterpenoid	Geographical origin of studied material			
	Moldavian [5]	Bulgarian [5–7]	Spanish [8–12]	Italian [12]
Teucrin A	+	+		+
Teucrin B = Dihydroteugin [13]	+	+	+	
Teucrin E	+	+	+	
Teucrin F	+			+
Teucrin G	+			+
Teucrin H1 = Teuflidin [10]			+	
Teucrin H2 = Teuchamaedryn B [10]		+	+	
Teuflin = Teuchamaedryn A [10]		+	+	+
Teuchamaedrin C	+			
Teugin			+	
Teucroxide			+	
Chamaedroxide			+	
6-Epiteucrin A			+	
6α-Hydroxyteuscordin	+			
Isoteuflidin			+	
Teucvin				+
Teucvidin				+

Pharmacology and Uses

Teucrium chamaedrys has been used since antiquity [19,20]. In folk medicine, the herb has served as a diuretic, as an agent against obesity, hemorrhoids and wounds, and as an expectorant, tonic, stomachic agent and cholagogue [2,3,21]. In 1986 and 1990, the French health authorities listed the flowering aerial parts of *T.chamaedrys* as a selected herbal drug, for which marketing licences could be obtained on the basis of adapted documentation and an abridged application. Permitted indications were the traditional uses as a symptomatic agent in mild diarrhea, as local agent for buccal hygiene, and as an adjuvant in weight-losing regimens [4,22]. However, the marketing licences of French herbal preparations containing *T.chamaedrys* were suspended in 1992, after their use had been associated with various cases of acute hepatitis (see the section on hepatic reactions).

Extracts from *T.chamaedrys* were reported to inhibit the growth of tissue cultures of HeLa cells, the growth of the mycelium of *Neurospora crassa* as well as the growth of roots of *Allium cepa* [23]. Two diterpenoids occurring in *T.chamaedrys*, teucvin and teucvidin, did not show antitumor activity against P388 lymphocytic leukemia in mice [24]. Teucvin has been reported to be a potent amoebicidal agent [25]. The antifeedant activity of teucrin A and some other diterpenoids occurring in *T.chamaedrys* against larvae of *Spodoptera littoralis* and *Heliothis armigera* was discussed by Simmonds et al. [26].

Adverse Reaction Profile

In 1992, the French health authorities suspended the marketing licence of herbal preparations containing *T.chamaedrys*, after the use of such preparations had been associated with numerous cases of acute hepatitis [27]. See the section on hepatic reactions for a detailed discussion.

Gastrointestinal Reactions

In clinical studies, the use of *T.chamaedrys* has been occasionally associated with symptoms of gastrointestinal intolerance, such as dyspepsia, stomach pain, and nausea [20].

Hepatic Reactions

Castot and Larrey [20] reviewed 26 French cases of hepatitis following the use of capsules or herbal teas containing *T.chamaedrys*. Ten of these cases were also the subject of separate, more detailed case reports [21,28–31]. As far as Castot and Larrey [20] could ascertain, the herb had been ingested in normal daily doses between 450 and 1600 mg per day. Acute cytolytic hepatitis with mimimal cholestasis developed after 2–18 weeks (mean 9 weeks) and was characterized by jaundice and high levels of aminotransferases (ALT, AST). Among the initial symptoms were weakness, abdominal pain, nausea or vomiting, fever (with or without pruritus), and hepatomegaly. Occasionally, blood hypereosinophilia or a decrease in prothrombin level was observed, and two patients had transient portal hypertension without encephalopathy. Liver biopsy samples revealed centrolobular or panlobular hepatocyte necrosis. Patients recovered within 1.5 and 6 months after withdrawal, but in 12 cases accidental rechallenge resulted in prompt recurrence of the hepatitis. No relationship could be established between the severity of the reaction and the daily dose level or the duration of treatment. The frequency of the adverse effect during the first trimester of 1992 was estimated at 1 case in about 4000 months of treatment.

Most of the cases reviewed by Castot and Larrey [20] did not have a very serious final outcome. In one patient, however, inflammatory lesions could still be demonstrated by a liver biopsy performed two years after the acute episode, and a biopsy sample taken from another patient (following reintroduction of the wall germander) showed signs suggestive of active chronic hepatitis. Severe cases have also been reported by other authors. Dao et al. [32] observed acute hepatitis with signs of portal hypertension in a 54-year-old woman after 4 months of wall germander's use; the hepatitis progressed to liver cirrhosis during seven additional months of use. Mostefa-Kara et al. [33] described a case of fatal hepatitis in a 68-year-old woman following accidental readministration; necropsy revealed massive hepatic necrosis. Ben Yahia et al. [34] reported the presence of serum anti-nuclear and anti-smooth muscle antibodies in two patients, who developed hepatitis after 6 to 7 months of treatment with the wall germander.

To evaluate the molecular mechanism of the hepatotoxicity, Loeper et al. [35,36] investigated the lyophilisate of a tea prepared from blooming aerial parts in mice under different conditions. Following intragastric administration of 0.8, 1.25 and 2.5 g/kg body weight, serum ALT activity increased to 16-, 110- and 656-fold the control value, respectively. The two higher doses resulted in midzonal eosinophilic hepatocyte necrosis. This hepatotoxicity could also be produced by intragastric administration of 0.125 g/kg of an enriched fraction, which contained the same level of furano neo-clerodane diterpenoids as 1.25 g/kg of the lyophilisate. There was a tendency of hepatic glutathione to decrease at 2–5 hours and to increase at 24 hours after a dose of 1.25 g/kg of the lyophilisate. The increase in serum ALT activity could be enhanced by inducers of the 3A family of cytochrome P-450 (dexamethasone and clotrimazole) and prevented by pretreatment with cytochrome P-450 inhibitors, including a specific inhibitor of the A3 family (troleandomycin). Toxicity was also increased by pretreatment with phorone (a depletor of hepatic glutathione), whereas it could be attenuated by inducers of microsomal epoxide hydrolase (clofibrate and butylated hydroxyanisole). These findings suggest that the hepatotoxicity of *T.chamaedrys* resides in one or more reactive metabolites of its furanoditerpenoids and that these metabolites can be detoxified by glutathione conjugate formation and probably also by epoxide hydrolase.

In their review of French cases of hepatotoxicity following the use of wall germander, Castot and Larrey [20] state that substitution of *T.chamaedrys* with another species was excluded but they do not make clear how this was established. The issue of a possible exchange is an important one, not in the least because the related *Teucrium canadense* L. (American germander) has been widely used in the United Kingdom to replace *Scutellaria lateriflora* in commercial skullcap materials and products [37]. As was reviewed in the previous volume of this book series, skullcap preparations have been repeatedly associated with hepatotoxicity [38]. Anderson [37] knows of one UK case of skullcap-related hepatotoxicity, in which the incriminated material definitely came from *T.canadense*, and she considers it likely that other British cases also involved *Teucrium* rather than *Scutellaria*. In view of this unpublished information, it would seem important to establish beyond doubt that the French cases of wall germander toxicity were due to *T.chamaedrys* and not to *T.canadense*.

Since *T.canadense* may share the hepatotoxicity of *T.chamaedrys*, it seems interesting to compare the chemical composition of both species. Anderson et al. [39] identified hydrocarbons, stigmasterol, sitosterol, the triterpene β-amyrin, oleanolic acid, and triglycerides (with lauric, myristic and palmitic acids as main fatty acids) as constituents of the whole herb of *T.canadense*. Bruno et al. [40] isolated eight different neo-clerodane diterpenoids from its aerial parts (Table 2). As there is some evidence to suggest that the hepatotoxicity of *T.chamaedrys* originates from its diterpenoid fraction (see above), the presence of these latter compounds seems to be of particular interest.

Furanoditerpenoids occur not only in *Teucrium chamaedrys* and *Teucrium canadense* but also in related *Teucrium* species [41,42]. It is therefore remarkable that the problems with *Teucrium chamaedrys* have raised so few questions about the safety of numerous other *Teucrium* species which are or have been used medicinally as well (Table 3).

Table 2. Neo-clerodane diterpenoids in the aerial parts of *T.canadense* [40]

Diterpenoid	Concentration (mg/g)
Teuflin	0.10
Isoteuflin	2.69
Teucvin	2.31
Teucvidin	0.31
Teuscorodal	0.13
(12R)-Teupolin I	0.015
12-Epiteupolin II	0.018
18-Acetylmontanin D	0.013

Table 3. Medicinal *Teucrium* species other than *T.chamaedrys* and *T.canadense* [1,2,14,43]

Teucrium africanum Thunb.
Teucrium aureum Schreb.
Teucrium botrys L.
Teucrium capense Thunb.
Teucrium chamaepitys L. = *Ajuga chamaepitys* Schreb.
Teucrium creticum L.
Teucrium cubense Jac.
Teucrium flavum L.
Teucrium fruticans L.
Teucrium incanum Aitch et Hemsl.
Teucrium iva L. = *Ajuga iva* Schreb.
Teucrium marum L. = *Teucrium maritimum* Lam.
Teucrium montanum L.
Teucrium polium L.
Teucrium riparium Hochst.
Teucrium scordium L.
Teucrium scorodonia L.
Teucrium stocksianum Boiss.
Teucrium villosum Forst. = *Teucrium inflatum* Swartz.

Drug Interactions

See the section on hepatic reactions.

Fertility, Pregnancy and Lactation

No data have been recovered from the literature.

Mutagenicity and Carcinogenicity

No data have been recovered from the literature.

References

1. Hoppe HA (1975) Drogenkunde. Band 1. Angiospermen. 8. Auflage. Berlin: Walter de Gruyter, pp.1066–1067
2. List PH, Hörhammer L (1979) Hagers Handbuch der Pharmazeutischen Praxis. Vierte Neuausgabe. Sechster Band. Chemikalien und Drogen, Teil C: T-Z. Berlin: Springer-Verlag
3. Launert E (1981) Hamlyn guide to edible and medicinal plants of Britain and Northern Europe. London: Hamlyn, p.170
4. Anonymous (1986) Avis aux fabricants concernant les demandes d'autorisation de mise sur le marché de specialités pharmaceutiques à base de plantes. Fascicule spécial no.86/20 bis. Paris: Direction de la Pharmacie et du Médicament, Ministère des Affaires Sociales et de l'Emploi
5. Papanov GY, Malakov PY (1980) Furanoid diterpenes in the bitter fraction of *Teucrium chamaedrys* L. Z Naturforsch 35b: 764–766
6. Gács-Baitz E, Kajtár M, Papanov GY, Malakov PY (1982) Carbon-13 NMR spectra of some furanoid diterpenes from *Teucrium* species. Heterocycles (Sendai) 19:539–550
7. Malakov PY, Papanov GY (1985) Teuchamaedrin C, a neo-clerodane diterpenoid from *Teucrium chamaedrys*. Phytochemistry 24:301–303
8. Savona G, García-Alvarez MC, Rodríguez B (1982) Dihydroteugin, a neo-clerodane diterpenoid from *Teucrium chamaedrys*. Phytochemistry 21:721–723
9. Eguren L, Perales A, Fayos J, Rodríguez B, Savona G, Piozzi F (1982) New neoclerodane diterpenoid containing an oxetane ring isolated from *Teucrium chamaedrys*. X-ray structure determination. J Org Chem 47:4157–4160
10. Fernández-Gadea F, Pascual C, Rodríguez B, Savona G (1983) 6-Epiteucrin A, a neo-clerodane diterpenoid from *Teucrium chamaedrys*. Phytochemistry 22:723–725
11. Garcia-Alvarez MC, Lukacs G, Neszmelyi A, Piozzi F, Rodríguez B, Savona G (1983) Structure of teucroxide. Application of natural-abundance ^{13}C-^{13}C coupling constants observed via double-quantum coherence. J Org Chem 48:5123–5126
12. Rodríguez M-C, Barluenga J, Savona G, Piozzi F, Servettaz O, Rodríguez B (1984) Isoteuflidin, a neo-clerodane diterpenoid from *Teucrium chamaedrys*, and revised structures of teucrins F and G. Phytochemistry 23:1465–1469
13. Rodríguez M-C, Barluenga J, Pascual C, Rodríguez B, Savona G, Piozzi F (1984) Neo-clerodane diterpenoids from *Teucrium chamaedrys*: the identity of teucrin B with dihydroteugin. Phytochemistry 23:2960–2961
14. Grzybek J (1968) Phytochemical characteristics of the species of genus *Teucrium* L. germander indigenous in Poland. Part I. Free sugars and flavonoids. Dissertationes Pharmaceuticae et Pharmacologicae 20:563–572
15. Grzybek J (1969) Phytochemical characteristics of the native *Teucrium* L. species. Part II. The remaining identified compounds. Dissertationes Pharmaceuticae et Pharmacologicae 21:253–260
16. Gross G-A, Lahloub MF, Anklin C, Schulten H-R, Sticher O (1988) Teucrioside, a phenylpropanoid glycoside from *Teucrium chamaedrys*. Phytochemistry 27:1459–1463
17. Harborne JB, Tomás-Barberán FA, Williams CA, Gil MI (1986) A chemotaxonomic study of flavonoids from European *Teucrium* species. Phytochemistry 25:2811–2816
18. Chialva F, Gabri G, Liddle PAP, Ulian F (1982) Qualitative evaluation of aromatic herbs by direct headspace GC analysis. Applications of the method and comparison with the traditional analysis of essential oils. J High Resolut Chromatogr Chromatogr Commun 5:182–188

19. Larrey D (1992) Hépatotoxicité: la phytothérapie aussi. Gastroenterol Clin Biol 16:913–915
20. Castot A, Larrey D (1992) Hépatites observées au cours d'un traitement par un médicament ou une tisane contenant de la germandrée petit-chêne. Bilan des 26 cas rapportés aux Centres Régionaux de Pharmacovigilance. Gastroenterol Clin Biol 16:916–922
21. Larrey D, Vial T, Pauwels A, Castot A, Biour M, David M, Michel H (1992) Hepatitis after germander (*Teucrium chamaedrys*) administration: another instance of herbal medicine hepatotoxicity. Ann Intern Med 117:129–132
22. Anonymous (1990) Avis aux fabricants concernant les demandes d'autorisation de mise sur le marché des médicaments à base de plantes. Fascicule spécial no. 90/22 bis. Paris: Direction de la Pharmacie et du Médicament, Ministère des Affaires Sociales et de la Solidarité
23. Grzybek J (1971) Biological activity of the extracts from native species of *Teucrium* L. Dissertationes Pharmaceuticae et Pharmacologicae 23:163–171
24. Nagao Y, Ito N, Kohno T, Kuroda H, Fujita E (1982) Antitumor activity of *Rabdosia* and *Teucrium* diterpenoids against P388 lymphocytic leukemia in mice. Chem Pharm Bull (Tokyo) 30: 727–729
25. Node M, Sai M, Fujita E (1981) Isolation of the diterpenoid teuflin (6-epiteucvin) from *Teucrium viscidum* var. *miquelianum*. Phytochemistry 20:757–760
26. Simmonds MSJ, Blaney WM, Ley SV, Savona G, Bruno M, Rodríguez B (1989) The antifeedant activity of clerodane diterpenoids from *Teucrium*. Phytochemistry 28:1069–1071
27. Anonymous (1992) Dossier Technique destiné à la presse profesionnelle médicale et pharmaceutique. Objet: Médicaments à base de germandrée-petit-chêne. Paris: Ministère de la Santé et de l'Action Humanitaire
28. Pauwels A, Thierman-Duffaud D, Azanowsky JM, Loiseau D, Biour M, Levy VG (1992) Hépatite aigue à la germandrée petit-chêne. Hépatoxicité d'une plante medicinale. Deux observations. Gastroenterol Clin Biol 16:92–95
29. Mattei A, Bizollon T, Charles J-D, Debat P, Fontanges T, Chevallier M, Trepo C (1992) Atteinte hépatique associée à la prise d'un produit de phytothérapie contenant de la germandrée petit-chêne. Quatre cas. Gastroenterol Clin Biol 16:798–800
30. Legoux J-L, Maitre F, Labarrière D, Gargot D, Festin D, Causse X (1992) Hépatite cytolytique et germandrée petit-chêne: un nouveau cas avec réintroduction. Gastroenterol Clin Biol 16:813–815
31. Diaz D, Ferroudji S, Heran B, Barneon G, Larrey D, Michel H (1992) Hépatite fulminante à la germandrée petit-chêne. Gastroenterol Clin Biol 16:1006–1007
32. Dao T, Peytier A, Galateau F, Valla A (1993) Hépatite chronique cirrhogène à la germandrée petit-chêne. Gastroenterol Clin Biol 17:609–610
33. Mostefa-Kara N, Pauwels A, Pines E, Biour M, Levy VG (1992) Fatal hepatitis after herbal tea. Lancet 340:674
34. Ben Yahia M, Mavier P, Métreau J-M, Zafrani ÉS, Fabre M, Gatineau-Saillant G, Dhumeaux D, Mallat A (1993) Hépatite chronique active et cirrhose induites par la germandrée petit-chêne. Trois cas. Gastroenterol Clin Biol 17:959–962
35. Loeper J, Descatoire V, Lettéron P, Moulis C, Degott C, Pessayre D (1993) Mechanism for the hepatotoxicity of germander (*Teucrium chamaedrys*), a plant responsible for an epidemic of hepatitis in France. J Hepatol (Amsterdam) 18 (Suppl.1):S74
36. Loeper J, Descatoire V, Letteron P, Moulis C, Degott C, Dansette P, Fau D, Pessayre D (1994) Hepatotoxicity of germander in mice. Gastroenterology 106:464–472
37. Anderson LA (1994) Personal communication, April 13, 1994. London: Medicines Control Agency
38. De Smet PAGM. *Scutellaria* species. In: De Smet PAGM, Keller K, Hänsel R, Chandler RF, ed. (1993) Adverse Effects of Herbal Drugs. Volume 2. Heidelberg: Springer-Verlag, pp.289–296
39. Anderson LA, Doggett NS, Ross MSF (1979) Preparative HPLC of the lipid fraction of *Teucrium canadense* L. J Liq Chromatogr 2:455–461
40. Bruno M, Piozzi F, Savona G, De La Torre MC, Rodríguez B (1989) *Neo*-clerodane diterpenoids from *Teucrium canadense*. Phytochemistry 28:3539–3541

41. Piozzi F (1981) The diterpenoids of *Teucrium* species. Heterocycles 15:1489–1503
42. Piozzi F, Rodríguez B, Savona G (1987) Advances in the chemistry of the furanoditerpenoids from *Teucrium* species. Heterocycles 25:807–841
43. Penso G (1983) Index Plantarum Medicinalium Totius Mundi Eorumque Synonymorum. Milano: Organizzazione Editoriale Medico Farmaceutica, p. 944

Tripterygium Species

P.A.G.M. De Smet

Botany

Plants belonging to the genus of *Tripterygium* (Celastraceae) are perennial vines. At least three representatives of this genus are found in China [1]:

- *Tripterygium wilfordii* Hook.f., which is grown in the southeastern part. It is called Leigongteng or Lei Gong Teng (Thunder God vine), Mang Cao (rank grass), Caichongyao or Huangteng [2,3].
- *Tripterygium hypoglaucum* (Levl.) Hutch., which occurs in the southwestern area. Folk names are Kunmingshanhaitang, Diaomaocao (the herb that causes hair falling), or Liufangteng [4].
- *Tripterygium regelii* Sprague et Tak., which is found in the northeast.

The roots of the two former species serve as important sources of Chinese herbal drugs [3,4].

Chemistry

Tripterygium wilfordii has been found to contain various alkaloids, diterpenoids, triterpenoids, and other substances [2,5,6].

Beroza [7–10] isolated five ester alkaloids from the roots and designated these as wilforine, wilfordine, wilforgine, wilfortrine, and wilforzine. Alkaline saponification of these alkaloids yielded wilfordic acid (from wilforine, wilforgine, and wilforzine) and hydroxywilfordic acid (from wilfordine and wilfortrine) [11]. Chinese researchers subsequently reported the presence of related alkaloids, such as euonine [6,12], wilforidine [13] and wilfornine [14]. The roots of *T.wilfordii* also contain the macrocyclic spermidine alkaloids celacinnine, celabenzine, and celafurine [15,16].

Takaishi et al. [17] isolated two highly esterified sesquiterpene alkaloids, triptofordinine A-1 and A-2, from the leaves of *T.wilfordii* var. *regelii*.

Kupchan et al. [18] reported the isolation of two diterpenoid triepoxides from the roots, triptolide and tripdiolide, together with the companion ketone triptonide. These substances were obtained in low yields of 0.001% each [18], but a recent textbook claims, on the basis of a Chinese reference, that triptolide contents up to 0.02% are possible, when the roots are collected in the fall [6]. Among the nume-

Adverse Effects of Herbal Drugs, Vol. 3
(ed. by P.A.G.M. De Smet, K. Keller, R. Hänsel, R.F. Chandler)
© Springer-Verlag Berlin Heidelberg 1997

numerous other diterpenoids in *T.wilfordii* are triptonolide, triptophenolide and its methyl ether, neotriptophenolide, triptolidenol, isoneotriptophenolide, triptonoterpene and its methyl ether [2,6]; triptonoterpenol, neotriptonoterpene, triptonodiol, and neotriptonolide [6]; 16-hydroxytriptolide [19,20], tripchlorolide [20,21], triptriolide [20], and tripterifordin [22]. Matlin et al. [23] isolated triptolide chlorohydrin from a crude aqueous/ethanolic extract of *T.wilfordii* roots but concluded that this was an artefact formed at some stage of the extraction process.

Recently, Zhang et al. [24] recovered triptolide, tripdiolide, triptonide, triptolidenol, 16-hydroxytriptolide, tripchlorolide, and triptriolide from the leaves of *T.wilfordii*, together with the novel diterpenoids tripdioltonide and 13,14-epoxide 9,11,12-trihydroxytriptolide.

Due to the very low yield of diterpenoids, alternative sources have been sought. Van Tamelen and co-workers [25] reported the total synthesis of l-triptolide and l-triptonide. They also synthesized racemic triptolide and triptonide [26], as did Buckanin et al. [27]. The production of triptolide and tripdiolide by plant tissue culture of *T.wilfordii* was investigated by Kutney et al. [28,29].

T.wilfordii also yields numerous triterpenoids, such as wilforlide A, wilforlide B, triptotriterpenic acid A, triptotriterpenic acid B, triptotriterpenoidal lactone A, triptodihydroxy acid methyl ester, 3,24-dioxo-friedelan-29-oic acid, tripterygone, $2\alpha,3\alpha,24$-trihydroxy-Δ^{12}-ursene-28-oic acid, 3-epikatonic acid, orthosphenic acid, polpunonic acid, salaspermic acid, and the red colored pigment tripterine (= celastrol) [2,6,30,31].

Other substances recovered from T.*wilfordii* are dulcitol [3,5], the lignan (-)-syringaresinol [32], and the norsesquiterpene wilforonide [2]. Xia et al. [33] isolated 1,8-dihydroxy-4-hydroxymethyl-anthraquinone from the stem and leaves.

The chemical composition of *T.hypoglaucum* shows similarities to that of *T.wilfordii* [4,5,34,35]. Among the constituents which have been reported so far are the alkaloids wilfordine, wilfortrine and euonymine [6]; the diterpenoids triptolide [4,34], triptonoditerpenic acid [36], triptoditerpenic acid and hypodiolide [37]; and dulcitol [4].

The roots of *T.regelii* yield several triterpenoids, such as regelin, regelinol, regelide, wilforlide A [1], regelin C, regelin D, regelindiol A and regelindiol B [38]. The bark of this species was reported to contain primisterine, which is a methylester of celastrol [39].

Takaishi et al. [40–42] described the presence of 11 new sesquiterpenes (named triptofordins) in the leaves of *T.wilfordii* Hook.f. var. *regelii* Makino. They also isolated 23 sesquiterpenes named triptogelins in the achenes of this plant [43–46].

See also the section on pharmacology and uses for information on the chemistry of ready-to-use preparations.

Pharmacology and Uses

The powdered root of *T.wilfordii* has been used since ancient times in China as an insecticide [1–3,47]. The isolated alkaloids also show insecticidal activity, whereby wilforine, wilfordine, wilforgine, and wilfortrine are much more toxic to insects than wilforzine [7,8,10].

There is also a longstanding tradition of using the root of *T.wilfordii* in Chinese folk medicine [2,35,48,49]. Because of its toxicity, however, the root does not seem to have gained much importance in Chinese medical practice until recent decades, when western-trained physicians started to evaluate its efficacy in rheumatoid arthritis and other immune-related diseases [2,22,47]. For medicinal use of *T.wilfordii*, root xylem is obtained after stripping off two layers of cortices which are believed to contain most of the toxic substances of the plant (cf. the introduction of the adverse reaction profile). The root xylem is dried and cut into small pieces and is then processed to obtain a crude or refined preparation [2]. Crude preparations include an aqueous decoction and an ethanolic elixir, the daily doses of which correspond to 15–25 g and 2–4 g of the root cuttings, respectively [2,3]. An ethanolic extract further treated with ethyl acetate may also be employed [5]. According to Su et al. [50], triptolide may act as a major standard of controlling the quality of ethyl acetate extracts of *T.wilfordii*.

Among the refined preparations are those designated as "glycoside(s)" [6,51], "polyglycosides" [52], "multi-glycosides" [2], or "total glycosides" [5]. Neither the contents nor the exact way of processing emerge unambiguously from the consulted literature. According to Qian [2], the "multi-glycosides" of *T.wilfordii* are also known as GTW, and they are prepared by the Institute of Dermatology, Chinese Academy of Medical Sciences. The xylem cuttings are first extracted with water, then with chloroform and finally GTW is separated by column chromatography, with a yield of 1 mg from 25 g of xylem. Qian [2] adds that GTW is commercially available as tablets, each containing 10 mg. The recommended dose for the treatment of rheumatoid arthritis and skin diseases is 60–90 mg per day for an adult of 60 kg body weight. Qian [2] considers the term "multi-glycosides" an inappropriate one as it merely implies that the drug contains "glycosides" whereas these are not necessarily the active principles. Lan et al. [53] purchased GTW from the Taizhou Pharmaceutical Factory; they describe the same extraction procedure as Qian but claim that 1 mg of the extract is equivalent to 2.5 g of crude xylem. Tao and co-workers [52] also obtained "polyglycosides" from the Taizhou Drug Factory, Jiangsu Province, under the code name of T2; this T2 preparation was later designated as a mixture of compounds extracted with ethanol from the woody portion of the roots of *T.wilfordii* [48]. Matlin et al. [23] describe the "total glycoside" extract as a water-soluble fraction from an alcoholic extract of the plant; they add that there is no chemical evidence supporting the presence of glycosides. For this reason, this monograph systematically puts terms like "glycosides" between quotation marks.

Among the numerous ailments, in which preparations from the root of *T.wilfordii* have been tested clinically with more or less success, are rheumatoid arthritis [51,54–56], ankylosing spondylitis [54,56], systemic lupus erythematosus [57,58], discoid lupus erythematosus [58,59], Henoch-Schönlein purpura, Behçet's syndrome, erythema nodosum, erythema multiforme, dermatitis herpetiformis, psoriasis, Sweet's syndrome, lepra reactions, erythroderma, palmoplantar pustulosis, and recurrent aphthous ulcers [3,5,60,61].

According to Li [62], the root of *T.wilfordii* is also employed in China as a substitute for or supplement to the steroid treatment of certain glomerular diseases. He claims that the drug may be beneficial in minimal change nephrosis, endocapillary glomerulonephritis and mesangial proliferative glomerulonephritis, whereas it is ineffective in focal segmental glomerulonephrosis, extracapillary glomerulonephritis and mesangiocapillary glomerulonephritis. Li [62] also ascribes beneficial effects to the root in certain types of secondary glomerulonephritis, in particular purpuric nephritis and lupus nephritis. An association between the ingestion of *Tripterygium wilfordii* and resolution of severe lupus nephritis in a young Chinese woman was recently reported by Kao et al. [63], while favourable effects in children with an idiopathic nephrotic syndrome were described by Jiang [64].

The root of *T.wilfordii* is also investigated in China as an antifertility agent for males [2] and as a drug for the treatment of menorrhagia [55]. Details about the antifertility effects of the crude drug and its constituents are presented in the section about fertility, pregnancy and lactation of the adverse reaction profile.

The beneficial effects of *T.wilfordii* in rheumatoid arthritis are superior to those of non-steroidal anti-inflammatory drugs [61]. In 1989, the Chinese Medical Journal published a double-blind placebo-controlled cross-over trial involving 70 Chinese patients with active rheumatoid arthritis, who had not responded to non-steroidal anti-inflammatory drug treatment for at least 2 months. Active treatment consisted of "glycosides" from *T.wilfordii*, taken orally in a dosage of 60 mg daily. An improvement in symptoms started as early as the first 1–4 weeks (i.e. earlier than with synthetic slow-acting or immunosuppressive antirheumatic agents), and the full therapeutic effect became evident after 12 weeks. Parallel to the clinical improvement, laboratory examinations showed reductions of the erythrocyte sedimentation rate (ESR), C-reactive protein (CRP), immunoglobulin (IgG, IgM, and IgA) levels, and rheumatoid factor (RF) titer [52]. These observations suggest that *T.wilfordii* has immunosuppressive properties, which might account for its therapeutic effectiveness in rheumatoid arthritis and could also be useful for other indications, such as clinical organ transplantation [47,61].

In vitro experiments in search of an immunosuppressive mechanism of action have shown that *T.wilfordii* inhibits the antigen- and mitogen-stimulated proliferation of T and B cells, the interleukin 2 (IL-2) production and IL-2 responsiveness by T cells, and the IgG production by B cells [47,48]. It was also reported that *T.wilfordii* suppresses the *in vitro* production of IgG, IgM and prostaglandin E_2 by human peripheral blood mononuclear cells (PBMC) obtained from normal individuals and patients with rheumatoid arthritis. These findings suggested that the drug may have both anti-inflammatory and immunomodulating actions [65]. Ye [66] likewise observed inhibitory effects of *T.wilfordii* on the *in vitro* production of IgG and IgM by PBMC. The drug acted both on monocytes and lymphocytes, but more strongly on the latter. This observation appeared to differ from the reported actions of gold and penicillamine. Jiang et al. [67] found that *T.wilfordii* markedly suppressed the activation and proliferation facets of human T lymphocytes *in vitro*.

The immunosuppressive potential of *T.wilfordii* has also been evaluated *in vivo*. Gu et al. [61] reported that the drug is a potent immunosuppressive inhibitor of the development of collagen-induced arthritis in mice. The effects of *T.wilfordii* in this animal model of human rheumatoid arthritis were, in some but not all respects, similar to those reported for cyclosporine A.

Zhang et al. [49] evaluated *T.wilfordii* in the MRL-*lpr/lpr* mouse, an animal model of autoimmune diseases such as systemic lupus erythematosus. They observed a marked prolongation of survival and a significant suppression of proteinuria, and suggested that the drug could potentially be useful for patients with systemic lupus erythematosus or nephrotic syndrome. Gu et al. [68] likewise observed beneficial effects of *T.wilfordii* in MRL-*lpr/lpr* mice. The drug reduced arthritis severity and proteinuria and it prolonged survival, which findings were consistent with reported decreases of proteinuria in Chinese patients with systemic lupus erythematosus. *T.wilfordii* did not appear to be immunosuppressive in the MRL-*lpr/lpr* mouse model, as it did not reduce anti-DNA, anti-type II collagen antibody levels or RF titers [68]. In Chinese patients with systemic lupus erythemasosus, however, the clinical response to the drug was accompanied by decreases in serum antinuclear antibody titers and increases in serum complement (C3) levels, which observations are suggestive of immunosuppressive properties [57,61].

Anti-inflammatory properties have been ascribed to the total alkaloid fraction of *T.wilfordii* [5]; "glycosides" [5]; the diterpenoids triptolide [20], tripdiolide [20], triptonide [20], triptolidenol [20], 16-hydroxytriptolide [19,20], tripchlorolide [20,21], and triptriolide [20]; the triterpenoids triptotriterpenic acid B [30], orthosphenic acid [30], and celastrol [69]; but not to dulcitol [5].

Immunosuppressive activities have been reported for the total alkaloid fraction of *T.wilfordii* [5]; the alkaloids wilfortrine [12], euonine [12], and wilfornine [14]; "glycosides" [5]; the diterpenoids triptolide [20], tripdiolide [20], triptonide [20], triptophenolide [70], triptolidenol [20], 16-hydroxytriptolide [19,20], and tripchlorolide [20,21]; the triterpenoid celastrol [69]; but not to the diterpenoid triptriolide [20].

Zheng [20] compared anti-inflammatory and immunosuppressive actions, as well as certain safety factors, of seven different diterpenoids from *T.wilfordii*, using croton oil-induced ear swelling and hemolysin-antibody formation mouse models. His rankings are summarized in Table 1.

T.wilfordii also has an antineoplastic action [3]. Kupchan et al. [18] found that an ethanolic extract of the root showed significant activity *in vivo* against L-1210

Table 1. Anti-inflammatory action (AA), immunosuppressive action (IA) and certain safety factors (CSF) of seven different diterpenoids from *T.wilfordii*, as assayed by Zheng [20] in croton oil-induced ear swelling and hemolysin-antibody formation mouse models

Diterpenoid	Code	AA (TI*)	IA (TI*)	CSF (of IA)
Triptolide	T10	yes (17)	yes (13.7)	>1
Tripdiolide	T8	yes (7.3)	yes (8.8)	>1
Triptonide	T7	yes (5.9)	yes (7.5)	>1
Triptolidenol	T9	yes (9.6)	yes (30.7)	7.1
16-Hydroxytriptolide	L2	yes (6.6)	yes (15.8)	3.6
Tripchlorolide	T4	yes (9.0)	yes (16.7)	5.1
Triptriolide	T11	yes (> 19)	no	>1

* TI = Therapeutic index

and P-388 leukemias in the mouse and *in vitro* against cells derived from human carcinoma of the nasopharynx. They identified triptolide and tripdiolide as major active constituents. In contrast, triptonide was without antileukemic activity [71]. Triptolide (0.2 and 0.25 mg/kg i.p.) was later reported to prolong the survival of L-615-bearing mice [72]. Antitumoral activity has also been attributed to the triterpenoids regelin and regelinol, which occur in the roots of *T.regelii* [1]. Takaishi et al. [73] examined the inhibitory effects of triptofordins from *T.wilfordii* var. *regelii* and related sequiterpenes from *Euonymus sieboldianus* against the induction of Epstein-Barr virus early antigen activation by 12-O-tetradecanoylphorbol-13-acetate (TPA). Both triptofordin F-2 and triptogelin A-1 were shown to have strong inhibitory activity in this model. This research group also attributed strongly inhibitory effects to triptogelin A-1 on the mouse skin tumor promotion induced by TPA [74].

The ethanolic extract of the root of *T.wilfordii* and its diterpenoid constituent tripterifordin showed significant anti-HIV activity *in vitro* [22]. The triterpenoid salaspermic acid, which can be isolated from the chloroform-soluble fraction of the root, also has anti-HIV properties [75].

The root of *T.hypoglaucum* also shows anti-inflammatory, immunosuppressive and antineoplastic activities. Among its medical uses in China are the treatment of rheumatoid arthritis, lupus erythematosus, psoriasis, erythema nodosum, chronic nephritis, and lepra reactions [4,5,76]. Its antifertility effects on males are also under investigation [34].

Pharmacokinetics

Although the literature about *T.wilfordii* is extensive, no reports about the pharmacokinetics of its major constituents have been unearthed.

Adverse Reaction Profile

According to a Chinese textbook, the root bark of *T.wilfordii* is more toxic than the root core (cf. the section on general animal data), and the fresh root bark is claimed to be more toxic than root bark stored for one year [3]. In order to minimize ill effects, two cortical layers should be removed completely and only the remaining xylem should be used. This root xylem is dried and cut and can then be processed to obtain crude preparations, such as aqueous decoctions and alcoholic extracts, or refined preparations, such as the alkaloids and the "glycosides" of the plant [2,3,5]. The alkaloids are not used clinically, because they have no well-defined therapeutic indications and show marked adverse effects. The "glycosides" are claimed to contain only minute amounts of toxic alkaloids and have less adverse effects than crude extracts. They are commercially available as tablets containing 10 mg of extract each, which are mostly prescribed in doses of 1–1.5 mg/kg per day [2,5,53]. Tao et al. [77] studied a dosage regimen of 30 mg per day for 12 weeks; clinical results in rheumatoid arthritis were similar to those of 60 mg per day, while dermatological and gastrointestinal side effects were milder and had lower incidences.

General Animal Data

The acute LD$_{50}$ of a root decoction of *T.wilfordii* in mice was determined to be 18.4–26.6 g/kg orally and 4.8 g/kg intraperitoneally, whereas LD$_{50}$ values for the root bark and root core were 3.9 and 7.2 g/kg intraperitoneally, respectively [3].

In an early study in rats, subcutaneous administration of a decoction of the root xylem for up to 68 days produced degenerative changes in the spleen, kidney, heart and liver, and congestion of the central nervous system and the gastrointestinal tract were also observed [2]. Zhang et al. [78] later studied the acute and subacute toxicity of an aqueous decoction prepared from the root bark of *T.wilfordii* (corresponding to 1 g of drug per ml). Ingestion of single doses of 10.0–33.8 g/kg revealed an LD$_{50}$ of 21.6 g/kg in rats. The animals showed anorexia, reduced activity and weight loss, with cyanosis of extremities and diarrhea in severe cases. The rats which succumbed died after a moribund stage associated with flaccid paralysis of the muscles. Some of them showed massive hemorrhage and coagulation necrosis in the outer medulla of the kidney, and lesions in other organs were similar to those seen in the subacute experiment. This experiment lasted for 14 days and involved the repeated ingestion of 13.3–30.0 g/kg. This resulted in marked atrophy of the spleen and thymus with necrosis in most of the lymphocytes in these organs and in the axillary lymph nodes. The changes were more pronounced in areas of the spleen where B lymphocytes reside, such as the germinal center of the Malpighian body and the splenic cord. Varying degrees of degeneration and necrosis were also observed in other vital organs. There were striking changes in the myocardial structure and enzyme activity, and massive hemorrhagic necrosis was seen in the outer medulla of the kidney. There were also changes in the liver but these were comparatively slight compared to those in the heart and kidney. The authors suggested a cytotoxic action analogous to that of an immunosuppressive agent as the mechanism of these pathological changes.

The acute oral LD$_{50}$ of "glycosides" of *T.wilfordii* in mice was estimated as 158 ± 14 mg/kg [2]. Intraperitoneal administration of 30–60 mg/kg of "total glycosides" for 5 days produced atrophy of the thymus in young mice [60]. Dietary feeding of "glycosides" to rats for 30–80 days in approximate daily doses of 30–120 mg/kg produced lethargy, decreased food intake and decreased body weight growth, particularly in the high dose group fed for a longer period of time. Individual rats in the high dose group had diarrhea and cachexia, followed by death. Histological examination of the treated rats showed damage to the seminiferous tubules or to the endometrium and myometrium, but their hematology and liver and kidney functions were not significantly different from those of controls. Dogs treated with "glycosides" at doses of 10–15 mg/kg daily for 14.5 months showed decreased food intake and a decreased WBC count. Histological findings were similar to those seen in rats [2]. In addition to loss of appetite, loss of body weight and leukopenia, thrombocytopenia was also observed in these animal experiments [6].

The acute LD$_{50}$ of triptolide in mice was found to be 0.8 mg/kg i.v. and 0.9 mg/kg i.p.. When dogs were given triptolide at 20–160 µg/kg i.v. per day for 7 days, no toxicity was found after 20 µg/kg per day. Doses of 40–80 µg/kg produced reversible toxic effects, such as gastrointestinal tract reactions, leukopenia, ECG changes and SGPT elevation. At the dose level of 160 µg/kg, triptolide was fatal with body weight loss, leukopenia, mycoardial degeneration, focal necrosis of the liver, decreased erythrocyte count, and bone marrow depression [2,79].

The intragastric LD$_{50}$ of triptophenolide in mice was more than 30 mg/kg [70], while the LD$_{50}$ of dulcitol in mice was over 7 g/kg [4].

T.hypoglaucum owes its vernacular name, Diaomaocao, which means the herb that causes hair falling, to the fact that its branches and leaves cause hair loss, when they are eaten by cows, sheep and other domestic animals [4]. According to a Chinese textbook, the root bark of this species is more toxic than the peeled root. In mice, a decoction of the peeled root showed an LD$_{50}$ of 64–68 g/kg intragastrically, whereas the LD$_{50}$ of a decoction of the root bark was about 41 g/kg [4].

General Human Data

T.wilfordii can cause fatal poisoning by accidental ingestion or overdosage, and its leaves and roots have been used for suicidal or homicidal intents [78]. A Chinese textbook states that poisoning following oral ingestion of 2–3 pieces of leaf has been reported and that 7 tender buds (around 12 g) or 30–60 g of the root bark are fatal [3]. Autopsy of patients poisoned by *T.wilfordii* has revealed extensive gastrointestinal hemorrhage, myocardial hemorrhage, congestion in the liver and lungs, and renal tubular necrosis. Death following high doses may be caused by myocardial damage, whereas the slower death which is associated with lower doses may be due to renal failure [3,78,80].

Guo et al. [54] treated 133 patients with rheumatoid arthritis or ankylosing spondylitis with a tincture prepared from the root of *T.wilfordii*. Daily doses of 15–30 ml (corresponding to 1.8–3.6 g of the crude drug) for periods varying from 2 months to 2 years produced gastrointestinal disturbances (gastric discomfort, anorexia, diarrhea, nausea, vomiting), mucocutaneous reactions (perioral blistering, oral mucosal ulcers, sore throat, conjunctivitis, mild hair loss, cracks and occasional petechial hemorrhage of the skin, skin pigmentation) and menstrual disturbances (hypermenorrhea, oligomenorrhea, and amenorrhea). The occurrence of 5 pyogenic infections and 1 viral infection with herpes zoster raised the question, whether the drug had lowered the resistance of these patients to infectious diseases by acting as an immunosuppressive agent.

It is generally believed that "glycosides" of *T.wilfordii* have less and milder side effects than the more crude preparations [2,5,51,60]. In one study, 1–1.5 mg/kg of "glycosides" per day in 3 divided doses was given to 200 patients with dermatological disorders for 10 days to 3 months. This regimen produced gastrointestinal disturbances in 10–20% of the patients (stomachache, anorexia, nausea, xerostomia, and burning sensation in the oesophagus). Dizziness, fatigue, drowsiness and chloasma occurred in a few patients, and 8 users experienced reversible leukopenia [60]. In a placebo-controlled double-blind trial on the effects of "glycosides" in rheumatoid arthritis, 4 of 35 patients did not complete a treatment course of 60 mg per day for 12 weeks because of adverse reactions. The 27 patients who took the drug for 12 weeks showed skin rash and cheilosis (15 patients), diarrhea (6 patients), abdominal pain (2 patients), anorexia (2 patients), amenorrhea (5 of 16 female patients aged < 50 years), and postmenopausal vaginal bleeding (1 of 10 female patients ≥ 50 years). No dropouts related to adverse effects were seen in a second group of patients, who received 60 mg per day for 4 weeks. The 25 patients who completed this course had skin rash and cheilosis (7 patients), diarrhea (2 patients) and amenorrhea (1 of 18 female patients aged < 50 years) [52].

Because of the toxic potential of *T.wilfordii*, Chinese authors advise against its use in hepatic diseases, renal diseases, cardiac diseases, pulmonary diseases, gastric diseases, splenic diseases, hypertension, leukopenia, thrombocytopenia, anemia, active peptic ulcer, and sensitive diathesis, pregnancy and breast-feeding. In addition, the drug should be administered with caution to children and patients of child-bearing age [3,52,54,56,60].

Among Chinese practitioners, *T.hypoglaucum* is reputed to have a lower incidence of side effects than *T.wilfordii* but also a lower therapeutic effectiveness [34]. The most common side effects of *T.hypoglaucum* are gastrointestinal symptoms (gastric pain, nausea, vomiting, diarrhea or constipation, and decrease of appetite). Other side effects include oligomenorrhea, amenorrhea, facial pigmentation, leukopenia and subcutaneous hemorrhage [4].

Cardiovascular Reactions

The use of *T.wilfordii* by experimental animals or human beings can result in serious myocardial damage (see the sections on general animal data and on general human data). For instance, Zhang et al. [78] observed striking changes in myocardial ultrastructure and enzyme activity in rats poisoned with the root bark. They add that a sustained and serious hypotension is an early feature commonly seen in patients intoxicated with *T.wilfordii*, and also refer to early Chinese studies, in which dogs poisoned with the drug manifested hypotension and bradycardia as well as ECG changes of the ST segment and T wave. According to Liao [3], human cases of atrioventricular block have occurred following parenteral administration.

Yu [51] observed one case of palpitation in 144 patients with rheumatoid arthritis, who were treated with "glycosides", but it remained unclear whether this was a side effect. Su et al. [50] found in a clinical study on the antirheumatic effects of the ethyl acetate extract of *T.wilfordii* and its isolated component triptolide that triptolide could impair some patients' hearts

Central Nervous System Reactions

An early experiment has shown that severe degenerative changes in the neurons of the CNS may be found in dogs exposed to Lei Gong Teng but such effects were not observed in toxicological experiments in rats. Clinical information concerning maintenance of consciousness in patients poisoned by Lei Gong Teng just before death suggests that the drug does not exert notable injurious effects on the CNS [78].

Dizziness, fatigue, and drowsiness occur in some patients [5,55] but it is not always clear whether these effects are related to the treatment [51].

Dermatological Reactions

Reported cutaneous reactions to *T.wilfordii* include eczematoid dermatitis, pigmentation and xerosis of the skin, pruritus, perioral herpes simplex, ulcers on lips, and alopecia [5,55].

In a clinical study on 144 patients with rheumatoid arthritis, "glycosides" produced skin rash in 23 patients, mostly on the face and neck. The lesions were millet-sized, pinkish, slightly itching, and tended to ulcerate on scratching; some were macular. The rash sometimes subsided spontaneously. After weeks of treatment, exposed skin, such as on the face and hands, and especially around the fingernails, began to become pigmented. The color was brownish or darkish-gray but gradually faded even though the drug was continued [51]. In another clinical study, skin rash tended to develop into erosion and scarring, and it was also observed that the nails could become thin, softened and friable [52].

Endocrinological Reactions

See the section on fertility, pregnancy and lactation.

Gastrointestinal Reactions

Among the most common adverse effects of "glycosides" and other *Tripterygium* preparations are gastrointestinal disturbances, including nausea, vomiting, anorexia, burning sensation of the lower portion of the esophagus, xerostomia, diarrhea, and constipation. Most of these symptoms subside spontaneously and it is usually not necessary to discontinue the drug [5,51,55,57].

Haematological Reactions

Leukopenia and thrombocytopenia are sometimes observed [6,51,58,62] but it is said that these effects usually revert to normal after discontinuation of therapy [5]. In a study on 144 patients with rheumatoid arthritis, "glycosides" produced leukopenia in nine patients and trombocytopenia in two patients. Both leukocytes and thrombocytes returned to normal during treatment, and only two cases were found with WBC counts under $3000/mm^3$ [51]. In another clinical study on 698 cases of rheumatoid arthritis, treatment with "glycosides" led to leukopenia with a WBC count below $3000/mm^3$ in fifteen patients (2.1%), whereas five patients (0.7%) developed thrombocytopenia without a bleeding tendency [2].

Qin et al. [57] observed a moderate anticoagulant activity in patients with systemic lupus erythematosus, who were treated with crude preparations from the roots and stems without the cortex (equivalent to 30–45 g of *T.wilfordii* per day).

Tao et al. [52] reported a case of reversible aplastic anemia which developed together with feverishness in a 27-year-old male patient who had been treated wrongly with 180 mg of "glycosides" for two weeks.

Hepatic Reactions

T.wilfordii can affect the liver of experimental animals and human beings (see the sections on general animal data and general human data). Shu et al. [55] observed occasional elevation of SGPT which returned to normal after cessation of the medication (a wine prepared from the whole root). Guo et al. [56] observed an elevated SGPT value in one of 59 long-term users of a tincture prepared from the root; the value normalized after treatment was stopped.

Ocular Reactions

Conjunctivitis has been observed in association with the use of a root tincture [54].

Oropharyngeal Reactions

Reported oropharyngeal reactions to *T.wilfordii* are pharyngeal pain, sensation of dryness in the mouth, and ulcers on the mucosa of the oral cavity [55].

Renal Reactions

The use of *T.wilfordii* by experimental animals or human beings can lead to severe nephrotoxicity (see the sections on general animal data and on general human data). For instance, acute kidney failure was observed in 1 or 2 of 44 patients with psoriasis who were treated once daily with a decoction prepared from 12–15 g of the root of *T.wilfordii*. In the laboratory, mice treated with 1 ml of a root decoction (corresponding to 1 g of the root) by gavage died within 8 days, and autopsy revealed narrowing and occlusion of the glomerular capillaries, epithelial granulation, and partial necrosis of the distal tubules [6].

Zhang et al. [78] tested a root bark extract in rats in repeated oral doses of 13.3–30.0 g/kg body weight, and observed necrotic renal changes accompanied by a striking increase of BUN, beginning from the 4th day of the experiment. Zhang et al. [78] add that urinary abnormalities and deterioration of renal function are often encountered in intoxicated patients with a protracted course, suggesting that acute renal failure may be the main cause of death in these cases.

Kidney damage was also observed by Wang and Yuan [58], who treated patients with systemic or discoid lupus erythematosus with tablets each containing 5 g of crude *T.wilfordii* in a dosage of three tablets three times per day.

Drug Interactions

Although the literature about *T.wilfordii* is quite extensive, there appear to be no published studies or reports which specifically address the issue of drug interactions between *T.wilfordii* and other herbal and non-herbal drugs.

Fertility, Pregnancy and Lactation

Female rats fed a laboratory diet containing "glycosides" (approximate dose of 30 mg/kg body weight per day) for 35 or 80 days developed a disturbed estrous cycle, decreased uterine weight and degenerative changes in the endometrium and myometrium; the menstrual cycle became irregular in 80–90% of the animals, and uterus weights were 28–43% less than those of untreated controls [2,6].

In clinical practice, treatment with "glycosides" or other *Tripterygium* preparations can induce irregular menstruation and amenorrhea in females [51,55,57], and the amenorrhea can be accompanied by an increased degree of vaginal atrophy [4,55]. Guo et al. [56] observed amenorrhea in 14 of 15 young female users (aged 20 to 40 years), who took a tincture prepared from the dried root of *T.wilfordii* for a protracted period. In the double blind study by Tao et al. [52], 60 mg of "glycosides" per day produced amenorrhea in 5 of 16 female patients aged < 50 years, who took "glycosides" for 12 weeks, compared to 1 of 18 female patients aged < 50 years, who took the drug for 4 weeks. In addition, Tao et al. [52] observed one case of postmenopausal vaginal bleeding in 10 female patients ≥ 50 years who were treated for 12 weeks.

Gu [81] studied endocrinological changes in female patients, who developed amenorrhea following therapy with "glycosides". FSH and LH concentrations began to rise after 2–3 months and reached menopausal levels at 4–5 months of treatment, while the levels of E2 began to drop after 3–4 months and had become very low after 5 months.

Amenorrhea due to therapeutic doses of "glycosides" usually seems to subside upon cessation of treatment [5,51,52,81], but this may not always be the case with more crude preparations, such as wine prepared from the whole dried root of *T.wilfordii* [55].

In female rats, "glycosides" given orally in daily doses of 50 mg/kg on days 1–4 or 7–9 of pregnancy had neither an anti-implantation effect nor an early pregnancy termination effect [82]. Yet the general toxic effects of *T.wilfordii* preparations on the reproductive system preclude administration to pregnant women, and these preparations should be administered with caution to children and people of child-bearing-age [60].

Male reproductive organs are affected even more strongly by *Tripterygium* "glycosides" than female organs [6]. In male rats fed a laboratory diet containing "glycosides" (approximate dose of 30 mg/kg body weight per day) for 35 or 80 days, marked damages to the seminiferous tubule were seen together with a decrease in the serum testosterone level in the 80-day group [2]. When rats were given "glycosides" by gastric tube at a dose of 10 mg/kg per day, 6 times a week, fertility began to decrease at the end of the 4th week and all the animals had become infertile after 8 weeks. At that time, there was a dramatic decrease in the density and, particularly, the motility of the spermatozoa. Blood testosterone levels, testicular weight and the histology of pituitary and hypothalamus were normal, and in most rats the histology of the testis and epididymis was normal as well. In individual rats, exfoliated cells (mainly spermatids and occasionally pachytene spermatocytes) were found in the tubular lumen. Very infrequently were damages seen in the seminiferous tubules, i.e., some depopulated tubules with a single layer of spermatogonia and Sertoli cells found adjacent to the apparently undamaged tubules [2,82].

Studies of the ultrastructure of the testis and epididymis of treated rats showed changes in the Sertoli cells, and deformed late spermatids with deformed acrosomal vesicles were commonly observed. Condensation of the nuclear material into small clumps and dilatation of the perinuclear space were often seen in the early and mid-spermatids. No perceptible changes were observed in the Leydig cells. It is therefore believed that "glycosides" damage mainly the epididymal spermatozoa and to a lesser extent, the spermatogenic cells. However, a testicular effect was also present, as morphological alterations did occur in the seminiferous tubules of some rats. The spermatogenic cell types most sensitive to the effect of "glycosides" appeared to be the spermatids and the pachytene spermatocytes [2].

The antispermatogenic activity of "glycosides" of *T.wilfordii* was reported to be similar to that of gossypol. After oral administration of "glycosides" at a dose of 30 mg/kg in the diet for 80 days, male rats showed degenerative changes in the seminiferous tubule and the sperm, with lowered number of spermatocytes. The seminiferous tubule became atrophic, and a decreased plasma testosterone level was observed [6].

The reproductive toxicity of *Tripterygium* "glycosides" in rats is said to be higher than in mice [6]. In one study, administration of "glycosides" to adult male mice by gastric gavage at a dose of 20 mg/kg per day (6 days a week, for 8 weeks) suppressed the motility and density of spermatozoa and increased the percentage of malformed spermatozoa in the cauda epididymis [2].

Zheng [83] reported that the immunosuppressive and antifertility activity of *Tripterygium* diterpenes are inseparable. Six of the seven diterpenes that were tested in mice showed antifertility activity in dosages < 1/40 of their LD_{50} values. The lowest dosages with antifertility activity were 5–28 times lower than those needed for anti-inflammatory activity and 5–12 times lower than those needed for immunosupresssive activity. Total dosages necessary for effective immunosuppression were 0.9–1.8 times the total dosages needed for effective antifertility.

Matlin et al. [23] showed by step-wise fractionation that the antifertility effects of "glycosides" from *T.wilfordii* can be accounted for by triptolide, tripdiolide and closely related diterpenes, including a chlorohydrin apparently formed as an artefact during the processing of the crude plant material. Tripdiolide was evidently the main antifertility component responsible for the activity seen in the aqueous phases. The minimum effective dose of pure tripdiolide required to fully inhibit fertility in male rats was less than 5.6 µg per rat per day.

In a general toxicity study in mice, weight growth, birth rate and litter size were decreased when both male and female animals were fed simultaneously with dietary "glycosides" [82]. In another mouse study, alkaloids produced stronger damage to the testes than "glycosides". When the mice reproduced after cessation of "glycosides", no malformation was found in the offspring [51].

Qian et al. [84] reported that the infertility effect of "glycosides" in rats after administration of 10 mg/kg per day by gastric gavage (6 times a week for 10 weeks) was reversible. The fertility of the treated rats began to recover 4 weeks after the withdrawal of the "glycosides" and was fully restored 1 week later. The histology of the testis was normal in 8 of the 10 treated rats, while minor changes were observed in the seminiferous epithelium of the remaining two. Lan et al. [53] also administered "glycosides" to male rats in a dosage of 10 mg/kg a day (for 8 weeks). Mating ability and fertility was tested after 6 weeks of treatment; fertility was significantly inhibited but mating ability was not affected.

Lan et al. [53] found that "glycosides" affected the survival of Sertoli and Leydig cells of rats in vitro. Sertoli cells were much more sensitive than Leydig cells. Exposure to 1–20 µg/ml of "glycosides" did not produce significant changes in the HCG-stimulated testosterone production of Leydig cells, but Sertoli and Leydig cells died when exposed to a dose of 30 µg/ml of "glycosides" for 24 hours. Lan et al. [53] caution that "glycosides" may cause irreversible infertility and the loss of sexual behavior, if administered for a long time or at a high dosage level. They cite evidence from rat experiments that "glycosides" can cause degenerative changes in the seminiferous epithelium in doses of 20–30 mg/kg per day and atrophy of the seminiferous epithelium as well as a decrease of the testosterone plasma level, when doses of 30–120 mg/kg per day are tested. They also refer to clinical data that the testicular volume may decrease in a few patients after long-term treatment with crude extracts of *T.wilfordii* and "glycosides". It has also been reported that antifertility doses do not affect the testosterone level in man and that "glycosides" did not affect the sexual behavior of 26 fertile men after treatment with 20 mg per day for 4–6 months.

Ye [85] compared the antifertility activity of "glycosides" in rats with that of the constituent T4 (= tripchlorolide). The dosages of the "glycosides" and T4 were 10 mg/kg per day and 0.05 mg/kg per day, respectively, fed for 7 weeks by gastric tube. The "glycosides" produced damage to the testis and epididymal tubes; deformed sperms and exfoliated cells (mainly spermatids and occasionally pachytene spermatocytes) were found in the tubular lumen of the epididymis. T4 mainly caused damage to the spermatozoa in the epididymis without discernible changes in the seminiferous tubules, epididymal epithelia, Leydig cells or Sertoli cells.

To assess the antifertility potential of *Tripterygium hypoglaucum*, Qian et al. [86] treated male rats with 1 g/kg per day of an alcoholic root extract by gastric gavage (6 times per week, for 6 weeks). This regimen effectively reduced fertility without producing significant changes in the Leydig or Sertoli cells.

In clinical practice, *Tripterygium* preparations can produce oligospermia and azoospermia (after two months or more) and a decrease in the size of the testis (after more prolonged treatment), reportedly without affecting libido or potency

[2]. In addition, "glycosides" extracted from the root of *T.wilfordii* were associated with gynecomastia in 2 of 40 male users [51].

Qian et al. [87] observed reduced density and zero motility of spermatozoa in 11 male patients with rheumatoid arthritis, who had taken "glycosides" at a low dose level of 20–30 mg/day (regular dose is 1 mg/kg per day) for 1.5–5 months. The patients showed normal serum levels of testosterone and LH, but their serum FSH level was significantly higher than in the control group (7.4 ± 5.1 IU/l compared to 2.9 ± 1.3 IU/l), even though it was within the normal range. No significant effects on libido or potency were reported. Normal sperm density and motility were observed in two additional patients, who had ceased to take "glycosides" for 2–4 months after having taken them at the same low dose level for 2–2.5 months.

Qian et al. [34] also evaluated the effects of *Tripterygium hypoglaucum* on the fertility of twelve male patients with rheumatoid arthritis who had taken 15 g of the root xylem as a decoction for 2–48 months (with an additional patient using this preparation for over ten years). Sperm concentration and motility were significantly reduced but libido, potency and testicular volume were reported to be normal, and mean testosterone, FSH and LH levels were not affected. The antifertility effects appeared to be reversible in 8 subjects tested 6–12 months after they had stopped taking the drug.

See also the section on mutagenicity and carcinogenicity.

Mutagenicity and Carcinogenicity

Although the literature about *T.wilfordii* is quite extensive, no reports about the mutagenicity or carcinogenicity of the crude drug or its isolated constituents have been unearthed.

In vitro experiments with *T.hypoglaucum* have shown that this plant can give positive results in the Ames test and that it can induce sister chromatid exchanges in human peripheral lymphocytes. *In vivo*, an aqueous root extract from *T.hypoglaucum* administered intraperitoneally to mice had similar effects on C-mitosis frequency and the size of micronuclei in bone marrow cells as colchicine. These latter observations suggest that the plant may induce aneuploidy [88].

References

1. Hori H, Pang G-M, Harimaya K, Iitaka Y, Inayama S (1987) Isolation and structure of regelin and regelinol, new antitumor ursene-type triterpenoids from *Tripterygium regelii*. Chem Pharm Bull 35:2125–2128
2. Qian SZ (1987) *Tripterygium wilfordii*, a Chinese herb effective in male fertility regulation. Contraception 36:335–345
3. Liao N-G (1987) Leigongteng. In: Chang H-M, But PP-H, red. Pharmacology and Applications of Chinese Materia Medica. Singapore: World Scientific Publishing, pp.1201–1207
4. Deng W-L (1987) Kunmingshanhaitang. In: Chang H-M, But PP-H, red. Pharmacology and Applications of Chinese Materia Medica. Singapore: World Scientific Publishing, pp.793–797

5. Xu W-Y, Zheng J-R, Lu X-Y (1985) Tripterygium in dermatologic therapy. Int J Dermatol 24:152–157
6. Tang W, Eisenbrand G (1992) Chinese drugs of plant origin. Chemistry, pharmacology, and use in traditional and modern medicine. Heidelberg: Springer-Verlag, pp.989–996
7. Beroza M (1951) Alkaloids from *Tripterygium wilfordii* Hook. – wilforine and wilfordine. J Am Chem Soc 73:3656–3659
8. Beroza M (1952) Alkaloids from *Tripterygium wilfordii* Hook: wilforgine and wilfortrine. J Am Chem Soc 74:1585–1588
9. Beroza M (1953) Alkaloids from *Tripterygium wilfordii* Hook. The structure of wilforine, wilfordine, wilforgine and wilfortrine. J Am Chem Soc 75:44–49
10. Beroza M (1953) Alkaloids from *Tripterygium wilfordii* Hook. Isolation and structure of wilforzine. J Am Chem Soc 75: 2136–2138
11. Beroza M (1963) Alkaloids from *Tripterygium wilfordii* Hook. The chemical structure of wilfordic and hydroxywilfordic acids. J Org Chem 28:3562–3564
12. Zheng YL, Xu Y, Lin JF (1989) Immunosuppressive effects of wilfortrine and euonine. Acta Pharm Sin 24:568–72
13. He Z-S, Hong S-H, Li Y, Sha H, Yu X-G (1985) Structure of a new alkaloid wilforidine from *Tripterygium wilfordii*. Acta Chim Sin 43:593–596
14. Deng F-X, Cao J-H, Xia Z-L, Lin S, Wang X-Y (1987) Studies on the sesquiterpene alkaloids of *Tripterygium wilfordii* Hook. f. Acta Bot Sin 29:523–526
15. Kupchan SM, Hintz HPJ, Smith RM, Karim A, Cass MW, Court WA, Yatagai M (1974) Celacinnine, a novel macrocyclic spermidine alkaloid prototype. J Chem Soc Chem Comm pp.329–330
16. Kupchan SM, Hintz HPJ, Smith RM, Karim A, Cass MW, Court WA, Yatagai M (1977) Macrocyclic spermidine alkaloids from *Maytenus serrata* and *Tripterygium wilfordii*. J Org Chem 42:3660–3664
17. Takaishi Y, Ujita K, Noguchi H, Nakano K, Tomimatsu T, Kadota S, Tsubono K, Kikuchi T (1987) Structures of triptofordinine A-1 and A-2 determined by two-dimensional NMR spectroscopy. Highly esterified sesquiterpene alkaloids from *Tripterygium wilfordii* Hook fil. var. *regelii* Makino. Chem Pharm Bull 35:3534–3537
18. Kupchan SM, Court WA, Dailey RG Jr, Gilmore CJ, Bryan RF (1972) Triptolide and tripdiolide: novel antileukemic diterpenoid triepoxides from Tripterygium wilfordii. J Am Chem Soc 94:7194–7195
19. Ma PC, Lu XY, Yang JJ, Zheng QT (1991) 16-Hydroxytriptolide, a new active diterpene isolated from Tripterygium wilfordii. Acta Pharm Sin 26:759–763
20. Zheng J (1991) Screening of active anti-inflammatory, immunosuppressive and antifertility components of Tripterygium wilfordii. III. A comparison of the anti-inflammatory and immunosuppressive activities of 7 diterpene lactone epoxide compounds in vivo. Acta Acad Med Sin 13:391–397
21. Lu X (1990) The isolation and structure of tripchlorolide (T4) from Tripterygium wilfordii. Acta Acad Med Sin 12:157–161
22. Chen K, Shi QA, Fujioka T, Zhang D-C, Hu C-Q, Jin J-Q, Kilkuskie RE, Lee K-H (1992) Anti-AIDS agents, 4. Tripteriforidin, a novel anti-HIV principle from *Tripterygium wilfordii*: isolation and structural elucidation. J Nat Prod 55:88–92
23. Matlin SA, Belenguer A, Stacey VE, Qian SZ, Xu Y, Zhang JW, Sanders JKM, Amor SR, Pearce CM (1993) Male antifertility compounds from Tripterygium wilfordii Hook f. Contraception 47:387–400
24. Zhang CP, Lu XY, Ma PC, Chen Y, Zhang YG, Yan Z, Chen GF, Zheng QT, He CH, Yu DQ (1993) Studies on diterpenoids from leaves of *Tripterygium wilfordii*. Acta Pharm Sin 28:110–115
25. Van Tamelen EE, Demers JP, Taylor EG, Koller K (1980) Total synthesis of l-triptonide and l-triptolide. J Am Chem Soc 102:5424–5425
26. Van Tamelen EE, Leiden TM (1982) Biogenetic-type total synthesis of (±)-triptonide and (±)-triptolide. J Am Chem Soc 104:1785–1786

27. Buckanin RS, Chen SJ, Frieze DM, Sher FT, Berchtold GA (1980) Total synthesis of triptolide and triptonide. J Am Chem Soc 102:1200–1201
28. Kutney JP, Beale MH, Salisbury PJ, et al. (1980) Tripdiolide from tissue culture of *Tripterygium wilfordii*. Heterocycles 14:1465–1467
29. Kutney JP, Hewitt GM, Kurihara T, et al. (1981) Cytotoxic diterpenes triptolide, tridiolide, and cytotoxic triterpenes from tissue cultures of *Tripterygium wilfordii*. Can J Chem 59:2677–2683
30. Zhang CP (1989) Studies on triterpenoids of total glucosides of *Tripterygium wilfordii* (T II). Acta Acad Med Sin 11:322–325
31. Zhang D-M, Yu D-Q, Xie F-Z (1991) The structure of tripterygone. Acta Pharm Sin 26:341–344
32. Bryan RF, Fallon L (1976) Crystal structure of syringaresinol. J Chem Soc Perkin Trans 2:341–345
33. Xia ZL, Huang SQ, Chen JY, Deng FX (1989) A new anthraquinone compound from the stem and leaves of *Tripterygium wilfordii* Hook f. China J Chin Materia Medica 14:675–676 and 703
34. Qian S-Z, Hu Y-Z, Wang S-M, Luo Y, Tang A-S, Shu S-Y, Zhou J-W, Rao T-Y (1988) Effects of *Tripterygium hypoglaucum* (Lévl.) Hutch on male fertility. Adv Contracep 4:307–310
35. Zhou B-N (1991) Some progress on the chemistry of natural bioactive terpenoids from Chinese medicinal plants. Mem Inst Oswaldo Cruz 86 (Suppl 2):219–226
36. Zhang L, Zhang ZX, An DK, Kong C (1991) Studies on the chemical constituents of *Tripterygium hypoglaucum* (Lévl) Hutch. Acta Pharm Sin 26:515–518
37. Zhang L, Zhang ZX, Sheng LS, An DK, Lu Y, Zheng QT, Wang SC (1992) Study on the chemical constituents of *Tripterygium hypoglaucum* (Lévl.) Hutch. Acta Pharm Sin 28:32–34
38. Pang G-M, Zhao C-J, Hori H, Inayama S (1989) Studies on new triterpenoids of *Tripterygium regelii*. Acta Pharm Sin 24:75–79
39. Hegnauer R (1964) Chemotaxonomie der Pflanzen. Band 3: Dicotyledoneae: Acanthaceae – Cyrillaceae. Basel: Birkhäuser Verlag, pp.398–399
40. Takaishi Y, Ujita K, Nakano K, Murakami K, Tomimatsu T (1987) Sesquiterpene esters from *Tripterygium wilfordii* Hook fil. var. regelii, structures of triptofordins A-C-1. Phytochemistry 26:2325–2329
41. Takaishi Y, Ujita K, Kida K, Shibuya M, Tomimatsu T (1987) Polyhydroxyagarofuran derivatives from *Tripterygium wilfordii* H. Phytochemistry 26:2581–2584
42. Takaishi Y, Ujita K, Nakano K, Tomimatsu T (1988) Structural elucidation of triptofordins F-1, F-2, F-3, and F-4, new sesquiterpenes polyesters from *Tripterygium wilfordii* Hook fil. var. regelii Makino. Chem Pharm Bull 36:4275–4283
43. Takaishi Y, Noguchi H, Murakami K, Nakano K, Tomimatsu T (1990) Sesquiterpene esters, triptogelin A-1-A-4, from *Tripterygium wilfordii* var. regelii. Phytochemistry 29:3869–3873
44. Takaishi Y, Tokura K, Tamai S, Noguchi H, Nakano K, Tomimatsu T (1991) Sesquiterpene esters from Tripterygium wilfordii. Phytochemistry 30:1561–1566
45. Takaishi Y, Tokura K, Tamai S, Ujita K, Nakano K, Tomimatsu T (1991) Sesquiterpene polyol esters from *Tripterygium wilfordii* var. regelii. Phytochemistry 30:1567–1572
46. Takaishi Y, Tamai S, Nakano K, Murakami K, Tomimatsu T (1991) Structures of sesquiterpene polyol esters from *Tripterygium wilfordii* var. regelii. Phytochemistry 30:3027–3031
47. Li X-W, Weir MR (1990) Radix *Tripterygium wilfordii* – a Chinese herbal medicine with potent immunosuppressive properties. Transplantation 50:82–86
48. Tao X, Davis LS, Lipsky PE (1991) Effect of an extract of the Chinese herbal remedy *Tripterygium wilfordii* Hook f on human immune responsiveness. Arthritis Rheum 34:1274–1281
49. Zhang X-Y, Tsuchiya N, Dohi M, Yamamoto K, Ishihara K, Okudaira H, Ito K, Miyamoto T (1992) Prolonged survival of MRL-*lpr/lpr* mice treated with *Tripterygium wilfordii* Hook-f. Clin Immunol Immunopathol 62:66–71

50. Su D, Song Y, Li R (1990) Comparative clinical study of rheumatoid arthritis treated by triptolide and an ethyl acetate extract of Tripterygium wilfordii. Chin J Modern Develop Trad Med 10:144–146 and 131
51. Yu D-Y (1983) Clinical observation of 144 cases of rheumatoid arthritis treated with glycoside of Radix Tripterygium wilfordii. J Tradit Chin Med 3:125–129
52. Tao X-L, Sun Y, Dong Y et al. (1989) A prospective, controlled, double-blind, cross-over study of *Tripterygium wilfordii* Hook f in treatment of rheumatoid arthritis. Chin Med J 102:327–332
53. Lan Z-J, Gu Z-P, Lu R-F, Zhuang L-Z (1992) Effects of multiglycosides of *Tripterygium wilfordii* (GTW) on rat fertility and Leydig and Sertoli cells. Contraception 45:249–261
54. Guo J-L, Yuan S-X, Wang X-C, Xu S-X, Li D-D (1981) *Tripterygium wilfordii* Hook f in rheumatoid arthritis and ankylosing spondylitis. Preliminary report. Chin Med J 94:405–412
55. Shu H-Y, Liu P-L, Huang G-Y (1984) Effects of *Tripterygium wilfordii* on the menstruation of 50 patients suffering from rheumatoid arthritis – with a summary of its therapeutic effects in 12 cases of menorrhagia. J Trad Chin Med 4:237–240
56. Guo J-L, Gao Z-G, Zang A-C, Bai R-X (1986) Radix Tripterygium wilfordii Hook f in rheumatoid arthritis, ankylosing spondylitis and juvenile rheumatoid arthritis. Chin Med J 99:317–320
57. Qin W-Z, Liu C-H, Yang S, et al. (1981) *Tripterygium wilfordii* Hook f in systemic lupus erythematosus. Report of 103 cases. Chin Med J 94:827–834
58. Wang BX, Yuan ZZ (1989) A tablet of *Tripterygium wilfordii* in treating lupus erythematosus. Chin J Modern Develop Trad Med 9:407–408 and 389
59. Qin W-Z, Zhu G-D, Yang S-M, Han K-Y, Wang J (1983) Clinical observations on *Tripterygium wilfordii* in treatment of 26 cases of discoid lupus erythematosus. J Trad Chin Med 3:131–132
60. Tripterygium Wilfordii Hook f Research Group (1984) Studies on total glycosides of *Tripterygium wilfordii* Hook f in dermatoses. Chin Med J 97:667–670
61. Gu W-Z, Brandwein SR, Banerjee S (1992) Inhibition of type II collagen induced arthritis in mice by an immunosuppressive extract of *Tripterygium wilfordii* Hook f. J Rheumatol 19:682–688
62. Li L-S (1989) Medical progress in China. An overview of nephrology in China. Chin Med J 102:488–495
63. Kao NL, Richmond GW, Moy JN (1993) Resolution of severe lupus nephritis associated with *Tripterygium wilfordii* Hook F ingestion. Arthritis Rheum 36:1751–1752
64. Jiang X (1994) Clinical observations on the use of the Chinese herb *Tripterygium wilfordii* Hook for the treatment of nephrotic syndrome. Pediatr Nephrol 8:343–344
65. Tao X-L, Dai H, Ye W, Zhang N-Z (1989) The effect of T_2 on in vitro PGE_2, IgG and IgM production of PBMC of normal individuals and patients with RA. Arthritis Rheum 32 (suppl): S131
66. Ye WH (1990) Mechanism of treating rheumatoid arthritis with polyglycosides of Tripterygium wilfordii Hook (T II). III. Study on inhibitory effect of T II on in vitro Ig secreted by peripheral blood mononuclear cells from normal controls and RA patients. Acta Acad Med Sin 12:217–222
67. Jiang M et al. (1992) The effect of glycoside *Tripterygium wilfordii* Hook F on the immune regulatory function of T lymphocyte. Nat Med J China 72:473–475 and 509–510
68. Gu W-Z, Banerjee S, Rauch J, Brandwein SR (1992) Suppression of renal disease and arthritis, and prolongation of survival in MRL-*lpr* mice treated with an extract of *Tripterygium wilfordii* Hook f. Arthritis Rheum 35:1381–1386
69. Xu WM, Zhang LX, Cheng ZH, Cai WZ, Miao HH, Pan DJ (1991) Inhibitory effect of tripterine on activities of IL-1, IL-2 and release of PGE2. Acta Pharm Sin 26:641–645
70. Yu DF, Hu BH, Chen GP, Yang CX, Yang J, Xu JY, Li LZ (1990) Structure revision of triptophenolide. Acta Pharm Sin 25:929–31
71. Kupchan SM (1976) Novel plant-derived tumor inhibitors and their mechanisms of action. Cancer Treatment Rep 60:1115–1126

72. Zhang T-M, Chen Z-Y, Lin C (1981) Antineoplastic action of triptolide and its effect on the immunologic functions in mice. Acta Pharmacol Sin 2:128–131
73. Takaishi Y, Ujita K, Tokuda H, Nishino H, Iwashima A, Fujita T (1992) Inhibitory effects of dihydroagarofuran sesquiterpenes on Epstein-Barr virus activation. Cancer Lett 65:19–26 and 67:215
74. Ujita K, Takaishi Y, Tokuda H, Nishino H, Iwashima A, Fujita T (1993) Inhibitory effects of triptogelin A-1 on 12-O-tetradecanoylphorbol-13-acetate-induced skin tumor promotion. Cancer Lett 68:129–133
75. Chen K, Shi Q, Kashiwada Y, et al (1992) Anti-AIDS agents, 6. Salaspermic acid, an anti-HIV principle from *Tripterygium wilfordii*, and the structure-activity correlation with its related compounds. J Nat Prod 55:340–346
76. Chen M-F, Zhang Q-Y, Yao J, Wu Z-Y, Shen R, Wang X-Y, Zhang H-X, Zhu J-G, Zhen Z-H, Chen J-Z (1983) Treatment of chronic nephritis with *Tripterygium hypoglaucum*. A clinical and experimental study. J Trad Chin Med 3:219–222
77. Tao X, Sun Y, Zhang N (1990) Treatment of rheumatoid arthritis with low doses of multiglycosides of *Tripterygium wilfordii*. Chin J Mod Develop Trad Med 10:289–291, 261–262
78. Zhang Y-G, Huang G-Z, Wang H-J, Wu Z-B, Xing S-L (1984) An experimental pathological study of acute Lei Gong Teng (*Tripterygium wilfordii* Hook) intoxication in rats. Acta Acad Med Wuhan 4:75–81
79. Cheng Y-L, Ye J-R, Lin D-J; Lin L-J, Zhu J-N (1981) Some toxicities of triptolide in mice and dogs. Acta Pharmacol Sin 2:70–72
80. Zhang Y-G, Huang G-Z (1988) Poisoning by toxic plants in China. Report of 19 autopsy cases. Am J Forens Med Pathol 9:313–319
81. Gu CX (1989) Cause of amenorrhea after treatment with *Tripterygium wilfordii* F. Acta Acad Med Sin 11:151–153
82. Qian S-Z, Zhong C-Q, Xu Y (1986) Effect of *Tripterygium wilfordii* Hook.f. on the fertility of rats. Contraception 33:105–110
83. Zheng J (1991) Screening of active anti-inflammatory, immunosuppressive and antifertility components of *Tripterygium wilfordii*. IV. A comparison of the male antifertility activities of 7 diterpene lactone epoxide compounds. Acta Acad Med Sin 13:398–403
84. Qian S-Z, Zhong CQ, Xu Y (1986) Studies on the reversibility of the antifertility effect of *Tripterygium wilfordii* Hook. f. (GTW) in male SD rats. Adv Contracep 2:298
85. Ye W (1991) Antispermatogenic effects of multiglycosides of Tripterygium wilfordii and monomer T4 in the testes and epididymal spermatozoa of rats. Acta Acad Med Sin 13:235–240
86. Qian S-Z, Wang S-M, Wang Y, Xu Y (1988) Studies of the effect of *Tripterygium hypoglaucum* (Level.) Hutch on the fertility of male rats. Adv Contracep 4:53–54
87. Qian S-Z, Zhong C-Q, Xu N, Xu Y, Ni L-Q, Feng G-Z (1986) The antifertility effect of total glycosides of *Tripterygium wilfordii* Hook.f. (GTW) in men. Adv Contracep 2:253–254
88. Wang X, Zhuo R, He Z (1993) Aneuploidy induction by water extract from *Tripterygium hypoglaucum* (Level) Hutch in mouse bone marrow cells. Mutagenesis 8: 395–398

Valeriana Species

R. Bos, H.J. Woerdenbag, P.A.G.M. De Smet and J.J.C. Scheffer

Botany

The genus *Valeriana* belongs to the Valerianaceae and contains about 230 species. The majority of representatives of this genus is distributed over the temperate regions of the Old World, but they also occur in Central and South America. This monograph will focus on the three most important species that play a role in herbal medicine: *Valeriana officinalis* L. s.l., *V. wallichii* DC. and *V. edulis* Nutt. ssp. *procera* F.G. Meyer [1].

V. officinalis L. s.l. (valerian) is listed in the European Pharmacopoeia. In Europe this species is cultivated on a large scale for the preparation of pharmaceuticals, prepared from the roots and rhizomes [2]. *V. officinalis* is a collective term; hence the addition s.l. (sensu lato). Five subspecies are distinguished within the species: *V. sambucifolia*, *V. procurrens*, *V. collina*, *V. exaltata*, and *V. pratensis*. The subspecies differ morphologically and cytologically, as well as in area of distribution [3]. Synonyms for *V. officinalis* L. are *V. alternifolia* Ledeb., *V. excelsa* Poir., and *V. sylvestris* Grosch. [4].

V. wallichii DC. (syn. *V. jatamansi* Jones), the Indian or Pakistani valerian, is listed in the Indian Pharmacopoeia. It is collected in the Himalayas [5].

V. edulis (syn. *V. mexicana* DC.) originates from Central America and is described in the Mexican Pharmacopoeia.

Chemistry

The roots and rhizomes of the three medicinally used *Valeriana* species show large differences with regard to their constituents. Dried roots and rhizomes of *V. officinalis* contain 0.5–2.0% (v/w) of essential oil, which is mainly composed of mono- and sesquiterpenoids. More than 150 compounds have been found in the oil so far. They include acyclic, monocyclic and bicyclic hydrocarbons, as well as oxygen-containing derivatives, such as alcohols, aldehydes, ketones, phenols, oxides and esters [2,6]. The composition of the oil is highly influenced by the origin of the plant material (genotype, soil and climate), and by the method of isolating the oil (from fresh or dried material, via extraction or distillation). Based on the principal component of the oil, four chemotypes can be distinguished within the species *V. officinalis*: the valeranone, valerianol, cryptofauronol and valerenal types [7–10].

The essential oil of *V. wallichii* (0.1–0.9% v/w) contains mainly the sesquiterpene alcohols patchouli alcohol and maaliol [11]. *V. edulis* hardly contains any essential oil. The volatile compounds that are obtained after distillation of the roots of this plant mainly include valeric, isovaleric and hydroxyvaleric acids, as well as several other decomposition products formed upon heating of valepotriates [3,6].

V. officinalis and *V. wallichii* have several constituents in common with Japanese valerian species. They include valeranone (jatamansone), faurinone, kessan, kessyl acetate, cryptofauronol, fauronyl acetate, maaliol and patchouli alcohol [12–20]. It has been found that the total terpene content in Japanese valerian species is 2 – 25 times higher than in European species [21].

In the 1960s, Thies and coworkers [22,23] isolated a novel group of natural products from subterranean parts of *V. wallichii*, and called these compounds valepotriates. Valepotriates are triesters of polyalcohols with an iridoid structure and possess an epoxy group (valeriana-epoxy-triesters). Differences are found in the number of hydroxyl groups, the type of ester groups, and the degree of saturation. As a result of dehydration or esterification of the various alcohol functions, species-dependent mixtures of valepotriates are yielded. Based on their chemical structure, valepotriates are divided into two main groups: the diene type (including valtrate, isovaltrate and acevaltrate) and the monoene type (including didrovaltrate and isovaleroxyhydroxydidrovaltrate (IVHD)) [3,11].

Valepotriates are unstable compounds: they are thermolabile and decompose under acid or alkaline conditions as well as in alcoholic solutions. After hydrolysis valeric and isovaleric acids are found among other compounds. The main decomposition products of the valepotriates are the yellow-colored baldrinals. Baldrinal originates from valtrate and acevaltrate; homobaldrinal from isovaltrate. The baldrinals are chemically reactive and may subsequently form polymers [3,24].

V. officinalis contains 0.8–1.7% of a mixture of valepotriates, consisting mainly of valtrate and isovaltrate in a ratio of 1:1–1:4 [2]. *V. wallichii* contains 1.8–3.5% of valepotriates. Next to valtrate and isovaltrate, didrovaltrate is also present in this species. Two chemotypes are distinguished for *V. wallichii*: the monoene and diene types [25]. *V. edulis* is the richest in valepotriates (8.0–12.0%). Valtrate, isovaltrate, acevaltrate, didrovaltrate and IVHD are present here [26,27]. Valerosidate, an iridoid glycoside, is found in *V. officinalis* (up to 1.5%) and in *V. wallichii* (up to 5%) [3]. Valepotriates are not only present in *Valeriana* species but also in *Centranthus* species. In addition, they do not occur exclusively in subterranean parts of the plants but also in the leaves of *Valeriana* and *Centranthus* species [28–33].

V. officinalis contains characteristic cyclopentane sesquiterpenes. In the essential oil valerenal, valerenol and its acetate, isovalerate and hexanoate esters, and small amounts of valerenic acid and valerenic acid methylester have been identified [20,34]. Important non-volatile cyclopentane sesquiterpenes are the valerenic acid derivatives: valerenic, acetoxyvalerenic and hydroxyvalerenic acids. The first two compounds are specific for *V. officinalis* [35], while the third one is probably formed when the root material is stored improperly, e.g. under too humid conditions. In that case hydroxyvalerenic acid is produced from acetoxyvalerenic acid. The content of valerenic acid derivatives ranges from 0.05% (in wild plants) to 0.9% (in cultivated strains) [2]. *V. wallichii* and *V. edulis* lack these cyclopentane sesquiterpenes.

In contrast to the valepotriates, the valerenic acid derivatives are chemically stabile. In the future, they may play an important role in the standardization of valerian preparations prepared from *V. officinalis* [34,36–38]. Using the guidelines of the German Pharmacopoeia (9th Edition), Schimmer and Röder [39] investigated valerian roots and valerian tincture. Valerenic acids were detected by TLC in 19 (out of 23) commercial plant drugs derived from *V. officinalis*. In two plant products containing extracts from *V. wallichii* DC. and *V. edulis* Nutt. ssp. *procera*, these compounds could not be detected. Valerenic acids were also detected in several self-prepared aqueous extracts and in commercial tinctures [39]. A disadvantage of this TLC method is that only valerenic acid derivatives can be assayed. An alternative may be found in an on-line HPLC method by which valerenic acid derivatives, valepotriates as well as the baldrinals can be detected in one run [24].

Finally, in the subterranean parts of *V. officinalis* a number of alkaloids (0.05–0.1%) occur: actinidine, 8-methoxyactinidine (valerianine) and naphthyridylmethylketone have been found as well as several other, yet unidentified, alkaloids [40–47]. Furthermore, isoferulic acid, γ-aminobutyric acid, free fatty acids and short-chain carboxylic acids have been isolated [2,48]. In the leaves of *V. officinalis*, the presence of four flavonoids has also been demonstrated [49]. From the roots of *V. wallichii*, two isomers of lanarine isovalerianate and 4-methoxy-8-pentyl-1-naphtolic acid have been isolated [50–52].

The differences in secondary metabolites between the three medicinally used *Valeriana* species imply that the pharmaceuticals prepared from the respective crude drugs also largely differ with regard to their chemical composition. In spite of that, legal demands do not exist on this point. However, several manufacturers have standardised their products either on valepotriates or on valerenic acid derivatives. Valerian preparations with a standardised valepotriate content are mostly prepared from *V. wallichii* and *V. edulis* because these species are relatively rich in valepotriates [53]. Those standardised on valerenic acid derivatives are made from *V. officinalis*.

Another important factor is the dosage form. When a herbal tea was prepared by extraction of valerian root with hot water, up to 60% of the valepotriates remained in the root material and only 0.1% could be recovered from the tea [54]. In another study using roots of *V. officinalis*, no valepotriates could be detected in the tea, whereas valerenic acid derivatives were present [24]. This leads to the conclusion that teas from *V. officinalis* root will be practically devoid of baldrinals [24,33,54]. For other valerian species (that are not commonly used in the form of a tea) no data are available on this point. However, as *V. wallichii* and *V. edulis* contain considerabley higher amounts of valepotriates than *V. officinalis*, it cannot be assumed that a tea prepared from *V. wallichii* and *V. edulis* will also be devoid of baldrinals.

Valerian tablets and capsules contained small amounts (≤ 1 mg) baldrinal a piece [24,33,54]. Tinctures prepared from *V. officinalis* were devoid of valepotriates already within three weeks after preparation, due to the low stability of these compounds in ethanolic solutions [24,31,54]. In view of this rapid degradation, it is surprising that no baldrinals could be recovered from commercially available tincture samples [24,33]. It is assumed that the baldrinals react further to form condensation products with other constituents from the tincture.

Pharmacology and Uses

Valerian root has already been used by the Greek and the Roman physicians as a diuretic, anodyne and spasmolytic agent. In the 17th century it was used to treat epilepsy. Its current use as a mild sedative dates back to the 18th century [48,55]. Valerian has often been used in conjunction with bromides, chloral hydrate, and phenobarbital, in the treatment of hysteria and other nervous conditions. It has also been used as a carminative [56]. Valepotriates have been applied to influence psychovegetative and psychosomatic disorders in cases of restlessness, agony and tension, as well as lack of concentration [3].

Nowadays, valerian preparations are used primarily to treat light forms of neurasthenia and emotional stress [57]. Further indications are disturbances in falling asleep and cramping pains in the gastro-intestinal tract, as a consequence of tension [3]. *V. wallichii* is used in Ayurvedic medicine [58], e.g. as a sedative.

In the past decades numerous studies have been directed to the pharmacology of valerian extracts and their isolated constituents, as reviewed in [32]. Originally, the essential oil and especially its constituents bornyl acetate and bornyl isovalerate were held responsible for the mild sedative properties of valerian preparations [59] but later this did not appear to account for the entire action of the drug. Although several alkaloids from valerian root have been found to exhibit sedative effects in rats [40,60–62], they are unlikely to play a significant role in the biological activity of valerian preparations because of their very low concentrations. Aqueous extracts of valerian roots only showed a sedative effect in laboratory animals at extreme doses [1].

After the characterization and demonstration of the biological activity of the valepotriates in the late 1960s and early 1970s, many investigators focused their attention on these substances. A mixture of various valepotriates, as present in an extract of *V. wallichii*, was found to have sedative properties in mice [63]. In addition, a spasmolytic effect of valepotriates on smooth muscle of the guinea pig was described [64,65]. A decrease of spontaneous locomotor activity of mice has also been noticed after administration of valepotriates [66,67]. In the perfused rat brain, changes in the electroencephalogram (EEG) have been found which were induced by valepotriates [68]. However, following oral administration of valepotriates, only a small fraction is absorbed. Therefore, no evidence exists that pharmacologically relevant concentrations are reached in the central nervous system after oral ingestion [3]. In a neurophysiological study with cats that were given valepotriates or valerian extract orally, no changes in the EEG were observed that could point to a central sedative effect. The muscle tonus of treated animals, however, became reduced [69]. It has been concluded by Krieglstein and co-workers [70,71] that valepotriates, valerenic acid, valeranone as well as the essential oil of valerian do not possess a central depressant action, because these substances were not found to induce a reduction of the glucose turn-over in the rat brain.

It has been demonstrated in the late 1950s and early 1960s that valerenic acid possesses spasmolytic properties and that valeranone has anticonvulsive, hypotensive and sedative effects [72–74]. Furthermore, the related species *Nardostachys jatamansi* DC., which was used in Asia for the treatment of nervous diseases, was shown to contain valeranone but lacked valepotriates. Later, the pharmacological properties of valeranone were confirmed, and valerenal and valerenic acid were also found to show central depressant and spasmolytic properties [75,76].

In the so-called 'syndrome test', in which a series of symptoms are observed in mice after administration of a test compound, a general depressant effect was found for several constituents of the essential oil of *V. officinalis* [75]. For valerenic acid, non-aspecific central depressant effects have been described following intraperitoneal administration to mice. At doses above 100 mg/kg body weight, effects were found in the rotarod test and in the traction test. Spontaneous locomotor activity of mice was reduced by a dose of 50 mg/kg of valerenic acid. At this dose a prologation of the barbiturate-induced sleeping time was found as well [76].

The psychotropic effects of "Hokkai-Kisso", i.e. roots of Japanese valerian, were compared with those of diazepam and imipramine. An orally administered ethanolic extract of valerian roots prolonged the hexobarbital-induced sleep, and decreased spontaneous ambulation in mice. In addition, the extract reversed reserpine-induced hypothemia in mice. These results indicate that valerian extract acts on the central nervous system and may be an antidepressant [77].

In another Japanese study, a correlation between the contents of the valepotriates and the pharmacological activity of various valerian roots was examined. Nepalese and Chinese valerian roots containing an appreciable quantity of valepotriates showed no sedative activity, while Japanese valerian roots containing less valepotriates inhibited stress-induced ulcer formation and prolonged hexobarbital-induced sleep in mice. When an extract of "Hokkai-Kisso" was fractionated and the effect of each of the fractions on the enhancement of hexobarbital-induced anesthesia was tested, kessyl glycol diacetate, kessyl glycol 8-acetate and kessyl glycol 2-acetate were obtained as active principles. The enhancement of hexobarbital-induced anesthesia by kessyl glycol diacetate was assumed to be due to its inhibitory effect on the central nervous system. However, kessyl glycol diacetate exhibited no inhibitory action on the stress-induced ulcer production [78].

Derivatives of kessoglycol, kessoglycol 2-acetate-8-acylates, kessoglycol 8-acylates, and kessoglycol 2,8-diacylates were prepared in order to examine their sedative effects in mice comparing with those of kessoglycol 2,8-diacetate. Using prolongation of hexobarbital-induced sleeping time, a structure-activity relationship of these compounds could not be established [79]. Kessoglycol 8-monoacetate had a sedative action and was more potent than kessoglycol diacetate [80].

In vitro, valerenic acid inhibited of the metabolism of the neurotransmitter γ-aminobutyric acid (GABA). This finding could be of interest for the *in vivo* situation, since high concentrations of GABA result in a depression of the central nervous system [81]. In another *in vitro* study directed to the interaction with GABA receptors in the rat brain, both the hydroalcoholic and the aqueous total extracts obtained from the roots of *V. officinalis* as well as the aqueous fraction derived from the hydroalcoholic extract showed affinity for the GABA-A receptor. This activity could be correlated to the sesquiterpenes or valepotriates. The lipophilic fraction of the hydroalcoholic extract as well as didrovaltrate showed affinity for the barbiturate receptor and, even if to a lesser extent, for peripheral benzodiazepine receptors. Apparently, the interaction of unknown constituents, present in total extracts, with GABA-A receptors may represent a molecular basis for the sedative effect observed both in man and experimental animals [82]. It has been shown that an aqueous extract of subterranean parts of *V. officinalis* induced the release of [^{3}H]-GABA in rat brain synaptosomes through the GABA-carrier by an exchange process [83,84]. It should be added, however, that the relevance of these *in vitro* data for the situation *in vivo* remains to be proven.

Recently, a commercially available valerian root extract prepared from *V. officinalis* and standardized on valerenic acid was shown to produce a moderate, dose-related sedation in mice following oral adminstration. Reduction in motility and an increase in the thiopental-induced sleeping-time were used as parameters and compared with diazepam and chlorpromazine. The extract showed only weak anticonvulsive properties [85].

Valerian root oil and pure volatile compounds (borneol, isoborneol, bornyl acetate and isobornyl acetate) are also used in aromatherapy. It has been suggested that a sedative effect, may arise from inhalation of the monoterpenes, but the only evidence for this comes from animal experiments [86].

In several clinical studies good results have been obtained with various valerian preparations, including mild sedation, decreased perceived sleep latencies and awakenings, and improved sleep [87-97]. It should, however, be noted that in general the quality of these studies was suboptimal, and that the exact chemical composition of the preparation used was often not clear.

Despite the fact that extensive research has been conducted on valerian, it is still unclear which compound(s) is (are) responsible for its sedative action [24,32]. It has been suggested that a combination of constituents is responsible for the effect and that degradation products of genuine constituents could also play a role [98]. However, it has been concluded by Hazelhoff [99] that the reputed tranquillizing effect of valerian preparations could be totally or primarily due to a peripheral effect (viz. spasmolysis) rather than to a real central effect [71].

Next to sedative and spasmolytic proporties, several other biological activities of *V. wallichii* are worth mentioning. An aqueous leaf extract showed antipyretic activity in rats [100]. The root oil of this plant possessed a weak antimicrobial and antimycotic effect [101]. In China, patients infected with *Rotavirus enteritis* (causing heavy diarrhea in children) were successfully treated with a preparation made from the herb of *V. wallichii*. The antipyretic and antidiarrheal effect of the herb was significant within 72 hours after the start of the treatment [102].

Pharmacokinetics

Valepotriates show a poor gastrointestinal absorption after oral administration [103,104]. Following oral administration of valtrate/isovaltrate to mice, 2% was degraded to baldrinal. In contrast to the valepotriates, the degradation product homobaldrinal was absorbed fairly well following oral application to mice. As much as 71% of the administered dose could be recovered from the urine in the form of baldrinal glucuronide. Since no unchanged homobaldrinal could be demonstrated in body fluids or in liver samples following oral administration, the compound appears to undergo a substantial first-pass metabolism [33].

After oral, intravenous or intraduodenal administration to mice, didrovaltrate was absorbed to a small extent in the unchanged form. The main part, however, was converted into a polymeric degradation product [105].

Adverse Reaction Profile

General Animal Data

Data on the toxicity of isolated constituents of valerian are confined to the mouse. After intraperitoneal injection the LD_{50} was 64 mg/kg body weight for valtrate, 125 mg/kg for didrovaltrate and 150 mg/kg for acevaltrate. Following oral administration no acute toxicity of valtrate, didrovaltrate and acevaltrate was found at doses up to 4600 mg/kg [63]. Valerenic acid, injected intraperitoneally, induced cramps at 150–200 mg/kg, while heavy convulsions were seen at 400 mg/kg. The latter dose appeared to be lethal at last [76].

General Human Data

No significant adverse reactions or side effects have been reported as a result of normal medication with valerian drugs [1,106]. The same was found in the clinical studies performed with valerian extracts, so far. The acute toxicity of valerian preparations is considered to be very low. However, studies directed to subchronical and chronical toxicity are still lacking and such studies are certainly warranted, especially because valepotriates and their degradation products, the baldrinals, may be capable of causing undesired effects (see under Mutagenicity and Carcinogenicity). In particular when valerian preparations are taken for a longer period of time, the absence of chronic risk data should be considered.

Allergic Reactions

Drugs that contain volatile oil may, in principle, cause allergy [3]. Allergic reactions have, however, never been described for *Valeriana* species.

Cardiovascular Reactions

At high doses, valerian is said to cause disturbance of the cardiac function [107] but no original references are given to support this.

Central Nervous System Reactions

Roth et al. [107] list several reactions of the central nervous system. However, original reference entries are not given. At high doses, valerian could cause depression of the central nervous system. Valerian oil may cause a reduced excitability of the brain and of the spinal cord. Light stupefaction may be caused by isovaleric acid. Furthermore, addiction to valerian, accompanied with headache, agitation, restlessness, insomnia and, probably as a secondary effect, disturbance of the cardiac function, is mentioned. However, there is insufficient evidence for providing valerian preparations – unless they provide a substantial amount of alcohol – with a warning label that they may affect driving ability [108], and a risk of addiction to valerian preparations is not documented.

Gastrointestinal Reactions

Because of the contact of the valepotriates and baldrinals with the gastrointestinal tract, a local mutagenic effect may not be excluded [33] (see also under Mutagenicity and Carcinogenicity).

According to Roth et al. [107], inhibition of the tonus and motility of the bowels has been found in frogs and rabbits, but no original references are cited.

Hematological Reactions

Cytotoxic effects of valepotriates with an epoxide moiety have been described on mouse bone marrow early progenitor cells *in vitro* [109] but such effects have not been found *in vivo* [110]. The latter finding was ascribed to the fact that the distribution of these compounds via the circulation is small, due to the large first-pass effect.

Hepatic Reactions

Valerian-containing products have at times been associated with hepatotoxic reactions but such products contained other herbal ingredients which could have been responsible (notably skullcap) [111–113]. However, mutagenic effects on the liver by valepotriates and baldrinals cannot be excluded (see under Mutagenicity and Carcinogenicity).

Drug Interactions

Valerenic acid, valeranone, the essential oil and extracts of valerian root have been shown to increase the barbiturate-induced sleeping-time in mice [62, 63, 74, 76, 100, 114]. This may indicate that the effect of central nervous depressants is amplified by valerian constituents.

In rotarod tests in mice, the genuine mixture of valepotriates from valerian root acted antagonistically against the hypnotic effect of ethanol. Anesthesia by ethanol was somewhat prolonged by large doses of this mixture. Large doses of valtrate shortened the ethanol anesthesia, whereas larger doses of acevaltrate prolonged it [115]. An antagonizing effect of valtrate during ethanol narcosis was also found in rats [117].

One double-blind study with volunteers has been directed to a possibly synergistic effect of the simultaneous consumption of valepotriates and alcohol. Oral administration of a mixture of valepotriates (valtrate, acevaltrate and didrovaltrate, 200–400 mg) was followed by a dose-dependent increase in the ability to concentrate. In combination with ethanol an expected reduction of efficiency was not observed. Valtrate, tested as a separate compound, did not influence the height and course of the blood alcohol curves [117].

Fertility, Pregnancy, and Lactation

A literature search did not reveal data showing that valerian or its isolated constituents influence fertility. Valerian preparations are considered safe for use during pregnancy and lactation [57,118]. According to an Australian Government Publishing Service publication valerian is placed in category A; "Drugs which have been taken by a large number of pregnant women and women of childbearing age without an increase in the frequency of malformations or other direct or indirect harmful effects on the fetus having been observed" [119].

In a recent study the effects of a valepotriate mixture on mothers and progeny were evaluated in rats. A 30-day administration of valepotriates did not change the average of estral cycle nor the number of estrous phases during this period. Also, there were no changes in the fertility index. Fetotoxicity studies and external examination did not show differences, although internal examination revealed an increase in number of retarded ossification after the highest doses employed (12 and 24 mg/kg). No changes were detected in the development of the offspring after treatment during pregnancy. As for temperature, valepotriates caused a hypothermizant effect in the mother after administration by the intraperitoneal route but not after oral administration. Generally, the valepotriates employed induced some alterations after administration by the intraperitoneal route, but doses given orally were innocuous to pregnant rats and their offspring [120]. The level of baldrinals in the test material was not determined, however.

Mutagenicity and Carcinogenicity

The valepotriates possess alkylating properties, for which the epoxy group is responsible. Cytotoxic properties against *in vitro* cultured tumour cells have been described for valepotriates. The mechanism of the cytostatic action is supposed to be based on an interaction of the valepotriates with thiol-containing enzymes [121]. The cytotoxic effects of the valepotriates on cultured hepatoma cells are counterated by compounds with free SH groups, such as cysteine and glutathione [122]. In addition, valepotriates inhibited the synthesis of DNA and proteins [123]. Cytotoxic properties are also known for baldrinals [33,123,124].

Valtrate and didrovaltrate have shown to have a strong cytotoxic action towards cultured hepatoma cells. Compounds with a free thiol group (e.g. glutathione) were able to antagonize the cytotoxic effect of valepotriates. This indicates that intracellular biological nucleophiles are able to protect the cells against the deleterious effects of the valepotriates by covalent and non-covalent binding [122]. Valepotriates inhibited the synthesis of both DNA and proteins in hepatoma cells [125]. Using scanning and transmission electron microscopy, morphological changes of hepatoma cells (form, size and surface area) as well as intracellular ultrastructural changes were found after incubation with both valtrate and didrovaltrate [123].

Valtrate, isovaltrate and dihydrovaltrate were mutagenic in *Salmonella typhimurium* strain TA 100 and in two *Escherichia coli* strains in the presence of a metabolic activation system [125]. The degradation products baldrinal and homobaldrinal were already mutagenic in the *Salmonella* strains TA 98 and TA 100 without metabolic activation. These compounds also showed a direct genotoxic activity in the SOS-chromotest [33,111,125,126].

It is unclear to what extent these toxic effects are relevant for humans, after ingestion of valepotriate-containing preparations. As already stated, valepotriates are hardly absorbed in their original form. In the gastrointestinal tract, baldrinals and possibly polymers are formed from the valepotriates. Subsequently, the baldrinals are rapidly glucuronidated in the liver. The metabolites which originate at this point are not mutagenic [36]. However, due to the contact of the valepotriates and baldrinals with the stomach and intestinal wall, the gastrointestinal tract and the liver are the primary target organs which may be exposed to mutagenic effects [33]. This may especially be true when valerian preparations are taken over a longer period of time, as is done quite often [1]. As yet, there is a lack of long-term studies on this subject. Therefore, the possible risks can not be excluded [3]. In the meantime, it would be prudent to prefer valerian preparations which are devoid of potentially hazardous valepotriates or baldrinals [36,38].

References

1. Hänsel R (1990) Pflanzliche Sedativa. Z Phytother 11:14–19
2. Bos R, Woerdenbag HJ, Hendriks H, Zwaving JH, Scheffer JJC, Wikström HV (1996) Seasonal variation of the essential oil, valerenic acid derivatives, and valepotriates in *Valeriana officinalis* roots. In preparation.
3. Steinegger E, Hänsel R (1992) Pharmakognosie, 5th edn. Berlin: Springer-Verlag, pp. 162–163, pp. 666–671
4. Penso G (1983) Index Plantarum Medicinalium Totius Mundi Eorumque Synonymorum. Milano: Organizzazione Editoriale Medico Farmaceutica, pp. 986–987
5. Evans WC (1989) Trease and Evans' Pharmacognosy, 13th ed. London: Baillière Tindall, pp. 525–528
6. Hendriks H, Bos R (1984) Essential oils of some *Valerianaceae*. Dragoco Rep (English ed.) 1:3–17
7. Bos R, Van Putten FMS, Hendriks H, Mastenbroek C (1986) Variations in the essential oil content and composition in individual plants obtained after breeding experiments with a

Valeriana officinalis strain. In: Brunke E-J, ed. Progress in Essential Oil Research. Berlin: Walter de Gruyter & Co., pp. 123–130
8. Hendriks H, Smith D, Hazelhoff B (1977) Eugenyl isovalerate and isoeugenyl isovalerate in the essential oil of Valerian root. Phytochemistry 16:1853–1854
9. Hazelhoff B, Smith D, Malingré ThM, Hendriks H (1979) The essential oil of *Valeriana officinalis* L. s.l. Pharm Weekbl 114:443–449
10. Hendriks H, Bruins AP (1980) Study of three types of essential oil of *Valeriana officinalis* L. s.l. by combined gaschromatographynegative ion chemical ionization mass spectrometry J Chromatogr 190:321–330
11. Bos R, Woerdenbag HJ, Hendriks H, Malingré TM (1992) Der indische oder pakistanische Baldrian. Z Phytother 13:26–34
12. Narayanan CS, Kulkarni KS, Viadya AS, Kanthamani S, Lakshmi Kumari G (1964) Components of indian Valerian root oil. Tetrahedron 20:963–968
13. Krepinsky J, Herout V, Sorm F (1959) Vergleichende Untersuchungen von Droge und von stabilisierten frischen Wurzelstöcken; Nachweis alphakessylalcohol in europäischem Baldrian. Collection Czech Chem Commun 24:1884–1896
14. Stoll A, Seebeck E, Stauffacher D (1957) Isolierung und Charakterisierung von bisher unbekannten Inhaltsstoffen aus dem Neutralteil des frischen Baldrians. Helv Chim Acta 136:1205–1229
15. Govindachari TR, Rajadurai S, Pai BR (1958) Struktur von Jatamanson Chem Ber 91:908–910
16. Hikino H, Hikino Y, Takeshita Y, Shirata K, Takemoto T (1963) The structure kessan, kessanol, valeranol, kanokonol, valeranone and kanokonol. Chem Pharm Bull 11:547;952;1207–1210;1210–1212
17. Rücker G, Kretzschmar U (1972) Patchouli-Alkohol und β-Patchoulen aus *Nardostachys chinensis* Planta Med 21:1–4
18. Hikino H, Hikino Y, Agatsuma K, Takemoto T (1968) Structure and absolute configuration of Faurinone. Chem Pharm Bull 16:1779–1783
19. Bos R, Hendriks H, Kloosterman J, Sipma G (1983) A structure of faurinone, a sesquiterpene ketone isolated from *Valeriana officinalis*. Phytochemistry 22:1505–1506
20. Woerdenbag HJ, Bos R, Scheffer JJC (1996) Valerian: quality assurance of the crude drug and its preparations. In: Houghton P, ed. Valerian. Medicinal and Aromatic Plants – Industrial Profiles. Amsterdam: Harwood Academic Publishers, in press
21. Suzuki H, Zhang BC, Harada M, Iida O, Satake M (1993) Quantitative studies on terpenes of Japanese and European valerians. Shoyakugaku Zasshi 47:305–310
22. Thies PW, Funke S (1966) Nachweis und Isolierung von sedativ wirksamen Isovaleriansäureestern aus Wurzeln und Rhizomen von verschiedenen Valeriana- und Kentranthus-Arten. Tetrahedron Lett 11:1155–1162
23. Thies PW (1966) Zur Konstitution der Isovalerensäureester Valepotriat, Acetoxyvalepotriat und Dihydrovalepotriat. Tetrahedron Lett 11:1163–1170
24. Bos R, Woerdenbag HJ, Hendriks H, Zwaving JH, De Smet PAGM, Tittel G, Wikström HV, Scheffer JJC (1996) Analytical aspects of phytotherapeutic valerian preparations. Phytochemical Analysis. 7:143–151
25. Wienschierz HJ (1978) Erfahrungen bei der Kultivierung von *Valeriana wallichi* (DC) in der Bundesrepublik Deutschland. Acta Horticulturae 73:315–321
26. Thies PW (1968) Die Konstitution der Valepotriate. Tetrahedron 24:313–347
27. Lorens M (1989) Untersuchungen zur Domestikation der mexikanischen Medizinalpflanze *Valeriana edulis* ssp. procera "Meyer". Technischen Universität München. Dissertation. Freising-Weihenstephan, Lehrstuhl für Gemüsebau
28. Funke ED, Friedrich H (1974) Valepotriate in oberirdischen und unterirdischen Organen von Valerianaceen. Phytochemistry 13:2023–2024
29. Hölzl J, Jurcic K (1975) Valepotriates in the leaves of *Valeriana jatamansi*. Planta Med 27:133–139

30. Funke ED, Friedrich H (1975) Valepotriate in oberirdischen Organen weiterer Arten der Valerianaceen. Planta Med 28:215–224
31. Petričič J (1979) Stability and estimation of valerian (Radix Valerianae) constituents. Acta Pharm Jugoslav 29:23–28
32. Houghton PJ (1988) The biological activity of valerian and related plants. J Ethnopharmacol 22:121–142
33. Dieckmann H (1988) Untersuchungen zur Pharmakokinetik, Metabolismus und Toxikologie von Baldrinalen. Dissertation. Berlin: Freie Universität
34. Bos R, Hendriks H, Bruins AP, Kloosterman J, Sipma G (1986) Isolation and identification of valerenane sesquiterpenoids from *Valeriana officinalis*. Phytochemistry 25:133–135
35. Hänsel R, Schulz J (1982) Valerensäuren und Valerenal als Leitstoffe des offizinellen Baldrians. Dtsch Apoth Ztg 122:215–219
36. Hänsel R (1992) Indischer Baldrian nicht empfehlenswert? Z Phytother 13:130–131
37. Bauer R, Czygan FCh, Franz G, Ihrig M, Nahrstedt A, Sprecher E (1994) Pharmazeutische Qualität, Standardisierung und Normierung von Phytopharmaka. Z Phytother 15:82–91
38. De Smet PAGM, Vulto AG (1988) Drugs used in non-orthodox medicine. In: Dukes MNG, Beely L (eds) Side Effects of Drugs – Annual 12. Amsterdam: Elsevier, 402–415
39. Schimmer O, Röder A (1992) Valerenic acid in commercial plant drugs and extracts prepared from the roots of *Valeriana officinalis* L. s.l. TLC studies using the guidelines of the German Pharmacopoeia. Pharm Ztg Wiss 137:31–36
40. Borkowski B, Lutomski J (1961) Die Gewinnung von Alkaloiden aus der getrockneten Wurzeln und Wurzelstöcken von *Valeriana officinalis* L. Pharm Zentralhalle 100:575–584
41. Torssell K, Wahlberg K (1967) Isolation, structure and synthesis of alkaloids from *Valeriana officinalis* L. Acta Chem Scand 21:53–62
42. Franck B, Petersen U, Hübner F (1970) Valerianin, ein tertiäres Monoterpen-Alkaloid aus Baldrian. Angew Chemie 82:875–876
43. Gross D, Edner G, Schütte HR (1971) Über monoterpenoide Valeriana-Alkaloide. Arch Pharm 304:19–27
44. Johnson RD, Waller GR (1971) Isolation of actinidine from *Valeriana officinalis*. Phytochemistry 10:3335–3339
45. Cionga E, Popesco V, Contz O, Boniforti L (1976) The alkaloids from *Valeriana officinalis*: identification of actinidine. Adv Mass Spectr Biochem 1:299–302
46. Buckova A, Eisenreichova E, Haladova M, Tomko J (1977) Alkaloids of the underground part of *Valeriana officinalis* L. Acta Fac Pharm 31:29–35
47. Janot MM, Guilhem J, Contz O, Verena G, Cionga E (1979) Contribution to the study of Valeriana alkaloids (*Valeriana officinalis* L.): Actinidine and naphthyridylmethylketone, new alkaloids. Ann Pharm Fr 37:413–420
48. Stoll A, Seebeck E (1957) Die Isolierung von Hesperitinsäure, Beheensäure und von zwei unbekannten Säuren aus Baldrian. Liebigs Ann Chem 603:158–168
49. Greger H, Ernet D (1971) Flavonoide und Systematik der Valerianaceae. Naturwissenschaften 58:416–417
50. Thies PW (1968) Über die Wirkstoffe des Baldrians; Linarin-isovalerianat, ein bisher unbekanntes Flavonoid aus *Valeriana wallichii* DC. Planta Med 16:361–371
51. Chari VM, Jardan M, Wagner H, Thies PW (1977) A ^{13}C-NMR study of the structure of an acyl-linarin from *Valeriana wallichii*. Phytochemistry 16:1110–1112
52. Pande A, Shukla YN (1993) Naphthoic acid derivative from *Valeriana wallichii* Phytochemistry 1993 5 1350–1351
53. Wichtl M (1989) Teedrogen, 2nd edn. Stuttgart: Wissenschaftliche Verlagsgesellschaft mbH, pp. 79–82
54. Hänsel R, Schulz J (1985) Beitrag zur Qualitätssicherung von Baldrianextrakten. 4. Mitt. Pharm Ind 47:531–533
55. Madaus G (1976) Lehrbuch der biologischen Heilmittel. Hildesheim: Georg Olms Verlag, pp. 2770–2777

56. Reynolds JEF, Prasad AB (ed) 1982 Martindale The Extra Pharmacopoeia. 28th edn. London: The Pharmaceutical Press, pp. 1768
57. Anonymous (1993) Farmacotherapeutisch Kompas. Amstelveen: Ziekenfondsraad, p.13
58. Kapoor LD (1990) CRC Handbook of Ayurvedic Medicinal Plants. Boca Raton: CRC Press, p. 330
59. Gstirner F, Kleinbauer E (1958) Zur pharmakologischen Prüfung der Baldrianwurzel. Pharmazie 13:415–436
60. Rabbeno A (1930) Sull' azione farmacologica del pirrole e dei pirrilalchilchetoni Nota III Richerche sul sistema nervoso isolato. Arch Int Pharmacodyn 36:172–204
61. Cionga E (1961) Betrachtung über die Baldrianwurzel. Pharmazie 16:43–44
62. Sándor P, Kovách AGB, Horváth KB, Szentpétery GB, Clauder O (1970) Pharmakologische Untersuchungen über die Wirkung von synthetischen α-Methyl-pyrryl-keton auf das Zentralnervensystem und den Kreislauf. Arzneimittelforsch 20:29–32
63. Von Eickstedt KW, Rahman S (1969) Psychopharmakologische Wirkungen von Valepotriaten. Arzneimittelforsch 19:316–319
64. Wagner H, Jurcic K (1979) Über die spasmolytische Wirkung des Baldrians. Planta Med 37:84–95
65. Hazelhoff B, Malingré TM, Meijer DKF (1982) Antispasmodic effects of *Valeriana* compounds. Arch Pharmacodyn Ther 257:274–87
66. Wagner H, Jurcic K, Schaette R (1980) Vergleichende Untersuchungen über die sedierende Wirkung von Baldrianextrakten, Valepotriaten und ihren Abbauprodukten. Planta Med 38:358–65
67. Hölzl J, Fink C (1984) Untersuchungen zur Wirkung der Valepotriate auf die Spontanmotilität von Mäusen. Arzneim Forsch/Drug Res 34:44–47
68. Fink C, Hölzl J, Rieger H, Krieglstein J (1984) Wirkungen von Valtrat auf das EEG des isoliert-perfundierten Rattenhirns. Arzneim Forsch/Drug Res 34:170–174
69. Holm E, Kowollik H, Reinecke A, von Henning GE, Behne F, Scherer HD (1980) Vergleichende neurophysiologische Untersuchungen mit Valtratum/Isovaltratum und Extractum Valerianae an Katzen. Med Welt 31:982–990
70. Krieglstein J, Grusla D (1988) Zentral dämpfende Inhaltsstoffe im Baldrian. Dtsch Apoth Ztg 128:2041–2046
71. Grusla D, Hölzl J, Krieglstein J (1986) Baldrianwirkung im Gehirn der Ratte. Dtsch Apoth Ztg 126:2249–2252
72. Stoll A, Seebeck E, Stauffacher D (1957) Isolierung und Charakterisierung von bisher unbekannten Inhaltsstoffen aus dem Neutralteil des frischen Baldrians. Helv Chim Acta 136:1205–1229
73. Arora RB, Arora CK (1963) Hypotensive and tranquillizing activity of jatamansone (valeranone), a sesquiterpene from *Nardostachys jatamansi* DC. Proceedings of the 2nd Int. Pharmacol. Meeting, Prague. Oxford: Pergamon Press, pp. 51–60
74. Rücker G, Tautges J, Sieck A, Wenzl H, Graf E (1978) Untersuchungen zur Isolierung und pharmakodynamischen Aktivität des Sesquiterpens Valeranon aus *Nardostachys jatamansi* DC. Arzneimittelforsch 28:7–13
75. Hendriks H, Bos R, Allersma DP, Malingré TM, Koster AS (1981) Pharmacological screening of valerenal and other components of essential oil of *Valeriana officinalis*. Planta Med 42:62–68
76. Hendriks H, Bos R, Woerdenbag HJ, Koster AS (1985) Central nervous depressant activity of valerenic acid in the mouse. Planta Med 51:28–31
77. Sakamoto T, Mitani Y, Nakajima K (1992). Psychotropic effects of Japanese valerian root extracts. Chem Pharm Bull 40:758–761
78. Hikino H, Hikino Y, Kobinata H, Aizawa A (1980) Sedative principles of valeriana roots. Shoyakugaku Zasshi 34:19–24
79. Takamura K, Kawaguchi M, Nabata H (1975) The preparation and pharmacological screening of kessoglycol derivative. Yakugaku Zasshi 95:1198–1204

80. Takamura K, Nabata H, Kawaguchi M (1975) The pharmacological action on the kessoglycol 8-monoacetate. Yakugaku Zasshi 95:1205–1209
81. Riedel E, Hänsel R, Ehrke G (1982) Hemmung des γ-Aminobuttersäureabbaus durch Valerensäurederivate. Planta Med 46:219–220
82. Mennini T, Bernasconi P, Bombardelli E, Morazzoni P (1993) In vitro study on the interaction of extracts and pure compounds from *Valeriana officinalis* roots with GABA, benzodiazepine and barbiturate receptors in rat brain. Fitoterapia 64:291–300
83. Santos MS, Ferreira F, Faro C, Rires E, Carvalho AP, Cunha AP, Macedo T (1994) The amount of GABA present in aqueous extracts of valerian is sufficient to account for [^{3}H]GABA release in Synaptosomes. Planta Med 60:475–476
84. Santos MS, Ferreira F, Cunha AP, Carvalho AP, Macedo T (1994) An aqueous extract of valerian influences the transport of GABA in synaptosomes. Planta Med 60:278–279
85. Leuschner J, Müller J, Rudmann M (1993) Characterisation of the central nervous depressant activity of a commercially available valerian root extract. Arzneim Forsch/Drug Res 43:638–641
86. Buchbauer G, Jäger W, Jirovetz L, Meyer F, Dietrich H (1992) Wirkungen von Baldrianöl, Borneol, Isoborneol, Bornylacetat und Isobornylacetat auf die Mobilität von Versuchstieren (Mäusen) nach Inhalation. Pharmazie 47:620–622
87. Standl R (1968) Untersuchungen mit einem aus der Baldrianwurzel gewonnenen Wirkstoff zur Sedierung von Zerebralsklerotikern. Z Geront 1:188–192
88. Dziuba K (1968) Erfahrungen mit dem Aequilans Valmane in ambulanter Praxis. Med Welt 35:1866–1868
89. Straube G (1968) Die Bedeutung der Baldrianwurzel in der Therapie. Therapie Gegenwart 4:555–562
90. Buchthala M (1968) Klinische Beobachtungen bei der Anwendung eines neuen Aequilans. Hippokrates 12:466–468
91. Hübler B (1969) Erfahrungen mit dem Aequilibrans Valmane als Zusatztherapeutikum bei vertabragenen Erkrankungen. Der Landarzt 45:1591–1594
92. Jauch H (1969) Valmane in der Geriatrie. Med Klin 64:437–439
93. Jansen W (1977) Doppelblindstudie mit Baldrisedon. Therapiewoche 27:2779–2786
94. Leathwood PD, Chauffard F, Heck E, Munoz-Box R (1982) Aqueous extract of valerian root (*Valeriana officinalis* L.) improves sleep quality in man. Pharmacol Biochem Behav 17:65–71
95. Leathwood PD, Chauffard F, Munoz-Box R (1983) Effect of *Valeriana officinalis* L. on subjective and objective sleep parameters. In: Sleep 1983. 6th Eur Congr Sleep Res. Basel: Karger, pp. 402–405
96. Lindahl O, Lindwall L (1989) Double blind study of a valerian preparation. Pharmacol Biochem Behav 32:1065–1066
97. Dreßing H, Riemann D, Löw H, Schredl M, Reh C, Laux P, Müller WE (1992) Baldrian-Melisse-Kombinationen versus Benzodiazepin, bei Schlafstörungen gleichwertig? Therapiewoche 42:726–736
98. Weiß RF (1990) Lehrbuch der Phytotherapie, 7th edn. Stuttgart: Hippokrates Verlag, pp. 350–354
99. Hazelhoff B (1984) Phytochemical and pharmacological aspects of valerian compounds with special reference to valepotriates. (Dissertation) Groningen: Rijksuniversiteit Groningen
100. Shrivastava SC, Sisodia CS (1970) Analgetic studies on *Vitex negundo* and *Valeriana wallichii*. Ind Vet J 47:170–175
101. Girgune JB, Jain NK, Grag BD (1980) Antimicrobial activity of the essential oil from *Valeriana wallichii* D.C. (Valerianaceae). Ind J Microbiol 20:142–143
102. Chen S, Xie X, Du B, Su Q, Wei Q, Wang Y, Li H, Wang Z, Wang Y, Cheng S, Pang Q, Wan X, Xu W, Wang C (1984) Infantile rotavirus enteritis treated with herbal *Valeriana jatamansi* (VJ). J Trad Chin Med 4:297–300

103. Schultz OE, Müller F (1960) Untersuchungen über Baldrian-Wirkstoffe mit dem Test nach Haffner. Arzneim Forsch/Drug Res 10:78–88
104. Takamura K, Kawaguchi M, Nabata H (1975) The preparation and pharmacological screening of kessoglycol derivative. Yakugaku Zasshi 95:1198–1204
105. Wagner H, Jurcic K (1980) In-vitro und in-vivo Metabolismus von ^{14}C-Didrovaltrat. Planta Med 38:366–376
106. Houghton P (1994) Valerian. Pharm J 253:95–96
107. Roth L, Daunderer M, Korman K (1984) Giftpflanzen – Pflanzengifte. Landsberg, München: Ecomed Verlagsgesellschaft mbH, pp. IV–1 V4–5
108. KNMP-Werkgroep Rijvaardigheid (1990) Geneesmiddelen en verkeersveiligheid. In: De Smet PAGM, Van Loenen AC, Offerhaus L, Van der Does E (eds). Medicatiebegeleiding. De medisch-farmaceutische achtergronden van verantwoord geneesmiddelengebruik. Houten: Bohn Stafleu Van Loghum, pp. 352–366
109. Tortarolo M, Braun R, Hübner GE, Maurer HR (1982) In vitro effects of epoxide-bearing valepotriates on mouse early hematopoietic progenitor cells and human T-lymphocytes. Arch Toxicol 51:37–42
110. Von der Hude W, Scheutwinkel-Reich M, Braun R, Dittmar W (1985) In vitro mutagenicity of valepotriates. Arch Toxicol 56:267–71
111. Miskelly F G, Goodyer LI (1992) Hepatic and pulmonary complications of herbal medicines. Postgrad Med J 68:935
112. Shepherd C (1993) Sleep disorders. Liver damage warning with insomnia remedy. Br Med J 306:1472
113. McGregor FB, Abernethy VE, Dahabra S, Cobden I, Hayes PC (1989) Hepatoxicity of herbal remedies. Br Med J 299:1156–1157
114. Takamura K, Kakimoto M, Kawaguchi M, Iwasaki T (1973) Pharmacological studies on the constituents of crude drugs and plants. I: Pharmacological action of *Valeriana officinalis*. J Pharm Soc Japan 93:599–606
115. Von Eickstedt KW, Rahman S (1969) Die Beeinflussung der Alkohol-Wirkung durch Valepotriate. Arzneim Forsch/Drug Res 19:995–997
116. Bräckow R, Von Eickstedt KW, Kühne U (1972) Beeinflussung der Aethanol-Narkose und des Aethanol-Blutspiegels durch Chlorprozamin und Valtratum. Arzneim Forsch/Drug Res 22:1977–1980
117. Mayer B, Springer E (1974) Psychoexperimentelle Untersuchungen zur Wirkung einer Valepotriatkombination sowie zur kombinierten Wirkung von Valtratum und Alkohol. Arzneim Forsch/Drug Res 24:2066–2070
118. Berglund F, Flodh H, Lundborg P, Prame B, Sannerstedt R (1984) Drug use during pregnancy and breast feeding. A classification system for drug information. Acta Obstet Gynecol Scand Suppl 126:1–55
119. Australian Drug Evaluation Committee (1989) Medicines in pregnancy. An Australian catagorization of risk. Canberra: Australian Governement Publishing Service.
120. Tufik S, Fujita K, De Lourdes Ventura Seabra M, Lobo LL (1994) Effects of a prolonged administration of valepotriates in rats on the mothers and their offspring. J Ethnopharmacol 41:39–44
121. Becker H, Chavedej S (1988) Valepotriates: production by plant cell cultures. In: Bajaj YPS, Biotechnology in Agriculture and Forestry, Vol. 4. Medical and Aromatic Plants I. Berlin, Springer-Verlag, pp. 294–309
122. Keochanthala-Bounthanh C, Haag-Berrurier M, Beck JP, Anton R (1990) Effects of thiol compounds versus cytotoxicity of valepotriates on cultured hepatoma cells. Planta Med 56:190–192
123. Keochanthala-Bounthanh C, Beck JP, Haag-Berrurier M, Anton R (1993) Effects of two monoterpene esters, valtrate and didrovaltrate, isolated from *Valeriana wallichii*, on the ultrastructure of hepatoma cells in culture. Phytother Res 7:124–127

125. Von der Hude W, Scheutwinkel-Reich M, Braun R (1986) Bacterial mutagenicity of the tranquilizing constituents of Valerianaceae roots. Mut Res 169:23–27
126. Bounthanh C, Bergmann C, Beck JP, Haag-Berrurier M, Anton R (1981) Valepotriates, a new class of cytotoxic and antitumor agents. Planta Med 41:21–28

Yohimbe Alkaloids – General Discussion

P.A.G.M. De Smet

Botany

General
Yohimbine and related indole alkaloids occur in a number of botanical species. Their presence in the rubiaceous genera of *Corynanthe* and *Pausinystalia* will be reviewed in separate contributions to this volume.

Yohimbine
Yohimbine is also found in several apocynaceous plants, such as *Aspidosperma quebracho-blanco* Schlecht., *Diplorhynchus condylocarpon* Pich., *Lochnera lancea* K.Schum., *Rauwolfia* spp. and *Vinca* spp. [1–3]. At one time, the reputed aphrodisiac action of *Alchornea floribunda* Muell.Arg. (Euphorbiaceae) was also attributed to yohimbine but careful follow-up analysis showed that this alkaloid is absent [4]. It was subsequently discovered that this latter plant contains the alkaloids alchorneine, isoalchorneine and alchorneinone [5,6].

Rauwolscine
Rauwolscine has also been isolated from *Rauwolfia canescens* L. [7].

Raubasine
Raubasine also occurs in *Rauwolfia serpentina* (L.) Benth. and *Vinca rosea* L. [8].

Chemistry

General
Yohimbe alkaloids can be divided on the basis of their structural skeleton into four categories, namely yohimbane, heteroyohimbane, corynane, and corynoxane alkaloids (Table 1).

Yohimbine belongs to the yohimbane derivatives. As this alkaloid has five asymmetric centers in its molecule, extensive isomerism can arise; several of the resulting isomers are found in nature (Table 2).

Table 1. Classification of yohimbe alkaloids according to their basic structural skeleton [1,2]

Basic skeleton	Examples
Yohimbane	yohimbine and its isomers (see Table 2)
Heteroyohimbane	raubasine*
Corynane	corynantheine, corynantheidine
Corynoxane	corynoxeine, corynoxine

* Raubasine is also known as ajmalicine, δ-yohimbine and tetrahydroserpentine [9,10]

Table 2. Yohimbine and naturally occurring stereoisomers [2,11]

Type	Name	Synonyms
Normal	yohimbine	quebrachine, aphrodine, corynine
	corynanthine	rauhimbine
	β-yohimbine	amsonine
Pseudo	pseudoyohimbine	ψ-yohimbine
Allo	alloyohimbine	
	rauwolscine	α-yohimbine, corynanthidine, isoyohimbine, mesoyohimbine
Epiallo	epi-3-α-yohimbine	isorauhimbine, epi-3-rauhimbine

Yohimbine

Several pharmacological reports about yohimbine do not specify whether the studied dose levels refer to yohimbine base or to the hydrochloride of this alkaloid. However, as 1 mg of yohimbine HCl corresponds to 0.907 mg of the free base [12], there is a 10% difference between these two possibilities.

Pharmacology and Uses

General

Weitzell et al. [13] studied the effects of yohimbine and five of its stereoisomers on noradrenergic neurotransmission in the pulmonary artery of the rabbit. Yohimbine, rauwolscine (= α-yohimbine) and β-yohimbine preferentially blocked the presynaptic α_2-adrenoceptor, whereby rauwolscine was even more selective than yohimbine. In contrast, corynanthine preferentially blocked the postsynaptic α_1-adrenoceptor. The difference in selectivity was primarily due to much higher presynaptic potencies of yohimbine, rauwolscine and β-yohimbine; the postsynaptic potency of corynanthine was not very different from that of the other alkaloids. Pseudoyohimbine and 3-epi-α-yohimbine were very weak antagonists at either receptor. These two alkaloids have the same 3α-configuration as reserpine (contrary to the 3β-configuration of the other alkaloids) and they were found to share with reserpine an impairing action on the vesicular storage of norepinephrine.

Evidence for the α_2-selectivity of rauwolscine and β-yohimbine and the α_1-selectivity of corynanthine has also been presented in other papers [8,14–17]. In one of these studies, β-yohimbine and dihydrocorynantheine showed high affinity for the α-adrenoceptor; both alkaloids were half as potent in this respect as yohimbine. β-Yohimbine had similar α_2-blocking selectivity as yohimbine, whereas dihydrocorynantheine was a selective α_1-antagonist. Dihydrocorynantheine was a rather weak inhibitor, however, because its α_1-blocking potency was slightly lower than that of yohimbine. Neither β-yohimbine nor dihydrocorynantheine showed β-blocking activities [17].

Angel et al. [18] compared the affinities of yohimbine and rauwolscine for α_{2A}- and α_{2B}-adrenoceptors and concluded that both alkaloids are non-selective α_2-antagonists. Demichel et al. [8] evaluated the pre- and postsynaptic α-blocking effects of yohimbine, corynanthine and raubasine in the isolated vas deferens of the rat and found that the ratio of presynaptic/postsynaptic blocking potency declined in the following order: yohimbine > raubasine > corynanthine.

In an early study by Creveling and co-workers [19], yohimbine and corynanthine stimulated the release of norepinephrine from the mouse heart (thus causing depletion of cardiac norepinephrine), while corynantheine, pseudoyohimbine, rauwolscine, and β-yohimbine were inactive.

Lambert et al. [11] reported that rauwolscine and β-yohimbine were relatively strong competitive antagonists of serotonin in the isolated fundal strip of the rat, just like yohimbine, whereas corynanthine and pseudoyohimbine were less potent, non-competitive antagonists. All these yohimbine isomers only showed weak or very weak inhibition of monoamine oxidase, serotonin uptake, acetylcholinesterase, and cholinergic activity. In the conscious dog, the relative potencies of yohimbine isomers in causing excitatory behavioral and cardiovascular effects were rauwolscine > β-yohimbine > yohimbine. Pseudoyohimbine and corynanthine were completely inactive.

Yohimbine

Yohimbine is predominantly an α_2-adrenoceptor antagonist. In contrast to classic α-antagonists (such as phentolamine and phenoxybenzamine), it is much more active at presynaptic α_2-adrenoceptors than at postsynaptic vascular α_1-adrenoceptors. This selectivity makes it a useful pharmacological probe to study adrenergic innervation. By inhibition of central α_2-adrenoceptors, yohimbine increases central epinephrine and norepinephrine turnover and thus results in increased sympathetic outflow. This activity is reflected by an increase in plasma free 3-methoxy-4-hydroxyphenylethyleneglycol (MHPG), the major metabolite of brain norepinephrine [14,20–25].

In addition to these α_2-adrenoceptor antagonistic properties, yohimbine can also interact with α_1-adrenoceptors. At high concentrations, it may have antiserotonergic and antidopaminergic actions but it remains to be demonstrated whether any of its autonomic or behavioral effects can be attributed to such actions. Yohimbine may also show local anesthetic activity, acetylcholinesterase inhibition, monoamine oxidase inhibition, an antidiuretic action, and calcium channel blocking effects. However, such actions appear to contribute little to the principal pharmacological effects of yohimbine. In other words, when the alkaloid is used as a pharmacological probe, the assumption of α_2-adrenoceptor selectivity seems justified provided that appropriate doses are chosen [23,26–29].

Major effects of yohimbine in intact animals and in man are cardiovascular symptoms, such as increases in blood pressure and heart rate, and psychic symptoms, such as anxiety (see the Adverse Reaction Profile). These effects are localized to actions in the central nervous system. Because of its ability to provoke anxiety, yohimbine has been used as a pharmacological tool in a dog model for testing antianxiety and antidepressant drugs [23].

Yohimbine has a long history of being promoted as an aphrodisiac. In the United States, the alkaloid may be used without a prescription as a purported aphrodisiac under its street name "yo-yo". In 1985, US researchers reported its free availability in bulk form through mail-order. There is no evidence, however, that the alkaloid has any power to arouse or increase sexual desire [24]. Although it has been suggested that it increases sexual arousal, Charney and Heninger [30] did not observe any change in sexual drive following the administration of yohimbine HCl (30 mg p.o.) to healthy volunteers. In the nineteeneighties, several placebo-controlled trials were published to support the view that treatment with yohimbine HCl may be effective in male patients with organic and/or psychogenic impotence. Beneficial effects were only noted in part of the patients and a latency period of 2–3 weeks was observed between the onset of therapy and an improvement of erectile function [31–33]. According to the Advisory Panel on Urology of the USP Dispensing Information, yohimbine HCl can be used to treat erectile impotence in oral doses of 5.4–6 mg three times a day. If side effects occur, dosage may be reduced in half, followed by gradual increases. A dose of 10 mg three times a day may be appropriate in some patients, but this regimen may increase the incidence of side effects [29]. It is not yet universally accepted, however, that yohimbine is an efficacious agent for the treatment of male impotence [34–37].

Morales et al. [20,21] reported an unexpected beneficial effect of yohimbine in diabetic patients with impotence, who suffered from incapacitating paresthesia of the lower limbs; four of six patients reported prompt relief from this symptom after the start of yohimbine therapy.

Yohimbine may be beneficial in the treatment of patients with autonomic insufficiency, which occurs frequently in diabetes mellitus and amyloidosis and less commonly as primary disorder in older individuals. In this condition, the autonomic nervous system is unable to regulate the body's hemodynamic response to postural and other stresses, and this results in marked functional impairment, primarily manifested as orthostatic hypotension [38]. According to Ahmad and Watson [39], the use of yohimbine in autonomic disorders associated with chronic postural hypotension should be reserved for patients with resistant symptoms.

Acute administration of yohimbine HCl (14 mg p.o.) was found to increase salivary flow in healthy volunteers [40]. This effect was also seen following oral administration of 10 mg to depressed patients who were suffering from dry mouth because of their therapy with tricyclic antidepressants [41]. Yohimbine has also been proposed as treatment of orthostatic hypotension secondary to tricyclic antidepressant use [42].

The clinical usefulness of yohimbine in the treatment of obesity has been studied but conflicting results have been reported [43,44]. Recently, yohimbine was reported to induce lipid mobilization in obese subjects [45].

Yohimbine has been used as a local anesthetic in ophthalmology [3]. Instillation of a 1% solution into the rabbit eye produced anesthesia for about 30 min [46].

Rauwolscine
In early animal studies, rauwolscine had similar adrenergic blocking activity and local anesthetic activity as yohimbine [7,47,48]. In anesthetized animals, the alkaloid showed a central vasomotor depressant action [49] and caused a marked fall of peripheral resistance through vasodilatation without significantly altering cardiac output [50].

Corynanthine
Rockhold and Gross [51] found that corynanthine and rauwolscine decreased arterial blood pressure in anesthetized rats. Corynanthine was more effective than rauwolscine after intravenous administration whereas their relative effectiveness was reversed following intraventricular application. In other words, corynanthine appeared more active peripherally and less active centrally than rauwolscine.

Corynanthine failed to mimic certain neurochemical and behavioral effects of yohimbine (increase of the concentration of brain serotonin and dose-dependent decreases of spontaneous locomotion and body temperature), when given to rats at the same dose levels of 5–20 mg/kg intraperitoneally [52].

Serle et al. [53] found that corynanthine reduced intraocular pressure in rabbits without inducing tachyphylaxis when administered twice daily for six weeks. They subsequently tested the effects of topical corynanthine tartrate in humans with symmetrical ocular hypertension. Although a 2% solution significantly reduced intraocular pressure for at least 8 hours in a single-dose trial, no reduction of intraocular pressure was produced, when the 2% concentration was applied topically 2–3 times daily for a total of 3 weeks. It would thus appear that the clinical usefulness of the alkaloid as an antiglaucoma drug is probably limited.

Corynantheidine
Corynantheidine was found to have sympathicolytic activity in animal experiments, such as hypotensive effects and antagonism of epinephrine-induced hypertension in the anesthetized rabbit [54].

Raubasine
The adrenolytic and sympathicolytic properties of raubasine have been described by many authors [8,55,56]. The alkaloid has been used as a peripheral and cerebral vasodilator in doses that varied widely from 1 mg to 20 mg 3–4 times daily [10]. In France, the alkaloid is still available in the form of combination products, which also contain dihydroergocristine or almitrine [42]. An intravenous dose of 20 mg to healthy volunteers resulted in a decrease in peripheral vascular resistance, accompanied by an increase in stroke volume and cardiac output and by a slight rise in systolic blood pressure [9]. In patients with obliterative arteriopathy, intravenous

treatment with 20 mg (as a single dose or daily for 14 days) produced no significant changes in heart frequency or blood pressure but the heart minute volume was increased [57]. Oral treatment with 90 mg of raubasine per day for 1–2 weeks reduced vascular resistance and systolic blood pressure in patients with cerebrovascular disorders [58].

Pharmacokinetics

Yohimbine

Owen et al. [59] studied the pharmacokinetic fate of oral yohimbine HCl in healthy male volunteers. An oral dose of 10 mg resulted in a rapid absorption (absorption half-life of 0.17 ± 0.11 h), and the alkaloid was eliminated very rapidly from the plasma with considerable interindividual variability (elimination half-life of 0.60 ± 0.26 h). Urinary excretion in unchanged form was not the major route of elimination, as the cumulative urinary excretion of yohimbine in 24 h was very low (0.35% ± 0.50%) and only an insignificant fraction was excreted after 24 h. The authors felt that hydrolysis of yohimbine to yohimbinic acid was unlikely to be a major metabolic route in man.

Guthrie et al. [12] compared the fate of 10 mg of yohimbine HCl in healthy young male subjects following intravenous and oral administration. The mean oral bioavailability of yohimbine was 33% but individual values varied from 7% to 87%. Considerable variability was also observed in other pharmacokinetic parameters. Intravenous administration was followed by very rapid distribution (half-life of approximately 6 min) and elimination (half-life of 0.68 h); the volume of distribution was rather small (0.26 ± 0.12 l/kg) and the clearance was 9.77 ± 4.46 ml/min per kg. After oral administration, absorption and elimination were very rapid (mean half-lives of approximately 7 min and 0.58 h, respectively), with peak plasma concentrations usually occurring within 10 to 45 min; both the volume of distribution (3.22 ± 3.57 l/kg) and the clearance (55.9 ± 65.1 ml/min per kg) were larger than after intravenous dosing.

The findings of Owen et al. [59] and Guthrie et al. [12] were corroborated by Hedner et al. [60], who studied the pharmacokinetics of yohimbine in 13 young healthy males. They gave yohimbine as HCl salt in an intravenous amount of 0.25 mg/kg (12 subjects) or 0.50 mg/kg (1 subject). After a rapid distribution phase of 3 min, the alkaloid was rapidly eliminated in most subjects (half-lives between 0.3 and 0.8 h), and only 0.5 to 1% of the administered dose was excreted renally as unchanged drug. One individual showed a markedly prolonged elimination half-life of 2.5 h, and his plasma clearance was much lower (20 l/h) than the clearance values found in the rest of the group (43–197 l/h).

Le Verge et al. [61] subsequently identified 11-hydroxy-yohimbine as a major metabolite of yohimbine in man, together with 10-hydroxy-yohimbine as a minor metabolite. They established, apparently in a single healthy volunteer, that the elimination half-life of the 11-hydroxy metabolite was much longer (6 h) than that of its parent compound.

In receptor binding studies, the affinity of 11-hydroxy-yohimbine for human α_2-adrenoceptors was 10 times lower than that of yohimbine, and 10-hydroxy-yohimbine even had less affinity than the 11-hydroxy congener. Yet both metabolites were found to have similar α_2-adrenoceptor antagonistic capacities (as measured by inhibition of epinephrine-induced platelet aggregation and inhibition of UK14304-induced antilipolysis in adipocytes) as their parent compound (UK14304 is a non-selective α_2-adrenoceptor agonist). An explanation for this discrepancy may be that yohimbine binds to a much higher degree to plasma proteins (82%) than the 11-hydroxy metabolite (43%) or 10-hydroxy metabolite (32%) [45].

Raubasine

Marzo et al. [55] observed peak plasma levels of 319 ± 33 ng/ml at 1 h after the oral administration of 0.24 mg/kg of ^{3}H-raubasine to healthy human volunteers. The cumulative urinary and fecal excretion over three days was 29% ± 3% and 24% ± 5%, respectively.

Adverse Reaction Profile

General Animal Data

General

Raymond-Hamet and Rothlin [62] determined intravenous LD$_{50}$ values of yohimbine, rauwolscine, β-yohimbine, alloyohimbine, corynanthine, and raubasine in the mouse, and reported that yohimbine was more toxic than all the other alkaloids (Table 3). Lambert and Lang [27] also found that yohimbine was more toxic to mice than corynanthine, but in their experiments yohimbine was less toxic than β-yohimbine (Table 3). Intraperitoneal injection of yohimbine (20–100 mg/kg) or β-yohimbine (10–50 mg/kg) produced body tremor, mild excitation, and occasion-

Table 3. LD$_{50}$ values and relative toxicity of yohimbine and related alkaloids in the mouse, as reported by different authors

Alkaloid	Raymond-Hamet and Rothlin [62] LD$_{50}$ i.v. (mg/kg)	Relative toxicity[1]	Lambert and Lang [27] LD$_{50}$ i.p. (mg/kg)[2]	Relative toxicity[1]
Yohimbine HCl	0.0173	–	40	–
Rauwolscine HCl	0.080	4.6x less toxic		
β-Yohimbine HCl	0.040	2.3x less toxic	24	1.7x more toxic
Alloyohimbine HCl	0.200	11.6x less toxic		
Corynanthine HCl	0.077	4.5x less toxic	185	4.6x less toxic
Raubasine HCl	0.040	2.3x less toxic		

[1] Toxicity of the alkaloid compared to toxicity of yohimbine
[2] Estimated from graphic representations in the original paper

ally convulsions rarely culminating in death. At lower doses, sedation and respiratory depression occurred. At all doses injected, there was a loss of general muscle tone. On the other hand, corynanthine caused only depression of motor activity and respiration without either convulsions or tremor, even at toxic doses > 100 mg/kg. Death from corynanthine apparently resulted from respiratory depression, since the mice were severely cyanosed at the terminal stages.

The subcutaneous LD_{50} of corynantheidine HCl in the mouse was 0.55 g/kg, compared to 0.25 g/kg for corynanthine. Corynantheine was somewhat more toxic than corynantheidine but less toxic than corynanthine in this assay, but in an intravenous study corynantheine HCl was more toxic than corynanthine HCl [63].

Yohimbine
Bourin et al. [64] reported that yohimbine had a subcutaneous LD_{50} of 40 mg/kg in mice. Quinton [65] found a similar subcutaneous LD_{50} of 43.9 mg/kg of yohimbine HCl (corresponding to 39.8 mg/kg of yohimbine base) in male mice. Death was preceded by intermittent bouts of clonic convulsions which were sometimes precipitated by external stimuli. Lower subcutaneous doses of 20 mg/kg of yohimbine HCl produced ptosis and slight sedation, lasting for 2 to 4 hours. Quinton adds that early workers observed hypertension, hyperventilation, salivation, diarrhea and symptoms of uneasiness, anxiety and increased alertness and reflex excitability in non-anesthetized animals. Higher doses of yohimbine produced muscle tremors, ataxia, excitement, and finally convulsions. This duality of central yohimbine effects was also observed by Lambert and Lang (see above).

General Human Data

Yohimbine
Systemic administration of yohimbine to human beings can cause a variety of cardiovascular, psychic and other adverse effects. In 1961, Holmberg and Gershon [66] reported one of the first detailed human studies of these effects in normal volunteers and mental hospital patients, such as schizophrenics. After a single intravenous dose of 0.5 mg/kg of yohimbine over 5 min, they observed facial flushing and an increase in heart rate (with 4 to 48 beats per min), followed by perspiration, salivation, lacrimation, pupillary dilatation and rises in systolic and diastolic blood pressure; sometimes, nausea and urgency of micturition and defecation occurred, and an erection was observed in 10–20% of the cases. In addition, the subjects showed various psychic changes, such as restlessness, impatience, irritability, and tremulousness. In some schizophrenic patients, intramuscular doses of 20–40 mg activated a more or less latent psychosis and induced hallucinations.

Other reported side effects of yohimbine include vomiting, diarrhea, piloerection, rhinorrhea, hot and cold flashes, dizziness, headache, and insomnia [22,24,29,41,42,67].

According to Margolis et al. [68], the use of an Afrodex capsule (containing 5 mg of yohimbine HCl, 5 mg of methyltestosterone, and 5 mg of nux vomica extract) three times a day produced side effects in 6.8% of 2000 patients. Among the reported side effects were nervousness, irritability, insomnia (50 times); headache (11 times); flushing (7 times); anorexia, nausea, gastric distress, diarrhea (34 times); vomiting (3 times); palpitations or tachycardia (10 times); dysuria (4 patients); back or genital pain (8 times); increased blood pressure (3 times); and miscellaneous effects such as dizziness and sweating (24 times). Most of these effects were transient or could be corrected by adjusting the dosage, but four patients discontinued the medication because of side effects (recurrence of peptic ulcer symptoms; testicular ache; increased blood pressure; unspecified intolerance). It should be noted that, when the study ended after 10 weeks, only 890 of the original 2000 patients were still included.

Morales et al. [20] treated 23 patients with organic impotence in a pilot study with 18 mg/day of yohimbine HCl p.o. One patient suffered from nausea and refused further therapy; two others complained of dizziness with or without nervousness but these effects disappeared after a reduction of the dose level to 6 mg/day whereafter the dose was gradually increased to 18 mg/day. Morales et al. [31,32] subsequently treated 100 patients with organic impotence and 48 patients with psychogenic impotence with 18 mg/day of yohimbine HCl p.o. for at least 10 weeks, apparently without observing serious undesirable effects. Susset et al. [33] treated 82 patients with organic and/or psychogenic impotence with yohimbine HCl at oral doses of 21.6 to 43.2 mg/day. Eight patients did not complete the study due to side effects at the lowest prescribed daily dose (21.6 mg/day); after these side effects failed to disappear at a dose level of 16.2 mg daily, these patients were omitted from the study. Of the remaining 71 patients, at least 4 stopped their medication due to side effects (which disappeared rapidly after termination of treatment). Side effects included anxiety (n=6), nausea (n=3), dizziness (n=3), increased frequency of urination (n=2), chills (n=2), headaches (n=2), and vomiting (n=1). However, none of the side effects was considered severe.

When yohimbine is given to healthy volunteers, a single oral dose of 10 mg is sufficient to increase plasma free 3-methoxy-4-hydroxyphenylethyleneglycol (MHPG), whereas a dose of 15–30 mg p.o. is usually needed to produce autonomic and/or psychic effects [22,30,40,41, 69–73]. The effects of relatively high single oral doses in healthy subjects have been studied by at least two research groups. Mattila et al. [74] observed increased systolic blood pressure, panic, discontentment, drowsiness, and passivity after the oral administration of 0.8 mg/kg of yohimbine base (in the form of its HCl salt). Henauer et al. [70] tested yohimbine HCl by mouth in nine healthy subjects, who received 0 mg, 30 mg and 60 mg on separate occasions. Both the 30 mg and 60 mg dose induced anxiety and increased systolic blood pressure, but the diastolic blood pressure was not influenced by either treatment. Pulse rate was increased in most subjects after 60 mg but only in two subjects after 30 mg or placebo.

Patients treated with certain drugs, such as tricyclic antidepressants, can be more sensitive to the effects of yohimbine than healthy volunteers (see the section on drug interactions). Yohimbine can also show enhanced activity in certain pathological conditions, such as hypertension, agoraphobia and panic attacks (see the sections on cardiovascular reactions and central nervous system reactions). Onrot et al. [75] challenged patients with autonomic failure characterized by orthostatic hypotension with 2.5 mg and/or 5 mg of yohimbine orally. The 5 mg dose significantly increased both systolic and diastolic blood pressure as well as heart rate. These cardiovascular parameters also tended to increase after a dose of 2.5 mg but these changes did not achieve statistical significance. Chronic yohimbine therapy was deemed unsuitable because of side effects in 4 of the 11 patients tested. One patient experienced nausea and vomiting after 5 mg, and also suffered from nervousness and irritability. These latter symptoms were also observed in two other patients, who had taken 2.5 mg or 5 mg. A fourth patient with mild dementia developed confusion and hallucinations after 5 mg.

According to text books, yohimbine is contra-indicated in patients with angina pectoris, cardiac disease, hypertension, and renal disease. Moreover, risk-benefit should be considered in patients with sensitivity to yohimbine, depression or another psychiatric illness, and hepatic function impairment. It would also be prudent to avoid the use of yohimbine during pregnancy or in children [29,37,42,67]. In view of these contra-indications, it is remarkable that yohimbe bark has been used in traditional medicine to treat angina and hypertension [76].

The course of accidental or intentional poisoning with yohimbine can vary considerably. Friesen et al. [77] merely observed vomiting, hypertension, tachycardia, tremors and anxiety of brief duration in a 62-year-old male, who had ingested approximately 200 mg of yohimbine. Linden et al. [24] described a 16-year-old girl, who experienced an acute dissociative state, weakness, paresthesias and loss of coordination following the ingestion of yohimbine at an estimated dose of 250 mg. Additional symptoms included memory disturbance, anxiety, headache, dizziness, tremors, substernal chest pain, nausea, diaphoresis, and intermittent palpitations. Upon physical examination, she was found to suffer from high blood pressure, sinus tachycardia, tachypnea, pallor, tremors, and an erythematous rash. The symptoms lasted approximately 36 hours but resolved spontaneously. Varkey [78] reported on a 38-year-old man with insulin-dependent diabetes, who developed various symptoms 25 hours after taking 350 mg of yohimbine: drowsiness, confusion, rigors, retrosternal pain, a drop in body temperature, atrial fibrillation and retrograde amnesia. Patscheider and Dirnhofer [79] attributed the death of a 2.5-year-old boy to the ingestion of 300 to 400 mg of yohimbine.

In 1989, the American Food and Drug Administration expressed the view that the Over The Counter use of yohimbine as an aphrodisiac would present a safety concern [34]. Earlier, the agency had stated that, even if the alkaloid were shown to be effective, individuals suffering from decreased libido and impaired sexual performance should not self-medicate but should seek treatment under professional guidance [80].

Raubasine
Intravenous administration of 10 mg can produce a weak feeling of heat [81]. Dizziness and a transient feeling of increased congestion of the blood, sometimes leading to unrest and fear, can occur following 20 mg intravenously [9,57].

In a six-months study on the combination of 20 mg of raubasine with 60 mg of almitrine bismesilate per day, 7 of 99 elderly patients with cognitive impairment dropped out because of vertigo, nausea, or epigastric pain (n=5), tiredness (n=1), and skin rash (n=1) [82]. The same dose regimen was also evaluated in 20 elderly patients for 13 months. One patient dropped out because of dizziness [83].

Allergic Reactions

Yohimbine

Sandler and Aronson [84] described a 42-year-old black male with a history of impotence and essential hypertension, who developed a generalized erythrodermic skin eruption, progressive renal failure, and a lupus-like syndrome. Symptoms started one day after ingesting three 5.4 mg tablets of yohimbine and consisted of fever, chills, malaise, and pruritic scaly skin. A one-week course of oral prednisone produced some clearing of the skin lesions but the changes recurred on cessation of the corticosteroid. Over the next two weeks, the patient developed progressive malaise, abdominal cramps, and a cold sensation in the fingers and toes. Examination after his admission to hospital revealed truncal erythroderma and desquamation of the hand palms. Blood chemistry screening revealed abnormal electrolyte, urea nitrogen and creatinine levels, whereas urinalysis showed proteinuria. The erythrocyte sedimentation rate was increased and antinuclear antibodies (ANA) testing was positive, whereas antidouble-stranded DNA was negative. The patient was started on aggressive hydration for his acute renal failure and received topical corticosteroids for his skin problems. Two weeks after admission, the patient was discharged with improved renal function but four months later he was readmitted for shortness of breath. Besides having maculopapular lesions on his trunk, legs, and arms, he was found to have pericardial and pleural effusions which were negative on Gram stain and culture. Pericardial biopsy revealed irregular fibrosis and patchy inflammation. The patient showed eosinophilia, an increased sedimentation rate and a positive ANA with negative antidouble-stranded DNA. Two weeks later, he was discharged in stable condition on an oral regimen of prednisone.

Cardiovascular Reactions

Yohimbine

Yohimbine is sometimes presented in the scientific literature [3] and in commercial sources [85] as a peripheral vasodilator, which can lower blood pressure. Yet it has been known since 1912 that yohimbine can produce sustained increases in blood pressure, when given orally or intramuscularly to man [23]. The reason for this remarkable discrepancy may be found in a key note paper by Gershon and Lang [86], who reported in 1962 that yohimbine produces a rise in blood pressure in conscious dogs, whereas it gives a fall in blood pressure in dogs anesthetized with various agents. This was an important finding because until that time the hemodynamic effects of yohimbine and other psychoactive indole alkaloids had been assessed in anesthetized or curarized animals [86]. The explanation for the different responses in conscious and anesthetized animals most probably lies in the fact that the pressor effects of yohimbine are due to a central site of action [23].

Goldberg et al. [87] determined the influence of several doses of yohimbine HCl on baseline blood pressure and heart rate and on physiologic and biochemical indices of sympathetic outflow. Cumulative administration of 0.016–0.125 mg/kg intravenously to normal volunteers produced dose-related rises in blood pressure (without altering heart rate) and enhanced various cardiovascular reflexes. It was also found that yohimbine HCl (0.125 mg/kg bolus injection followed by a continuous infusion of 0.001 mg/kg/min) induced a two-to-threefold rise in plasma norepinephrine, without changing plasma epinephrine or renin activity. Ex vivo platelet aggregation in response to epinephrine was inhibited during yohimbine.

As was pointed out in the section on general human data, at least 15 mg by mouth is usually needed to produce cardiovascular effects in healthy volunteers [e.g. 22]. Goldstein et al. [88] have reported, however, that patients with essential hypertension show larger increases in blood pressure and arterial norepinephrine than do normotensive controls following intravenous administration of yohimbine (0.125 mg/kg bolus followed by 0.001 mg/kg/min for 15 min). Excessive pressor responses did not occur in all hypertensive subjects but only in about 1/3 of the patients, in whom blood pressure often remained increased for up to several hours after stopping the yohimbine infusion. This subgroup also reacted with tachycardia, excessive catecholamine responses, and a variety of emotional experiences (such as euphoria, panic, a feeling of restraint and aggressive urge). Similar results were obtained in a follow-up study on the effects of oral yohimbine HCl (21.6 mg) in patients with essential hypertension, who had discontinued their antihypertensive medication at least 2 weeks before the study. Yohimbine increased systolic blood pressure, diastolic blood pressure, and mean blood pressure significantly, without changing heart rate. Three of the 25 patients, who tended to have especially large increases in blood pressure and plasma norepinephrine levels, showed emotional or behavioral changes (anxiety, tearfulness, panic). It was concluded that yohimbine should be administered with caution to patients with high blood pressure, especially in individuals with evidence of increased basal sympathetic outflow [36].

Increased sensitivity to the cardiovascular effects of yohimbine may also be expected in patients with autonomic failure [75] or agoraphobia and panic attacks [89], and in patients treated with tricyclic antidepressants or certain other drugs (see the section on drug interactions).

Rauwolscine
An intramuscular dose of 0.5 to 10 mg/kg augmented the blood pressure of unanesthetized rats with experimental renal hypertension [90].

Raubasine
Oral administration of 25 to 50 mg/kg of raubasine augmented the blood pressure of unanesthetized rats with experimental renal hypertension, whereas a lower dose of 5 mg/kg was inactive [90]. See also the section on general human data.

Central Nervous System Reactions

General
Corynanthine (25 mg/kg intraperitoneally) displayed a weak sedative action, as measured by prolongation of the hexobarbitone-induced loss of righting reflex in

mice, whereas neither yohimbine (5 mg/kg intraperitoneally) nor rauwolscine (5 mg/kg intraperitoneally) had such an effect [16].

Yohimbine

In the mouse, yohimbine can induce clonic seizures (see the section on general animal data). The dose level needed for this effect is much greater than that necessary for α_2-antagonism: the subcutaneous CD_{50} dose (dose required to produce seizures in half of the mice) was determined to be 25.5 mg/kg. The convulsant effects of yohimbine are not due to α_2-antagonism, as other α_2-antagonists (such as rauwolscine) were ineffective in doses up to 100 mg/kg. Yohimbine-induced seizures were attenuated by experimental GABA-mimetic agents and excitatory amino acid antagonists, which suggests that they are mediated through the impairment of GABA-ergic transmission as well as a possible endogenous enhancement of excitatory amino acid transmission [91].

Oral administration of yohimbine HCl (0.10 to 0.75 mg/kg) to bonnet macaques significantly increased episodes of motoric activation and affective response interspersed with intervals of behavioral enervation; there was no dose-response relationship [92].

In man, yohimbine causes a variety of psychic changes (see the section on general human data). Charney et al. [89] showed that yohimbine (20 mg orally) produced more robust behavioral and somatic effects in patients with agoraphobia and panic attacks than it did in healthy subjects. There was a significant correlation between patient-rated anxiety and yohimbine-induced rises in the plasma level of the norepinephrine metabolite MHPG, and patients experiencing frequent panic attacks had a greater plasma MHPG response to yohimbine than the healthy volunteers or patients having less frequent panic attacks. In an extension of this study, Charney et al. [93] found that yohimbine produced panic attacks in 1 of 20 healthy subjects and in 37 of 68 panic disorder patients. In the healthy volunteers, yohimbine did not significantly increase plasma cortisol levels, whereas such an effect could be observed in the patients who experienced a panic attack after yohimbine administration.

Price et al. [94] reported that challenge doses of 10–20 mg of yohimbine orally precipitated manic symptoms in three of seven depressed patients with a bipolar diathesis, compared with no cases among 48 unipolar patients.

Rauwolscine

According to Kohli and De [48], rauwolscine shares the central nervous system activity of yohimbine. Intraperitoneal injection of 10–20 mg/kg produced signs of psychic excitement in the guinea pig. In the rabbit, intraperitoneal injection of 20 mg/kg also produced psychic excitement and increased motor activity, whereas intravenous administration of 12–15 mg/kg produced clonic convulsions. Dunn and Corbett [91] did not observe clonic convulsions in mice, however, following treatment with rauwolscine in doses up to 100 mg/kg subcutaneously.

Raubasine

Fontaine [95] studied the effects of raubasine (15–30 mg/day for periods varying from less than 1 month to more than 3 months) in 50 patients with a cerebral vascular disorder. This regimen resulted in fits of psychic and psychomotoric excitation. In two cases, oneiric confusion developed which disappeared when the treatment was stopped and which did not reappear when the therapy was reintroduced at a moderate dose level.

Dermatological Reactions

Yohimbine

An erythematous rash may be among the symptoms of massive overdosing (see the section on general human data). In normal doses, yohimbine has been associated with a case of lupus-like skin problems (see the section on allergic reactions).

Endocrine Reactions

Yohimbine

In one study, oral administration of 30 mg of yohimbine HCl to healthy volunteers gave a modest increase in plasma cortisol [30] whereas in other studies oral doses of 20–30 mg had little or no effect on this parameter [96,97]. The cortisol response to 20 mg of yohimbine HCl by mouth was significantly greater in depressed patients, who had been free of antidepressants for at least three weeks, even though the MHPG responses in these patients were similar to those in healthy controls [97].

In rats, yohimbine (0.5–2.5 mg/kg intravenously) reduced levels of thyrotropin and growth hormone [23]. In monkeys, yohimbine (2.5 mg/kg infused intravenously) produced a rapid increase of serum prolactin levels, whereas a lower dose of 1 mg/kg did not produce such an effect; none of the two doses had a significant effect on serum growth hormone [98]. It should be noted that the doses used in this study were relatively large and that yohimbine can produce autonomic effects in man without changes in prolactin levels [23]. Mattila et al. [74] found that a high oral dose of yohimbine (0.8 mg/kg of the base in the form of the HCl salt) increased plasma prolactin concentrations in healthy human subjects without inducing a significant alteration in the growth hormone level.

At one time, it was claimed that yohimbine causes prolonged estrus or pseudopregnancy in intact adult female rats but not in hypophysectomized or castrate animals; however, subsequent work failed to confirm these results [26].

Haematological Reactions

Yohimbine
In healthy subjects, an oral dose of 8 or 12 mg of yohimbine selectively antagonized epinephrine-induced ex vivo platelet aggregation but did not influence collagen, arachidonic acid, or adenosine diphosphate-induced aggregation [73].

Raubasine
Neuman et al. [56] investigated the effect of raubasine (60 mg/day for 6 weeks) on platelet biological activity in 14 patients, most of whom had a cardiovascular disease and/or hyperlipoproteinemia. There were no effects on bleeding time but raubasine produced a reduction of ADP- and epinephrine-induced platelet aggregation, particularly in the cardiovascular patients.

Metabolic Reactions

Yohimbine
In early animal studies, yohimbine was found to inhibit epinephrine-induced hyperglycemia. Yohimbine was also reported to raise plasma insulin levels, to enhance the insulin release by epinephrine, and to potentiate the diabetogenic effects of streptozotocin in laboratory animals [23].

In a human study by Galitzky et al. [72], 12 mg/day of oral yohimbine for 14 days produced no significant changes in various blood parameters of 10 normal volunteers (such as glucose, insulin, non-esterified fatty acids, cholesterol, and triglycerides). An acute oral dose of 0.2 mg/kg did not affect plasma glucose or insulin but it produced significant rises in the plasma levels of non-esterified fatty acids. Others have also observed an increase in plasma free fatty acids following administration of yohimbine to normal volunteers [23].

Raubasine
Neuman et al. [56] observed no changes in the levels of blood glucose or plasma lipids in cardiovascular and/or hyperlipoproteinemic patients who were treated with 60 mg/day of raubasine for 6 weeks.

Espinoza and Westermann [99] did not find a negative effect of raubasine on the glycemic control of 31 diabetic patients, most of whom were given daily doses of 60 mg p.o. and 10–20 mg i.v.

Renal Reactions

Yohimbine
See the section on allergic reactions.

Raubasine
An intravenous dose of 10 mg was given to 15 patients with moderate to severe renal insufficiency without exacerbation of their renal insuffiency [81].

Respiratory Reactions

Yohimbine
Bronchospasm and increased mucus production developed in a 60-year-old man, who had been started on 16.2 mg of yohimbine HCl a day for impotence just prior to the onset of symptoms. A causal role of yohimbine was suggested by the temporal relationship and the absence of a history of bronchospastic disease [100].

Drug Interactions

General
In animal studies, yohimbine and rauwolscine antagonize the central hypotensive and sedative actions of clonidine more strongly than corynanthine [16,101].

Lambert and Lang [27] compared interactions of yohimbine, β-yohimbine, and corynanthine with amphetamine in the mouse. β-Yohimbine was found to potentiate amphetamine toxicity in a less marked way than yohimbine, whereas corynanthine markedly antagonized amphetamine toxicity. These opposite effects closely paralleled the ability of the different alkaloids to produce an anxiety-like state in the conscious dog.

Yohimbine
The ability of other drugs to potentiate the effects of yohimbine in the mouse was studied extensively by Quinton [65]. This author compared the toxicity of 20 mg/kg of yohimbine HCl subcutaneously with and without pretreatment with numerous agents (given orally 1 hr before the administration of yohimbine). Among the various substances that were found to increase the toxicity of yohimbine were:

– Tricyclic antidepressants (such as imipramine and amitriptyline);
– Neuroleptics with α-adrenergic blocking activity (such as chlorpromazine, promazine and chlorprotixene);
– Central nervous stimulants with sympathicomimetic properties (such as amphetamine, ephedrine and cocaine);
– α-Adrenoceptor blocking agents (phenoxybenzamine, phentolamine), bretylium and dihydroergotamine, when given in fairly high doses;
– Inhibitors of monoamine oxidase (such as tranylcypromine and phenelzine), but only within a few hours of administration;
– Antimuscarinic agents (atropine and atropine methonitrate), but only to some extent, when given in moderate to high doses.

No or an only slight increase in yohimbine toxicity was seen with reserpine, the adrenergic neurone blocker guanethidine, the β-adrenoceptor blocker pronethalol, promethazine, and lysergic acid diethylamide. Quinton [65] also reported that certain drugs were capable of reducing or abolishing the combined toxicity of yohimbine and imipramine, viz. reserpine, ganglion blocking agents, and the β-adrenoceptor blocker pronethalol.

Increased toxicity in the mouse by a combination of yohimbine with cocaine [19] or amphetamine [27] was also reported by other researchers. Bourin et al. [64] found that the central α_1-agonist adrafinil failed to protect mice against yohimbine-induced mortality, whereas the central α_2-agonist clonidine did. In the same model, three β-blocking agents with the capacity to cross the blood-brain barrier readily (propranolol, penbutolol and metoprolol) also provided protection, whereas the very slightly lipophilic β-blocker atenolol did not. In experiments by Liljequist et al. [102], yohimbine significantly suppressed ethanol-induced locomotor stimulation in mice. Others reported no or an attenuating influence of yohimbine on morphine effects in rodents [23]. In the conscious dog, neither levodopa nor lithium potentiated the cardiovascular and behavioral effects of yohimbine; levodopa showed partial inhibition of yohimbine effects [103,104]. In the same species, the cardiovascular effects of yohimbine were reduced by hexamethonium, phenoxybenzamine and reserpine [105].

– *Centrally active antihypertensives*
As was pointed out in the section on cardiovascular reactions, yohimbine is sometimes presented as a peripheral vasodilator, which can lower blood pressure and can thus potentiate other antihypertensives [3,85]. In reality, however, its α_2-adrenoceptor antagonistic properties will antagonize centrally active antihypertensives which owe their action to stimulation of central α_2-adrenoceptors (e.g. guanabenz and the methyldopa metabolite α-methylnorepinephrine) [24]. Yohimbine also antagonizes the hypotensive and sedative effects of clonidine [16,101], which have been traditionally attributed to central α_2-adrenergic effects. Recent studies suggest, however, that even though clonidine has sufficient α_2-adrenergic agonism to produce sedation, its hypotensive properties may be primarily due to stimulation of central I_1-imidazoline receptors. Since yohimbine reverses the hypotensive effect of clonidine in a biphasic manner, more than one receptor may be involved in this interaction [106]. Vice versa, the effects of yohimbine can be antagonized by clonidine. In one study of healthy volunteers, clonidine (0.1–0.2 mg) incompletely counteracted the effects of highly dosed yohimbine (0.8 mg/kg) on systolic blood pressure and it failed to block all the subjective and hormonal responses to yohimbine [74]. In another study of normal human subjects, 5 μg/kg of clonidine by mouth counteracted the anxiety, increases in plasma MHPG and blood pressure and other autonomic symptoms induced by 30 mg of oral yohimbine [69].

– *Tricyclic antidepressants*
Yohimbine should be administered with caution to patients undergoing concurrent treatment with tricyclic antidepressants or other drugs which interfere with neuronal uptake or metabolism of norepinephrine [29,36]. Tricyclic antidepressants have been shown to increase yohimbine toxicity in laboratory animals [65]. This potentiation seems to be of central origin as quaternary derivatives of imipramine and

amitriptyline appear to be inactive. Selective inhibitors of serotonin reuptake do not potentiate yohimbine toxicity to the same degree as do the tricyclic derivatives which inhibit norepinephrine reuptake [64].

There is substantial documentation that the interaction between yohimbine and tricyclic antidepressants also occurs in human patients. Clinical evidence that imipramine enhances the autonomic and central effects of yohimbine (increase in blood pressure, flushing, perspiration, nausea, tremor, restlessness) was already presented in 1961 by Holmberg and Gershon [66]. Charney et al. [107] reported 25 years later that yohimbine HCl (15 mg/day by mouth) induced increases in blood pressure and anxiety symptoms in two of twelve depressed patients treated with desipramine; five of the remaining ten patients reacted with anxiety symptoms or elevated blood pressure to a yohimbine HCl dosage of 30 mg/day. Lacomblez et al. [71] demonstrated that low oral doses of yohimbine (12 mg/day) not only corrected orthostatic hypotension but could also induce moderate hypertension in clomipramine-treated subjects with depression. Bagheri et al. [108] evaluated the pharmacokinetics and pharmacodynamic effects of yohimbine in depressed patients treated with a tricyclic antidepressant (amitriptyline or clomipramine). Contrary to findings in healthy volunteers, five out of nine patients who received an oral dose of 10 mg of yohimbine exhibited side effects, such as transient sensation of rhinorrhea (n=4), facial flush, tachycardia and nausea (n=3), tremor and sweating (n=2). The patients showed substantially higher plasma levels of yohimbine than a control group that had been treated with a slightly higher dose (12 mg of yohimbine). This finding clearly suggests the possibility of a pharmacokinetic interaction, the mechanism of which is yet unknown. No side effects were observed after oral administration of 4 mg of yohimbine to another group of ten depressed patients on amitriptyline or clomipramine. In an earlier study, Bagheri et al. [41] saw acute diarrhea (n=1) and headache with facial flush (n=1) in 20 depressed patients on tricyclic antidepressants following an acute oral dose of 10 mg of yohimbine. Another patient reacted with agitation, tremor, facial flush, sweating and vomiting. Treatment with 12 mg/day in divided doses produced transient rhinorrhea in seven of ten patients.

– *Other drugs (epinephrine, amobarbital, chlorpromazine, reserpine, atropine, benzodiazepines, Ditran, naloxone)*
Holmberg and Gershon [66] observed in psychiatric patients that epinephrine produced a greater increase in heart rate after yohimbine (0.5 mg/kg intravenously over 5 min) than it did alone and that certain effects of yohimbine (tremor, flushing and restlessness) became more marked when epinephrine was superimposed. Premedication with amobarbital abolished the yohimbine-induced subjective sensations and the increase in heart rate, and it attenuated the increase in blood pressure. Chlordiazepoxide also reduced anxiety and tension but to a lesser degree. Ingram [109] also evaluated drug interactions with yohimbine (0.5 mg/kg intravenously over 5 min) in psychiatric patients. Chlorpromazine enhanced the psychic and autonomic effects while reserpine and amobarbital blocked these responses. Atropine decreased the pressor response to yohimbine without altering other autonomic effects, and it seemed to depress the psychic effects only partially. Charney et al. [69] demonstrated in healthy subjects that pretreatment with diazepam (10 mg

by mouth) antagonized yohimbine-induced anxiety without attenuating increases in plasma MHPG, blood pressure, and autonomic symptoms. The combination of diazepam and yohimbine in healthy subjects was also evaluated by Mattila et al. [74]. An oral dose of yohimbine HCl (corresponding to 0.8 mg/kg of the base) prevented diazepam-induced poor coordination and heavy headedness and reduced diazepam-induced drowsiness without significantly affecting the plasma concentrations of diazepam; diazepam (0.3 mg/kg p.o.) did not antagonize the effects of yohimbine on systolic blood pressure or panic.

Charney et al. [96] investigated, whether yohimbine (30 mg p.o.) would influence pharmacological effects of alprazolam in healthy volunteers, because of evidence that alprazolam, in contrast to other benzodiazepines, may be effective in reducing panic attacks, Concomitant use of yohimbine antagonized alprazolam-induced decreases in blood pressure, plasma MHPG and plasma cortisol, and attenuated the alprazolam-induced increase in subjective ratings of drowsy and mellow. A significant pharmacokinetic interaction between the two drugs could not be observed.

Itil and Fink [110] reported that intravenous administration of yohimbine (0.01–0.50 mg/kg) to schizophrenics and other psychiatric patients decreased changes in consciousness induced by the anticholinergic psychotomimetic drug Ditran.

Charney and Heninger [30] established that the combination of naloxone HCl and yohimbine HCl (30 mg p.o.) produced more effects in healthy volunteers than the sum of the effects of the two drugs separately. Among the effects observed were full penile erection as well as increased nervousness, anxiety, tremors, palpitations, nausea, hot and cold flashes, and increased plasma cortisol concentrations. Naloxone did not alter plasma levels of yohimbine, and plasma MHPG concentrations following the combination were not different than those following yohimbine alone.

Corynanthine

The α_1-adrenoceptor-blocking agent corynanthine increased haloperidol-induced catalepsy in mice, with an ED_{50} value of 4.7 mg/kg intraperitoneally [111].

Lambert and Lang [27] state, without providing further detail, that corynanthine does not potentiate yohimbine toxicity.

Fertility, Pregnancy and Lactation

General

Rauwolscine, β-yohimbine, alloyohimbine, corynanthine and raubasine all produced an adrenolytic effect on the rabbit uterus similar to that of yohimbine [62].

Corynantheidine had no marked effect on the rabbit uterus but it antagonized the effects of epinephrine on this organ [54].

Yohimbine

In early animal studies, yohimbine blocked and reversed uterine contractions in response to epinephrine, and high doses had depressant effects on the uterus [23].

Intravenous perfusion of the α_2-adrenoceptor blocker yohimbine (0.03 mg/kg/min for 1h) inhibited uterine activity before and during labour in unanesthetized ewes. In contrast, treatment with the α_1-adrenoceptor blocker prazosin did not modify uterine activity either before or during labour, but this finding was not in agreement with observations in the rat [112]. Testing of the tocolytic effect of yohimbine on human myometrial strips showed that this α_2-blocking agent produced a highly significant decrease of uterine activity. A similar effect was obtained with the α_1-blocker prazosin and the non-selective α-blocker phentolamine [113].

A single dose of yohimbine (20 mg/kg intramuscularly) given to female rats on their 4th day of pregnancy altered neither the course of pregnancy nor litter size [114]. Other studies of the risk of yohimbine use during pregnancy are lacking, however, and it would be prudent to avoid the alkaloid during pregnancy [42].

Data about the use of yohimbine during lactation could not be retrieved from the literature.

Mutagenicity and Carcinogenicity

General
The literature has yielded no references on the mutagenicity or carcinogenicity of yohimbe alkaloids, except for one study on raubasine.

Raubasine
Raubasine did not show genotoxic activity, when tested in the SOS Chromotest (using *Escherichia coli* PQ37) in the absence or presence of a metabolic activator; mutagenicity testing of the alkaloid in yeast diploid cells (*Saccharomyces cerevisiae* strain XS2316) also gave negative results [115].

References

1. Poisson J (1964) Recherches récentes sur les alcaloïdes du Pseudocinchona et du Yohimbe. Ann Chim (Paris) 9:99–121
2. Manske RHF (1965) Alkaloids of *Pseudocinchona* and *Yohimbe*. In: Manske RHF, red. The Alkaloids – Chemistry and Physiology. Volume 8: The indole alkaloids. New York: Academic Press, pp.693–723
3. Hoppe HA (1975) Drogenkunde. Band 1. Angiospermen. 8. Auflage. Berlin: Walter de Gruyter
4. Raymond-Hamet, Goutarel R (1965) L'*Alchornea floribunda* Mueller Arg. doit-il à la yohimbine ses effets excitants chez l'homme? C R Acad Sc Paris 261:3223–3224
5. Khuong-Huu F, Leforestier J-P, Maillard G, Goutarel R (1970) L'alchornéine, alcaloïde dérivé de la tétrahydro-imidazo-[1.2a] pyrimidine, isolé de deux Euphorbiacées africaines, l'*Alchornea floribunda* Muell. Arg. et l'*Alchornea hirtella* Benth. C R Acad Sc Paris Série C pp.2070–2072
6. Khuong-Huu F, Le Forestier JP, Goutarel R (1972) Alchornéine, isoalchornéine et alchornéinone, produits isolés de l'*Alchornea floribunda* Muell. Arg. Tetrahedron 28:5207–5220
7. Kohli JD, Balwani JH, Ray C, De NN (1957) Pharmacological action of rauwolscine: Part 1 – Adrenergic blocking activity. Arch Int Pharmacodyn 111:108–121

8. Demichel P, Gomond P, Roquebert J (1981) Pre- and postsynaptic α-adrenoreceptor blocking activity of raubasine in the rat vas deferens. Br J Pharmacol 74:739–745
9. Hohnloser E (1967) Kreislaufanalytische Untersuchungen unter der Einwirkung des Rauwolfia-Alkaloids Raubasin. Arzneim Forsch 17:967–969
10. Wade A, Reynolds JEF, red. (1977) Martindale The Extra Pharmacopoeia. 27th edn. London: The Pharmaceutical Press, p.1806
11. Lambert GA, Lang WJ, Friedman E, Meller E, Gershon S (1978) Pharmacological and biochemical properties of isomeric yohimbine alkaloids. Eur J Pharmacol 49:39–48
12. Guthrie SK, Hariharan M, Grunhaus LJ (1990) Yohimbine bioavailability in humans. Eur J Clin Pharmacol 39:409–411
13. Weitzell R, Tanaka T, Starke K (1979) Pre- and postsynaptic effects of yohimbine stereoisomers on noradrenergic transmission in the pulmonary artery of the rabbit. Naunyn-Schmiedeberg's Arch Pharmacol 308:127–136
14. Timmermans PBMWM, Kwa HY, Van Zwieten PA (1979) Possible subdivision of postsynaptic α-adrenoceptors mediating pressor responses in the pithed rat. Naunyn-Schmiedeberg's Arch Pharmacol 310:189–193
15. Tanaka T, Starke K (1980) Antagonist/agonist-preferring α-adrenoceptors or α_1/α_2-adrenoceptors? Eur J Pharmacol 63: 191–194
16. Timmermans PBMWM, Schoop AMC, Kwa HY, Van Zwieten PA (1981) Characterization of α-adrenoceptors participating in the central hypotensive and sedative effects of clonidine using yohimbine, rauwolscine and corynanthine. Eur J Pharmacol 70:7–15
17. Ito Y, Yano S, Watanabe K, Yamanaka E, Aimi N, Sakai S-I (1990) Structure-activity relationship of yohimbine and its related analogs in blocking alpha-1 and alpha-2 adrenoceptors: a comparative study of cardiovascular activities. Chem Pharm Bull 38:1702–1706
18. Angel I, Niddam R, Langer SZ (1990) Involvement of alpha-2 adrenergic receptor subtypes in hyperglycemia. J Pharmacol Exp Ther 254:877–882
19. Creveling CR, Daly JW, Parfitt RT, Witkop B (1968) The chemorelease of norepinephrine from mouse hearts. IV. Structure-activity relationships. Reserpines and yohimbines. J Med Chem 11: 596–598
20. Morales A, Surridge DHC, Marshall PG, Fenemore J (1982) Nonhormonal pharmacological treatment of organic impotence. J Urol 128:45–47
21. Morales A, Surridge DH, Marshall PG (1982) Yohimbine for treatment of impotence in diabetes. N Engl J Med 305:1221
22. Charney DS, Heninger GR, Sternberg DE (1982) Assessment of α_2 adrenergic autoreceptor function in humans: effects of oral yohimbine. Life Sci 30:2033–2041
23. Goldberg MR, Robertson D (1983) Yohimbine: a pharmacological probe for study of the α_2-adrenoreceptor. Pharmacol Rev 35: 143–180
24. Linden CH, Vellman WP, Rumack B (1985) Yohimbine: a new street drug. Ann Emerg Med 14:1002–1004
25. Anonymous (1986) Yohimbine: time for resurrection? Lancet 2:1194–1195
26. Nickerson M (1949) The pharmacology of adrenergic blockade. Pharmacol Rev 1:27–101
27. Lambert GA, Lang WJ (1977) Interaction between yohimbine alkaloids and amphetamine in mice. Psychopharmacology 51:209–212
28. Watanabe K, Yano S, Horiuchi H, Yamanaka E, Aimi N, Sakai S (1987) Ca^{2+} channel-blocking effect of the yohimbine derivatives, 14β-benzoyloxyyohimbine and 14β-p-nitrobenzoyloxyyohimbine. J Pharm Pharmacol 39:439–443
29. Anonymous (1993) USP DI. Volume I – Drug Information for the Health Care Professional. 13th edn. Rockville: United States Pharmacopeial Convention, Inc., pp.2807–2808
30. Charney DS, Heninger GR (1986) α_2-Adrenergic and opiate receptor blockade. Synergistic effects on anxiety in healthy subjects. Arch Gen Psychiatry 43:1037–1041
31. Morales A, Condra M, Owen JA, Surridge DH, Fenemore J, Harris C (1987) Is yohimbine effective in the treatment of organic impotence? Results of a controlled trial. J Urol 137: 1168–1172

32. Reid K, Surridge DHC, Morales A, Condra M, Harris C, Owen J, Fenemore J (1987) Double-blind trial of yohimbine in treatment of psychogenic impotence. Lancet 2:421–423
33. Susset JG, Tessier CD, Wincze J, Bansal S, Malhotra C, Schwacha MG (1989) Effect of yohimbine hydrochloride on erectile impotence: a double-blind study. J Urol 141:1360–1363
34. Young FE (1989) Aphrodisiac drug products for over-the-counter human use. Final rule. Fed Reg 54:28780–28786
35. Thesen R, Schulz M, Braun R (1990) Ganz oder teilweise "negativ" bewertete Arzneistoffe. Pharm Ztg 135:1812–1814
36. Grossman E, Rosenthal T, Peleg E, Holmes C, Goldstein DS (1993) Oral yohimbine increases blood pressure and sympathetic nervous outflow in hypertensive patients. J Cardiovasc Pharmacol 22:22–26
37. Reynolds JEF, red. (1993) Martindale The Extra Pharmacopoeia. 30th edn. London: The Pharmaceutical Press, p.1428
38. Robertson D, Goldberg MR, Tung C-S, Hollister AS, Robertson RM (1986) Use of alpha$_2$ adrenoreceptor agonists and antagonists in the functional assessment of the sympathetic nervous system. J Clin Invest 78:576–581
39. Ahmad RAS, Watson RDS (1990) Treatment of postural hypotension. Drugs 39:74–85
40. Chatelut E, Rispail Y, Berlan M, Montastruc JL (1989) Yohimbine increases human salivary secretion. Br J Clin Pharmacol 28:366–368
41. Bagheri H, Schmitt L, Berlan M, Montastruc JL (1992) Effect of 3 weeks treatment with yohimbine on salivary secretion in healthy volunteers and in depressed patients treated with tricyclic antidepressants. Br J Clin Pharmacol 34:555–558
42. Anonymous (1993) Vidal 1993. Paris: Editions du Vidal, pp.354,474,726,1576–1577
43. Berlin I, Stalla-Bourdillon A, Thuillier Y, Turpin G, Puech AJ (1986) Absence d'efficacité de la yohimbine dans le traitement de l'obésité. J Pharmacol 17:343–347
44. Kucio C, Jonderko K, Piskorska D (1991) Does yohimbine act as a slimming drug? Isr J Med Sci 27:550–556
45. Berlan M, Le Verge R, Galitzky J, Le Corre P (1993) α_2-Adrenoceptor antagonist potencies of two hydroxylated metabolites of yohimbine. Br J Pharmacol 108:927–932
46. Hesse E, Langer J (1931) Zur Pharmakologie der Yohimbealkaloide. Med Klin 27:1536–1537
47. Kreitmar H (1928) Pharmakologischer Teil. Merck's Jahresbericht 24:22–26
48. Kohli JD, De NN (1956) Pharmacological action of rauwolscine. Nature (London) 177:1182
49. Tangri KK, Bhargava KP (1961) Central component of vasomotor activity of yohimbine and its stereo-isomer rauwolscine. Arch Int Pharmacodyn 130:266–279
50. Das NN, Dasgupta SR, Mukherjee KL, Werner G (1955) Haemodynamic effects of rauwolscine. J Indian Med Res 43:101–106
51. Rockhold RW, Gross F (1981) Yohimbine diastereoisomers: cardiovascular effects after central and peripheral application in the rat. Naunyn-Schmiedeberg's Arch Pharmacol 315:227–231
52. Papeschi R, Sourkes TL, Youdim MBH (1971) The effect of yohimbine on brain serotonin metabolism, motor behavior and body temperature of the rat. Eur J Pharmacol 15:318–326
53. Serle JB, Podos SM, Lustgarten JS, Teiṭelbaum C, Severin CH (1985) The effect of corynanthine on intraocular pressure in clinical trials. Ophthalmology 92:977–980
54. Paris R, Janot M-M, Goutarel R (1945) Sur quelques propriétés physiologiques et en particulier sur l'action sympathicolytique de la corynanthéidine. C R Soc Biol 139: 665–666
55. Marzo A, Ghirardi P, Alessio R, Villa A (1977) Absorption and excretion of ^{3}H-raubasine in human subjects and dogs. Arzneim Forsch 27:2343–2344
56. Neuman J, De Engel AMF, Neuman MP (1986) Pilot study of the effect of raubasine on platelet biological activity. Arzneim Forsch 36:1394–1398
57. Weidinger P (1970) Ergebnisse der klinischen Prüfung von Raubasin. Med Welt 10:403–408
58. Glocke M, Grübl M, Klein K, Teufel W (1976) Wirkungsnachweis von Raubasin aus einer neuen Rezeptur von Lamuran® Dragees. Med Klin 71:1564–1568

59. Owen JA, Nakatsu SL, Fenemore J, Condra M, Surridge DHC, Morales A (1987) The pharmacokinetics of yohimbine in man. Eur J Clin Pharmacol 32:577–582
60. Hedner T, Edgar B, Edvinsson L, Hedner J, Persson B, Petterson A (1992) Yohimbine pharmacokinetics and interaction with the sympathetic nervous system in normal volunteers. Eur J Clin Pharmacol 43:651–656
61. Le Verge R, Le Corre P, Chevanne F, Döe De Maindreville M, Royer D, Levy J (1992) Determination of yohimbine and its two hydroxylated metabolites in humans by high-performance liquid chromatography and mass spectral analysis. J Chromatogr 574:283–292
62. Raymond-Hamet, Rothlin E (1960) Toxicité et activité utéro-adrénalinolytique, d'une part de quelques stéréo-isomères de la yohimbine, d'autre part de la δ-yohimbine ou raubasine. Compt Rend Soc Biol (Paris) 154:2037–2039
63. Paris R, Janot M-M, Goutarel R (1945) Toxicité de la corynanthéidine, nouvel alcaloïde cristallisé des écorces de *Pseudocinchona africana* Aug.Chev. Compt Rend Soc Biol 139:663–664
64. Bourin M, Malinge M, Colombel M-C, Larousse C (1988) Influence of alpha stimulants and beta blockers on yohimbine toxicity. Progr Neuro-Psychopharmacol Biol Psychiat 12:569–574
65. Quinton RM (1963) The increase in the toxicity of yohimbine induced by imipramine and other drugs in mice. Br J Pharmacol 21:51–66
66. Holmberg G, Gershon S (1961) Autonomic and psychic effects of yohimbine hydrochloride. Psychopharmacologia 2:93–106
67. Anonymous (1993) Physicians' Desk Reference. 47th edn. Montvale: Medical Economics Company Inc., pp.929,1217 and 1739
68. Margolis R, Sangree H, Prieto P, Stein L, Chinn S (1967) Clinical studies on the use of Afrodex in the treatment of impotence: statistical summary of 4000 cases. Curr Ther Res 9:213–219
69. Charney DS, Heninger GR, Redmond Jr. DE (1983) Yohimbine induced anxiety and increased noradrenergic function in humans: effects of diazepam and clonidine. Life Sci 33:19–29
70. Henauer SA, Gillespie HK, Hollister LE (1983) Yohimbine and the model anxiety state. J Clin Psychiatry 45:512–515
71. Lacomblez L, Bensimon G, Isnard F, Diquet B, Lecrubier Y, Puech AJ (1989) Effect of yohimbine on blood pressure in patients with depression and orthostatic hypotension induced by clomipramine. Clin Pharmacol Ther 45:241–251
72. Galitzky J, Rivière D, Tran MA, Montastruc JL, Berlan M (1990) Pharmacodynamic effects of chronic yohimbine treatment in healthy volunteers. Eur J Clin Pharmacol 39:447–451
73. Berlin I, Crespo-Laumonnier B, Cournot A, Landault C, Aubin F, Legrand J-C, Puech AJ (1991) The α_2-adrenergic receptor antagonist yohimbine inhibits epinephrine-induced platelet aggregation in healthy subjects. Clin Pharmacol Ther 49: 362–369
74. Mattila M, Seppala T, Mattila MJ (1988) Anxiogenic effect of yohimbine in healthy subjects: comparison with caffeine and antagonism by clonidine and diazepam. Int Clin Psychopharmacol 3:215–229
75. Onrot J, Goldberg MR, Biaggioni I, Wiley RG, Hollister AS, Robertson D (1987) Oral yohimbine in human autonomic failure. Neurol 37:215–220
76. Anonymous (1990) Yohimbe. Lawrence Rev Nat Prod, March 1990
77. Friesen K, Palatnick W, Tenenbein M (1993) Benign course after massive ingestion of yohimbine. J Emerg Med 11:287–288
78. Varkey S (1992) Overdose of yohimbine. Br Med J 304:548
79. Patscheider H, Dirnhofer R (1973) Tödliche Vergiftung eines Kleinkindes durch Yohimbin. Beitr Gerichtl Med 30:336–344
80. Young FE, Heckler MM (1985) Aphrodisiac drug products for over-the-counter human use. Fed Reg 50:2168–2170
81. Giessauf W, Pogglitsch H (1970) Über die Wirkung von Raubasin auf die Nierenfunktion. Wien Med Wschr 120:291–293

82. Poitrenaud J, Piette F, Malbezin M, Sebban C, Guez D (1990) Almitrine-raubasine and cognitive impairment in the elderly: results of a 6-month controlled multicenter study. Clin Neuropharmacol 13 (Suppl 3):S100–S108
83. Guez D (1990) Longterm effects and safety of almitrine-raubasine in age-associated cognitive decline. Clin Neuropharmacol 13 (Suppl 3):S109–S116
84. Sandler B, Aronson P (1993) Yohimbine-induced cutaneous drug eruption, progressive renal failure, and lupus-like syndrome. Urology 41:343–345
85. De Smet PAGM, Smeets OSNM (1994) Potential risks of health food products containing yohimbe extracts. Br Med J 309:958
86. Gershon S, Lang WJ (1962) A psycho-pharmacological study of some indole alkaloids. Arch Int Pharmacodyn 135:31–56
87. Goldberg MR, Hollister AS, Robertson D (1983) Influence of yohimbine on blood pressure, autonomic reflexes, and plasma catecholamines in humans. Hypertension 5:772–778
88. Goldstein DS, Eisenhofer G, Garty M, Sax FL, Keiser HR, Kopin IJ (1989) Pharmacologic and tracer methods to study sympathetic function in primary hypertension. Clin Exp Theory Pract A11 (Suppl.1):173–189
89. Charney DS, Heninger GR, Breier A (1984) Noradrenergic function in panic anxiety. Effects of yohimbine in healthy subjects and patients with agoraphobia and panic disorder. Arch Gen Psychiatry 41:751–763
90. De Jongh DK, Van Proosdij-Hartzema EG (1955) Investigations into experimental hypertension. IV. The acute effects of *Rauwolfia* alkaloids on the blood pressure of rats with experimental renal hypertension. Acta Physiol Pharmacol Neerl 4:175–186
91. Dunn RW, Corbett R (1992) Yohimbine-induced seizures involve NMDA and GABAergic transmission. Neuropharmacol 31:389–395
92. Rosenblum LA, Coplan JD, Friedman S, Bassoff T (1991) Dose-response effects of oral yohimbine in unrestrained primates. Biol Psychiatry 29:647–657
93. Charney DS, Woods SW, Goodman WK, Heninger GR (1987) Neurobiological mechanisms of panic anxiety: biochemical and behavioral corellates of yohimbine-induced panic attacks. Am J Psychiatry 144:1030–1036
94. Price LH, Charney DS, Heninger GR (1984) Three cases of manic symptoms following yohimbine administration. Am J Psychiatry 141:1267–1268
95. Fontaine Ch (1968) Influence de la raubasine a doses fortes sur la réadaptation de malades atteints d'affections vasculaires cérébrales. Sem Hop 44:806–809
96. Charney DS, Breier A, Jatlow PI, Heninger GR (1986) Behavioral, biochemical and blood pressure responses to alprazolam in healthy subjects: interactions with yohimbine. Psychopharmacology 88:133–140
97. Price LH, Charney DS, Rubin AL, Heninger GR (1986) α_2-Adrenergic receptor function in depression. The cortisol response to yohimbine. Arch Gen Psychiatry 43:849–858
98. Gold MS, Donabedian RK, Redmond Jr. DE (1979) Further evidence for alpha-2 adrenergic receptor mediated inhibition of prolactin secretion: the effect of yohimbine. Psychoneuroendocrinology 3:253–260
99. Espinoza N, Westermann B (1967) Untersuchungen über den Einfluss von Raubasin auf den Kohlenhydratstoffwechsel von Diabetikern. Dtsch Med Wschr 92:1562–1564
100. Landis E, Shore E (1989) Yohimbine-induced bronchospasm. Chest 96:1424
101. Ortmann R, Mutter M, Delini-Stula A (1982) Effect of yohimbine and its diastereoisomers on clonidine-induced depression of exploration in the rat. Eur J Pharmacol 77:335–337
102. Liljequist S, Berggren U, Engel J (1981) The effect of catecholamine receptor antagonists on ethanol-induced locomotor stimulation. J Neural Transm 50:57–67
103. Sanghvi I, Urquiaga X, Gershon S (1971) Exploration of the anti-depressant potential of L-DOPA. Psychopharmacologia 20: 118–127
104. Geyer HJ, Sanghvi I, Gershon S (1973) Exploration of the anti-depressant potential of lithium. Psychopharmacologia 28:107–113
105. Lang WJ, Lambert GA, Rush ML (1975) The role of the central nervous system in the cardiovascular responses to yohimbine. Arch Int Pharmacodyn 217:57–67

106. Ernsberger P, Haxhiu MA, Graff LM, Collins LA, Dreshaj I, Grove DL, Graves ME, Schäfer SG, Christen MO (1994) A novel mechanism of action for hypertension control: moxonidine as a selective I_1-imidazoline agonist. Cardiovasc Drugs Ther 8:27–41
107. Charney DS, Price LH, Heninger GR (1986) Desipramine-yohimbine combination treatment of refractory depression. Implications for the β-adrenergic receptor hypothesis of antidepressant action. Arch Gen Psychiatry 43:1155–1161
108. Bagheri H, Picault P, Schmitt L, Houin G, Berlan M, Montastruc JL (1994) Pharmacokinetic study of yohimbine and its pharmacodynamic effects on salivary secretion in patients treated with tricyclic antidepressants. Br J Clin Pharmacol 37:93–96
109. Ingram CG (1962) Some pharmacologic actions of yohimbine and chlorpromazine in man. Clin Pharmacol Ther 3:345–352
110. Itil T, Fink M (1968) EEG and behavioral aspects of the interaction of anticholinergic hallucinogens with centrally active compounds. Progr Brain Res 28:149–168
111. Pichler L, Kobinger W (1985) Possible function of α_1-adrenoceptors in the CNS in anaesthetized and conscious animals. Eur J Pharmacol 107:305–311
112. Prud'Homme MJ (1988) Effect of α-adrenergic blocking agents on uterine activity in the ewe at the end of gestation. Acta Physiol Hungar 71:485–489
113. Lechner W, Daxenbichler G, Marth Ch (1987) Wehenhemmung mit α-Adrenorezeptorenblockern. Z Geburtshilfe Perinatol 191:102–104
114. Bovet–Nitti F, Bovet D (1959) Action of some sympathicolytic agents on pregnancy in the rat. Proc Soc Exp Biol Med 100: 555–557
115. Von Poser G, Andrade HHR, Da Silva KVCL, Henriques AT, Henriques JAP (1990) Genotoxic, mutagenic and recombinogenic effects of rauwolfia alkaloids. Mutat Res 232:37–43

Yohimbe Alkaloids – *Corynanthe* Species

P.A.G.M. De Smet

Botany

The genus of *Corynanthe* belongs to the Rubiaceae. The principal species of medicinal interest is *Corynanthe pachyceras* K.Schum., also known as *Pseudocinchona africana* A.Chev., *Pseudocinchona pachyceras* (K.Schum.) A.Chev. and *Pausinystalia pachyceras* (Schum.) De Wild. It serves as source plant of Pseudocinchonae africanae cortex [1–4].

Commercial yohimbe bark samples sometimes contain considerable amounts of this bark [5].

Chemistry

The bark of *Corynanthe pachyceras* yields 3.05–6.25% of total alkaloids [5]. Yohimbine is absent but numerous other yohimbe alkaloids have been identified: corynanthine (1.1%), rauwolscine (=α-yohimbine), β-yohimbine, corynanthidine, corynantheine, dihydrocorynantheine, corynantheidine (0.3%), corynoxeine and corynoxine [4,6–10].

Melchio et al. [11] examined the bark and leaves of *Corynanthe mayumbensis* (R. Good) N. Hallé (syn. *Pseudocinchona mayumbensis*) and extracted six heteroyohimbane alkaloids: epi-19 ajmalicine (= mayumbine), iso-3 epi-19 ajmalicine, rauniticine, iso-3 rauniticine, tetrahydroalstonine, and akuammigine.

The bark of *Corynanthe paniculata* Welwitsch contains 0.8% of yohimbine; it was also reported to yield the alkaloid paniculatine but this may be an impure substance [12].

Pharmacology and Uses

In Africa, the bark of *Corynanthe pachyceras* is used inter alia in fevers and malaria and also as aphrodisiac [1,3,4]; the stems, roots and leaves of the plant may serve similar purposes there [13].

An aqueous extract of bark of *Corynanthe pachyceras* showed the following sedative and cardiovascular effects in animal studies [4,14]:

- The extract reduced motility and amphetamine toxicity in the mouse, whereas it prolonged barbiturate-induced narcosis.
- The extract lowered blood pressure in rats and dogs.
- The extract supressed the inotropic and chronotropic effects of isoprenaline on the atrium of the rabbit heart in vitro.

See also the general discussion of yohimbe alkaloids elsewhere in this volume.

Adverse Reaction Profile

A general discussion of the adverse reaction profile of yohimbe alkaloids is presented elsewhere in this volume.

General Animal Data

The intravenous LD_{50} in the mouse of a dried aqueous extract from the bark of *Corynanthe pachyceras* (containing 3–3.2% of alkaloids) was reported to be 4.9 mg/kg [4].
See also the general discussion of yohimbe alkaloids elsewhere in this volume.

Fertility, Pregnancy and Lactation

See the general discussion of yohimbe alkaloids elsewhere in this volume.

Mutagenicity and Carcinogenicity

No data about the mutagenicity or carcinogenicity of *Corynanthe* alkaloids have been recovered from the literature.

References

1. Steinmetz EF (1976) Pseudocinchonae Africanae Arboris Cortex. Quart J Crude Drug Res 14:68
2. Penso G (1983) Index Plantarum Medicinalium Totius Mundi Eorumque Synonymorum. Milano: Organizzazione Editoriale Medico Farmaceutica, pp.271 and 712
3. Oliver-Bever B (1986) Medicinal plants in tropical West Africa. Cambridge: Cambridge University Press
4. Hänsel R, Keller K, Rimpler H, Schneider G, red. (1992) Hagers Handbuch der Pharmazeutischen Praxis. 5th edn. Vierter Band: Drogen A-D. Berlin: SpringerVerlag, pp.1029–1032
5. Hajonides van der Meulen Th, Van der Kerk GJM (1964) Alkaloids in *Pausinystalia yohimbe* (K. Schum.) ex Pierre. Part II. The isolation of a new alkaloid. Rec Trav Chim Pays-Bas 83:148–153
6. Raymond-Hamet (1933) Sur une nouvelle méthode d'extraction et de séparation des alcaloïdes du "Pseudocinchona africana" A.Chev. Bull Sci Pharm 40:523–527

7. Paris R, Janot M-M, Goutarel R (1945) Toxicité de la corynanthéidine, nouvel alcaloïde cristallisé des écorces de *Pseudocinchona africana* Aug.Chev. Compt Rend Soc Biol 139:663–664
8. Karrer P, Schwyzer R, Flam A (1952) Die Konstitution des Corynantheins und Dihydro-corynantheins. Helv Chim Acta 35:851–862
9. Hajonides van der Meulen Th, Van der Kerk GJM (1964) Alkaloids in *Pausinystalia yohimbe* (K. Schum.) ex Pierre. Part I. The paper-chromatographic identification of alkaloids occurring in some yohimbine-containing barks. Rec Trav Chim Pays-Bas 83:141–147
10. Manske RHF (1965) Alkaloids of *Pseudocinchona* and *Yohimbe*. In: Manske RHF, red. The Alkaloids – Chemistry and Physiology. Volume 8: The indole alkaloids. New York: Academic Press, pp.693–723
11. Melchio J, Bouquet A, Pais M, Goutarel R (1977) Alcaloides indoliques CVI (1), Identité de la mayumbine et de l'epi-19 ajmalicine. L'iso-3 rauniticine, un nouvel alcaloïde extrait du *Corynanthe mayumbensis* (R. Good) N. Hallé. Tetrahedron Lett 4:315–316
12. Le Hir A, Goutarel G, Janot M-M (1953) Extraction et séparation de la yohimbine et de ses stéréoisomères. Ann Pharm Franç 11:546–564
13. Iwu MM (1993) Handbook of African medicinal plants. Boca Raton: CRC Press
14. Gargallo JC (1972) Hypotensive and sedative Pseudocinchona africana extract. Chem Ab 76:90041k

Yohimbe Alkaloids – *Pausinystalia* Species

P.A.G.M. De Smet

Botany

The genus of *Pausinystalia* belongs to the Rubiaceae. The principal species of medicinal interest is *Pausinystalia yohimbe* (K. Schum.) Pierre ex Beille, sometimes spelled as *P.johimbe* or as *P.yohimba*. Another Latin binomial for this species is *Corynanthe yohimbe* K. Schum., sometimes spelled as *C.johimbe* [1–6]. Vernacular names are yohimbe, yohimbehe (E); Yohimbe (G); yohimbe, yohimbé, yohimbéhé (F) [2,7–9]. The commercially available plant part is the stem bark [10].

Another *Pausinystalia* species of medicinal interest is *Pausinystalia macroceras* (K.Schum.) Pierre ex Beille, also known as *Corynanthe macroceras* K. Schum. [11,12].

Chemistry

Total alkaloid levels in different parts of *P.yohimbe* were investigated by Paris and Letouzey [10]; they reported levels varying from 2.7% to 5.9% in the stem bark (Table 1). The following alkaloids have been recovered from the stem bark: yohimbine, rauwolscine (=α-yohimbine), β-yohimbine, alloyohimbine, pseudoyohimbine, raubasine (= ajmalicine), corynanthine, corynantheine, dihydrocorynantheine, and dihydrositsirikine [1,7–9,13–17].

Le Hir et al. [7] found 0.8% of yohimbine, 0.03% of β-yohimbine and 0.04% of pseudoyohimbine in a bark sample, which definitely originated from *Pausinystalia yohimbe*. Hajonides van der Meulen and Van der Kerk [14] also reported quantitative information about the concentrations of yohimbine and some other individual alkaloids in the stem bark of genuine *P.yohimbe* (Table 2). Other reported constituents of yohimbe bark are yohimbic acid, tannic acid, and a colouring agent [3].

Yohimbe bark preparations on the western health food market may not have the composition which is declared on the label. Recent analysis of yohimbe tablets from the United States merely showed caffeine and no yohimbine, even though the label claimed that 500 mg of yohimbe bark extract was present in each tablet [18]. The bark of *Corynanthe pachyceras* also serves as adulterant of genuine yohimbe bark [14].

Table 1. Total alkaloid percentages in different plant parts of *Pausinystalia yohimbe*, as reported by Paris and Letouzey [10]

Plant part	Total alkaloid percentages
Small roots	3.10–3.86
Bark of the large roots	4.70–5.06
Bark of the stem 1– 2 m aboveground	2.70–3.34
Bark of the stem 7–12 m aboveground	2.80–3.63
Bark of the stem 14–21 m aboveground	3.00–5.92
Bark of the large branches	1.80–2.82
Bark of the small branches	0.20–0.60
Leaves	0.07–0.14

Table 2. Weight percentages of alkaloids in two bark samples of *Pausinystalia yohimbe* (calculated on the dry bark), as reported by Hajonides van der Meulen and Van der Kerk [14]

	Sample A	Sample B
Total alkaloids	5.71%	5.29%
Yohimbine (impure)[1]	1.14%[2]	2.22%[2]
Rauwolscine	0.46%	0.39%
Pseudoyohimbine	0.36%	0.02%
Raubasine	0.08%	0.04%
Dihydrositsirikine[3]	0.12%	0.39%

[1] Approximate yield of yohimbine, as small amounts of α-yohimbine and β-yohimbine were also present in the fraction
[2] Recalculated from the originally reported values (which apparently related to precipitated hydrochloride) by multiplication with 0.9
[3] Originally described as "compound A" [14] and as "tetrahydro-desmethyl-corynantheine" [15]; later identified by Kutney and Brown [17] as the alkaloid dihydrositsirikine

Leboeuf et al. [11] studied the trunk bark of *Pausinystalia macroceras* and recovered 4% of total alkaloids. They isolated yohimbine as major alkaloid (2.4–2.6%), and demonstrated the presence of rauwolscine (0.32%), β-yohimbine (0.06%), corynanthine (0.2%) and raubasine (0.28%) as minor indole alkaloids. In addition, the bark yielded 0.28% of the levorotatory isomer of calycanthine, a quinoline dimeric tryptophane derived alkaloid.

Yohimbine has also been reported to occur in other *Pausinystalia* species, notably *P.angolensis* Wernham [1] and *P.trillesii* Beille [3,16].

Pharmacology and Uses

In Africa, the bark of *Pausinystalia yohimbe* is considered to be an aphrodisiac and a stimulant [5] and the bark of *P.macroceras* is applied there for similar purposes [11].

In western society, crude yohimbe bark and ready-to-use yohimbe preparations are promoted as health food products with aphrodisiac properties. The crude bark is used for making tea by simmering 5 to 10 teaspoons of the shaved material in one pint of water. Yohimbe bark may also be smoked with the purpose of producing "effortless seduction" or a hallucinogenic reaction [9,18–20].

In addition, yohimbe bark has been employed in traditional medicine to treat angina and hypertension [9]. This is a remarkable practice, since the major yohimbe alkaloid yohimbine is nowadays considered to be contra-indicated in patients with such diseases [21].

See also the general discussion of yohimbe alkaloids elsewhere in this volume.

Adverse Reaction Profile

A general discussion of the adverse reaction profile of yohimbe alkaloids is presented elsewhere in this volume.

General Human Data

In 1993, the American Food and Drug Administration reported that it was investigating serious adverse reactions to yohimbe products, including renal failure, seizures and death [22].

See also the general discussion of yohimbe alkaloids elsewhere in this volume.

Fertility, Pregnancy and Lactation

See the general discussion of yohimbe alkaloids elsewhere in this volume.

Mutagenicity and Carcinogenicity

See the general discussion of yohimbe alkaloids elsewhere in this volume.

References

1. Hajonides van der Meulen Th, Van der Kerk GJM (1964) Alkaloids in *Pausinystalia yohimbe* (K. Schum.) ex Pierre. Part I. The paper-chromatographic identification of alkaloids occurring in some yohimbine-containing barks. Rec Trav Chim Pays-Bas 83:141–147
2. Hoppe HA (1975) Drogenkunde. Band 1. Angiospermen. 8. Auflage. Berlin: Walter de Gruyter
3. List PH, Hörhammer L (1977) Hagers Handbuch der Pharmazeutischen Praxis. Vierte Neuausgabe. Sechster Band. Chemikalien und Drogen, Teil A: N-Q. Berlin: Springer-Verlag, pp.482–485
4. Pelletier SW (1983) Alkaloids – Chemical and biological perspectives. Volume one. New York: John Wiley & Sons, p.350
5. Oliver-Bever B (1986) Medicinal plants in tropical West Africa. Cambridge: Cambridge University Press
6. Thesen R, Schulz M, Braun R (1990) Ganz oder teilweise "negativ" bewertete Arzneistoffe. Pharm Ztg 135:1812–1814
7. Le Hir A, Goutarel G, Janot M-M (1953) Extraction et séparation de la yohimbine et de ses stéréoisomères. Ann Pharm Franç 11:546–564
8. Poisson J (1964) Recherches récentes sur les alcaloïdes du Pseudocinchona et du Yohimbe. Ann Chim (Paris) 9:99–121
9. Anonymous (1990) Yohimbe. Lawrence Rev Nat Prod, March 1990
10. Paris R, Letouzey R (1960) Répartition des alcaloïdes dans le yohimbe (Pausinystalia yohimbe) (K. Schum.) ex Pierre (Rubiacées). J Agr Trop Botan Appl 7:256–258
11. Leboeuf M, Cavé A, Mangeney P, Bouquet A (1981) Alcaloïdes du Pausinystalia macroceras. Planta Med 41:374–378
12. Penso G (1983) Index Plantarum Medicinalium Totius Mundi Eorumque Synonymorum. Milano: Organizzazione Editoriale Medico Farmaceutica, pp.271 and 712
13. Karrer P, Schwyzer R, Flam A (1952) Die Konstitution des Corynantheins und Dihydro-corynantheins. Helv Chim Acta 35:851–862
14. Hajonides van der Meulen Th, Van der Kerk GJM (1964) Alkaloids in *Pausinystalia yohimbe* (K. Schum.) ex Pierre. Part II. The isolation of a new alkaloid. Rec Trav Chim Pays-Bas 83:148–153
15. Hajonides van der Meulen Th, Van der Kerk GJM (1964) Alkaloids in *Pausinystalia yohimbe* (K. Schum.) ex Pierre. Part III. The structure of a new alkaloid. Rec Trav Chim Pays-Bas 83:154–166
16. Manske RHF (1965) Alkaloids of *Pseudocinchona* and *Yohimbe*. In: Manske RHF, red. The Alkaloids – Chemistry and Physiology. Volume 8: The indole alkaloids. New York: Academic Press, pp.693–723
17 Kutney JP, Brown RT (1966) The structural elucidation of sitsirikine, dihydrositsirikine and isositsirikine. Tetrahedron 22:321–336
18. De Smet PAGM, Smeets OSNM (1994) Potential risks of health food products containing yohimbe extracts. Br Med J 309:958
19 Mack RB (1985) Taljaribu kila dawa isifal: yohimbine intoxication. N Carolina Med J 46:229–230
20. Buffum J (1985) Pharmacosexology update: yohimbine and sexual function. J Psychoact Drugs 17:131–132
21. Anonymous (1993) USP DI. Volume I – Drug Information for the Health Care Professional. 13th edn. Rockville: United States Pharmacopeial Convention, Inc., pp.2807–2808
22. Department of Health and Human Services (1993) Unsubstantiated claims and documented health hazards in the dietary supplement marketplace. Rockville: Public Health Service, Food and Drug Administration, p.101

Zingiber Officinale

D. Corrigan

Botany

Zingiber officinale Roscoe, usually known as ginger, belongs to the family Zingiberaceae. The genus zingiber comprises some 80–90 species which are perennial aromatic herbs with fleshy rhizomes and tuberous roots. The chief commercial varieties of ginger are Chinese, Nigerian, Cochin and Jamaican, reflecting the fact that the plant is grown in areas as diverse as China, India [Cochin], Nigeria, Sierra Leone, Sri Lanka, Vietnam, Australia and Jamaica. Fresh ginger is sun-dried in the country of origin. It may or may not be peeled ['scraped'] to remove cork [1]. The official British Pharmacopoeia grade is defined as „the rhizome of *Zingiber officinale* Roscoe scraped or unscraped. It is known in commerce as unbleached ginger" [2].

Chemistry

Ginger is noted for its aroma and for its pungent flavour. The aroma is due to an essential oil, the content of which ranges from 0.25 to 3.3% v/w [1,3,4]. Macleod and Pieris [5] noted that the aroma volatiles, of which more than 200 have been identified [6], varied considerably depending on chemotaxonomic differences between cultivars and region of production [5]. The essential oil of fresh ginger has a high content of geranial [α-citral] and neral [β-citral] which gives a lemony aroma [1,5]. Some ginger oils have a camphoraceous smell attributed to the presence of cineole [1]. On drying, the monoterpene content declines and there is an increase in sesquiterpene content including in particular β-sesquiphellandrene (7–17%), β-bisabolene (5–12%), α-curcumene (6–19%) and α-zingiberene (20–30%) [3,4,5]. Among the other monoterpenes present are camphene, linalool and borneol, while also included in the sesquiterpene fraction [which makes up 30–70% of the oil] are E,E-α-farnesene, zingiberol, *cis*-sesquisabinene hydrate and zingiberenol [3–6].

The pungent oleoresin which can be obtained by extraction with acetone and subsequent evaporation of the solvent (*Oleoresina Zingiberis* BPC 1949) [7], constitutes between 4 and 7.5% w/w in the dried drug and up to 20% in fresh rhizomes [8]. The major pungent compounds are a homologous series of phenolic ketones called gingerols [9]. The oleoresin also contains shogaols formed by the dehydration of gingerols during storage or thermal processing. GC-MS has shown that ginger contains: [3]-, [4]-, [5]-, [6]-, [8]-, [10]- and [12]-gingerols, [3]-, [4]-, [5]-, [6]-, [8]-and [10]-shogaols, [4]-, [6]-, [8]- and [10]-gingerdiols, [6]-methylgingediol, [4]- and [6]-gingediacetates [10]. Other related compounds included paradols, zingerone, hexahydrocurcumin and O-methyl ether derivatives of these compounds [11]. Diarylheptenones such as gingerenones A, B and C have been isolated from aqueous ethanolic extracts of the rhizomes [12]. Among the other constituents of the rhizome are galanolactone, a diterpene [13], as well as 6-gingesulphonic acid isolated from the water soluble fraction [14]. Yoshikawa et al. [15] compared twenty different gingers of varying origin using HPLC. They found that Japanese ginger contained [6]-gingerol, 6-dehydrogingerdione and galanololactone, but this latter compound was not detected in imported ginger samples. They further noted that the [6]-gingerol and galanolactone content of fresh ginger decreased remarkably during the processing into Zingeribis Rhizoma. Three new monoacyldigalactosylglycerols called gingerglycolipids A, B and C were also elucidated [13]. Tanabe and coworkers [16] have isolated a diterpene, (E)-8β,17-epoxylabd-12-ene-15,6-dial, which they term ZT, from ginger. Fresh ginger contains a significant amount of a protease [17].

Pharmacology and Uses

Ginger is widely used as a spice [1]. As a medicine, ginger has been used for 2,500 years in China. It is an ingredient for almost half of all oriental herbal medicines, particularly those of Sino-Japanese origin [10]. Hikino [10] in his review noted that two forms of ginger are used, fresh (or air-dried) ginger and the processed form which involves steaming the root before drying. Hikino [10], while listing a large number of effects for both types, concluded that there were no essential differences in pharmacological action between the fresh and processed drug. However, Pancho et al. [18] compared the effects of fresh and processed ginger as well as [6]-gingerol (the major pungent principle of the fresh material) and [6]-shogaol (the major component of the processed drug) on norepinephrine- and $PGF_2\alpha$- induced contractions using mouse mesenteric veins. The methanol extract of fresh ginger and [6]-gingerol significantly potentiated the contractions due to $PGF_2\alpha$ but the processed ginger extract and [6]-shogaol strongly inhibited the $PGF_2\alpha$- induced contraction. Both gingerol and shogaol inhibited responses due to norepinephrine with shogaol showing the greater potency. However, both the fresh and processed ginger extracts showed no such inhibitory effects, indicating that other components of these extracts may have masked the effects of [6]-gingerol and [6]-shogaol.

Antiinflammatory activity equivalent to that of acetylsalicylic acid has been reported in the rat [19] as well as in vitro inhibition of prostaglandin release, which Mascolo [19] suggested correlated with the antipyretic activity noted by his group and that of Suekawa [20]. According to Kiuchi et al. [21] gingerols act as general inhibitors of lipoxygenases and hence affect prostaglandin synthetase activity in vitro. A series of papers by Srivastava [22–25] has dealt with the effect of ginger on arachidonic acid metabolism and also on its ability to inhibit platelet aggregation, while Backon [26] has drawn attention to the ability of the rhizome to inhibit thromboxane synthetase and raise prostacyclin levels without increasing PGE_2 or

PGF$_2\alpha$ levels. Srivastava [25] specifically notes that in a group of 7 women who ate 5 g of fresh ginger for 7 days mean thromboxane levels declined by almost 37%. Srivastava [27] links these effects to positive clinical findings in patients with rheumatoid arthritis who consumed 5 g of fresh or 0.5–1 g of dried ginger daily for three months. All of the patients (n=6) reported pain relief, better joint movement, a decrease in swelling and morning stiffness. The same author [28] has reported on 56 patients (28 with rheumatoid arthritis, 18 with osteoarthritis and 10 with muscular discomfort). More than 75% of the arthritis reported relief of pain and swelling, while all of the patients with muscular discomfort experienced pain relief. In all cases the ginger (1–2 g) was taken orally. Chang and But [29] include a reference to the successful use of ginger injections in 113 Chinese cases of rheumatic or chronic low back pain.

Backon [30] refers to the use of ginger by his group to treat burns, a use also referred to by Leung [31] based on his translation of a Chinese paper which describes the use of the juice of the fresh rhizome applied topically to treat 400–500 cases of burns.

Studies of antiserotonergic effects have given contradictory results, with some experiments (using guinea pig ileum) showing activity [13,32], while tests in a bovine platelet bioassay were negative [33]. Mustafa and Srivastava [34] found that in one patient 1.5–2 g of powdered ginger p. o. per day markedly reduced the frequency of migraine attacks.

Animal studies indicate cholagogic and antihepatotoxic effects [35,36]. A number of enzyme systems related to cholesterol and bile acid synthesis are affected by ginger, resulting in a lowering of cholesterol levels in animals [16,37–41].

Chang and But [29] include reports of improvement in cases of gastric and duodenal ulcers but patients were susceptible to relapse. There are also a number of reports of animal studies generally showing decreases in gastric secretion [29,42] and inhibition of HCl/ethanol-induced gastric lesions, an effect ascribed to zingiberene, [6]-gingerol and 6-gingesulphonic acid [14,42].

In Western medicine most attention has, in recent years, centred on ginger as an antiemetic. Studies in leopard and ranid frogs show that the gingerols and shogaols inhibited the emetic action induced by the oral administration of copper sulphate pentahydrate [44]. There have been nine studies of powdered ginger as an antiemetic in humans. Six of the studies reported positive effects [45–50], while three were negative [51–53]. Of the negative studies only one appears to have been a blind study and the criteria used, based on National Aeronautical and Space Administration (NASA) standardised motion sickness tests, were different to those used in the positive trials. None of the nine trials appear to have used a standardised ginger preparation which makes comparison of the outcomes difficult. Three of the positive studies related to motion sickness [45–47], two recommended the use of the plant to reduce or prevent post-operative vomiting after gynaecological surgery [48, 50] and one study investigated the value of ginger in hyperemesis gravidarum [49].

According to the British Herbal Compendium [54] ginger preparations are included in Schedule I of the General Sale List under the UK Medicines Act 1968, which means that preparations can, with reasonable safety, be sold other than under the supervision of a pharmacist. It also states that in Belgium, ginger may only be sold as a medicine with the indication ,,traditionally used in the symptomatic treatment of digestive disorders". In Germany the Kommission E Monograph states that the uses of ginger include dyspeptic complaints and prophylaxis of the symptoms of travel sickness.

Ginger shows modest antibacterial [19,29], antifungal [12,29], molluscicidal [55], and ascaricidal effects [23,29]. Antirhinoviral activity due to the sesquiterpenes has recently been reported [56].

Other effects which have been reported include hypoglycaemia in rabbits after oral dosing [19], increased catecholamine secretion due to zingerenone [57], while shogaol showed an intense antitussive effect in comparison with dihydrocodeine phosphate [20]. According to Sato et al., cited by Hikino [10], ginger extracts displayed significant antitumour activity against cultured human JTC-26 cancer cells and also against Sarcoma-180 ascites in mice. Ginger extracts inhibited DNA damage induced by lipid peroxidation and also suppressed the generation of active oxygen as well as linoleic acid oxidation [58]. In another study of the antioxidant effect, ginger rhizome gave an antioxidant index higher than butylated hydroxytoluene [59]. The US Food and Drug Administration [FDA] does not include Jamaican ginger as being generally safe and effective as an ingredient of smoking deterrent products [60].

Pharmacokinetics

Ding et al. [61] studied the pharmacokinetics of a bolus i. v. dose of 3 mg of [6]-gingerol per kg in cannulated rats. They found that gingerol was cleared very rapidly from plasma with a terminal half-life of 7.23 min and a total body clearance of 16.8 ml/min/kg. A two-compartment open model was found to describe the data adequately. Serum protein binding was 92.4% which was surprising given the rapid clearance from plasma. Given that it has been reported [20] that pharmacological effects were maintained up to 180 min after i. v. administration of a dose of 3.5 mg/kg, it was suggested by Ding et al. [61] that gingerol may be irreversibly sequestered in the tissues or that it may be effective at plasma concentrations lower than the limits of detection of the HPLC assay they used.

Adverse Reaction Profile

Ginger oil was granted Generally Recognised As Safe [GRAS] status by the Flavoring Extract Manufacturers Association [FEMA] in 1965 and is approved by the U.S. Food and Drug Administration [FDA] for food use [17]. The Council of Europe included ginger oil in the list of substances, spices and seasonings deemed admissible for use with a possible limitation of the active principle in the final product [62].

General Animal Data

Emig [63] administered up to 97 g of ginger by intragastric feeding to each of three rabbits over a 10 day period. One of the rabbits died due to causes other than ginger. The other rabbits showed no ill effects. Injection of a concentrated alcoholic extract [1 ml equivalent to 5 g of drug] into the marginal ear vein of the rabbit had no effect at a dose of 1 ml. The rabbit given 1.5 ml immediately became spastic, with a stimulated nervous system, pupils contracted at first then dilated and rapid respiration. After 24 hours the animal returned to normal. A third rabbit given 2 ml died immediately.

Mascolo [19] tested a concentrated ethanolic (80%) extract in mice dosed by gavage in volumes of 10 ml/kg. The extract was well tolerated orally up to a dose of 2.5 g/kg with no mortality or side effects except a mild diarrhoea in 2 animals. However doses of 3.0 and 3.5 g/kg of the extract caused 10–30% mortality due to involuntary contractions of skeletal muscle within 72 hours of administration. Other symptoms observed included gastrointestinal spasm, hypothermia, diarrhoea and anorexia [19]. The safety coefficient of the injection of fresh ginger in mice was determined to be more than 625 times higher than that of the clinical dose for an adult [29].

According to the monograph by Opdyke [64], both the acute oral LD_{50} value in rats and the acute dermal LD_{50} value in rabbits exceeded 5 g of ginger oil/kg body weight.

Suekawa et al. [20] reported LD_{50} values for [6]-gingerol and [6]-shogaol in mice. For [6]-gingerol the values for i. v., i. p. and p. o. administration were 25.5, 58.1 and 250.0 mg/kg respectively. For [6]-shogaol the corresponding values were 50.9, 109.2 and 687.0 mg/kg respectively. In the case of i. v. administration the animals died within 5 minutes but survivors showed sedation-like symptoms and began to recover gradually after about 30 minutes and were fully recovered after 2 hours. With the two other routes of administration the symptoms were similar to those after i. v. dosing but the time elapsing until death differed [20].

Tanabe and colleagues [16] performed an acute toxicity test with ZT on mice and reported that no deaths occurred at an oral dose of 25 mg/kg or at an intra-abdominal dose of 25 mg/kg.

Scott and Kennedy [65] detected aflatoxins in 8 out of 15 samples of ginger analysed. One sample contained 25 µg of aflatoxin B_1 and 15 µg of aflatoxin B_2 per kg.

General Human Data

A significant number of cases of „ginger paralysis" including fatalities were reported in the United States in 1930. Subsequent investigations showed that the ginger preparations consumed by the victims were contaminated with 2% tri- o-tolyl phosphate which was responsible for the paralysis [66].

No side effects were reported by Grontved and Hentzen [46, 47] in their two studies of ginger in vertigo and in seasickness. Srivastava and Mustafa [27, 28] in their separate studies of 7 and 56 patients who used up to 2 g of ginger daily for up to 2.5 years also recorded that no side effects were reported by any of the subjects. Bone et al. [48] and Phillips et al. [50] in their clinical trials of 1 g of ginger as a postoperative antiemetic, also noted a lack of side effects following use of ginger.

Cardiovascular Reactions

Emig [63] injected 5 ml of a concentrated ethanolic extract (equivalent to 25 g of drug) into the femoral vein of an anaesthesized dog. In addition to a marked increase in respiration, there was transient vagal inhibition followed by an increase in blood pressure and heart rate which continued to increase after vagal section. An alcoholic extract containing the resin was found to stimulate vasomotor and respiratory centres of anaesthesized cats. It also had a direct stimulant effect on the heart [29]. Zhu [29] found that the mean systolic and diastolic pressures of normal subjects given 1 g of fresh ginger to chew without swallowing were increased 11.2 and 14 mm Hg respectively but there was no significant change in pulse rate.

Shoji et al. [67] recorded a dose-dependent positive inotropic effect on isolated guinea pig atria treated with a methanol extract of the rhizome. This effect was subsequently ascribed to the gingerols. In further studies both [6]-shogaol and [6]-gingerol produced depressor responses on systemic blood pressure in rats at doses of 10–100 µg/kg [20]. At higher doses (0.5–1.0 mg/kg) a triphasic pattern was seen, consisting of an immediate fall, followed by a rise and another decrease [20]. The lower doses caused a decrease in heart rate and higher doses produced remarkable bradycardia after i. v. administration, possibly due to vagal stimulation. Suekawa [68] subjected [6]-shogaol to further studies in rats at a dose of 0.5 mg/kg i. v. and concluded that [6]-shogaol may cause a peripheral pressor response by releasing an unknown active substance from nerve ends via a calcium channel which is not affected by antagonists such as diltiazem and verapamil.

Central Nervous System Reactions

Emig [63] reported that in a dog injected with the equivalent of 7.5 g of drug as an ethanolic extract, the entire nervous system appeared to be stimulated. Both [6]-shogaol and [6]-gingerol administered i. v. (1.75–3.5 mg/kg) or p. o. (70–140 mg/kg) showed inhibition of spontaneous movement and enhancement of hexobarbital-induced sleep in mice [20]. [6]-Shogaol had a stronger effect than [6]-gingerol on the EEG of rats. Low amplitude fast waves appeared in the early stage following dosing and then a pattern of drowsiness of about 1 hour's duration in the cortical EEG. It must be noted, however, that none of the human studies with powdered ginger have reported any CNS effects following use of the rhizome [41–53].

Dermatological Reactions

Opdyke [64] in his monograph on ginger oil notes that the undiluted oil was not irritating to the skin of hairless mice. It was moderately irritating to intact or abraded rabbit skin when applied under occlusion for 24 hours. In humans there was no irritation after a 48 hour closed-patch test with 4% oil in petrolatum. A similar concentration was used to perform a sensitisation test on 25 volunteers with negative results although Tulipan [69] had noted that toiletries containing the essential oil might produce dermatitis in hypersensitive individuals. Stäger et al. [70] performed scratch tests with commercial spices, including ginger, in 70 patients with positive skin tests to birch and/or mugwort pollens and celery. Ginger elicited positive skin reactions in only three out of eleven patients whereas spices from the Apiaceae family, e. g. fennel, gave positive reactions in more than 24 patients. On the other hand Futrell and Rietschel [71] reported that in a group of fifty-five patients with suspected contact dermatitis, positive patch tests with spices at 10% and 25% concentrations in petrolatum were more common with ginger (seven patients) than with any of the other spices.

Yamamoto [72] reported that ingestion of ginger exacerbated symptoms in patients with acute inflammatory skin diseases.

Gastrointestinal Reactions

Liu and Ho [73] reported four cases of ginger-induced bezoar and cite a reference to a further three cases. The majority of cases involved preserved ginger root as a snack consumed by children and elderly edentulous patients. The cases presented with vomiting, constipation, abdominal distension and radiological evidence of dilated small bowel loops with fluid levels.

In his review on ginger, Awang [74] writes that heart burn is the most serious side effect noted. Stewart [53] states that three out of eight subjects given ginger reported gastric burning during a gastric emptying procedure. Desai and colleagues [75] examined the DNA content of gastric aspirates before and after intragastric infusions of 2, 4 or 6 g doses of ginger in human volunteers; 6 g or more of ginger caused a significant increase in exfoliation of gastric surface epithelial cells.

There are conflicting views on the effect of ginger on gastrointestinal motility in animal studies with some reports [20,76,77] showing no acceleration of gastrointestinal transport while others [78] suggest that shogaols and gingerols enhance intestinal transport. Phillips and co-workers [79] adressed the question of an effect of ginger on gastric emptying in 16 healthy volunteers during a randomised double-blind crossover study using a dose of 1 g of ginger, administered in capsule form to reduce the risk of oesophageal irritation. They found that ginger had no effect on gastric emptying, as measured using the oral paracetamol absorption model.

Haematological Reactions

Backon [80] has suggested that ginger may have adverse effects on bleeding time because it is such a powerful thromboxane synthetase inhibitor. Phillips et al. [50] noted that in the 40 women given a single 1 g dose of ginger as an antiemetic for day case laparoscopic gynaecological surgery, there appeared to be no subjective difference in intraoperative or postoperative bleeding between the treatment and placebo groups. Verma and co-workers [81] found that the consumption of 5 g of dry ginger in combination with a fatty meal by 10 healthy male volunteers significantly ($P < 0.001$) inhibited platelet aggregation by ADP and epinephrine compared to the placebo control group. More recently Lumb [82] administered 2 g of dried ginger capsules to eight male volunteers in a randomised double-blind placebo-controlled study. There were no differences between ginger and placebo in terms of bleeding time, platelet count, thromboelastography and whole blood platelet aggregometry. Lumb [82] concluded that the effect of ginger on thromboxane synthetase activity was either dose-dependent or occurred only with fresh ginger and that up to 2 g of dried ginger was unlikely to cause platelet dysfunction when used therapeutically.

Metabolic Reactions

According to Meghal and Nath [83], rats fed with suboptimal amounts of thiamine as well as ginger in their rations showed an increase in urinary and faecal excretion of thiamine up to the 4 th week, after which excretion decreased slightly. Ginger was one of a number of spices, which contain a thermostable anti-thiamine compound [84].

Henry and Pigott [85] investigated the effect of ginger on the resting metabolic rate of eight Caucasian subjects and found that ginger had no significant effect on the metabolic rate.

Renal Reactions

There have been claims in the older literature [86] that ginger might promote glomerulonephritis (Brights disease) in renal patients but this effect is not supported by any recent case report or study.

Drug Interactions

Using an *in situ* recirculating perfusion method, Sakai et al. [87] found that ginger extracts enhanced the absorption of sulphaguanidine from the rat small intestine by up to 150% compared to controls.

Fertility, Pregnancy and Lactation

Despite the fact that ginger has been subjected to a double-blind crossover clinical trial in hyperemesis gravidarum [49], no formal study of the effects of ginger on the outcome of pregnancy has been recovered from the literature. References cited by Perry [88] indicate that ginger is an emmenagogue, a term which is often used as an euphemism for an abortifacient. In the above-mentioned clinical trial, Fischer-Rasmussen and colleagues [49] reported on the outcome of pregnancy in the 27 women who completed the trial. One patient had a spontaneous abortion while a second had a legal abortion for non-medical reasons. The mean birth weight of the 25 living infants was 3585 g (range 2450–5150 g). The mean gestational age at delivery was 39.9 weeks (range 36–41). All infants were without deformities and discharged in good condition. All had Apgar scores of 9–10 after 5 min.

The German Kommission E Monograph states that ginger should not be used for vomiting in pregnancy [54].

Mutagenicity and Carcinogenicity

Kada et al. [89] pointed to the existence of an antimutagenic factor in ginger which reduced the number of His$^+$ revertants induced by the known mutagenic tryptophan pyrolysate incubated with *Salmonella* TA98 using S9 liver homogenate as activator. Further work by the same group showed that while *Z. officinale* was remarkably effective, Japanese ginger [*Z. mioga*] was only moderately effective. This latter plant was shown to be carcinogenic when pellets containing a methanol extract of it, bracken, *Z. officinale*, arginine and piperidine, were implanted in the urinary bladder of mice [91]. According to Morita et al. [90] *Z. officinale* was effective against mutagenic pyrolysis products from a number of amino acids as well as L-tryptophan.

Nakamura and Yamamato [92] found that the addition of *Z. officinale* juice to solutions of 2-(2-furyl)-3-(5-nitro-2-furyl)acryl amide (AF2) and N-methyl-N'-nitro-N-nitrosoguanidine (NTG) markedly increased the mutagenesis of these two chemicals in the Hs30 strain of *E. coli* B/r. After fractionation of the plant juice it was found that [6]-gingerol was a potent mutagen. They also found that ginger juice significantly suppressed mutagenesis by [6]-gingerol and also suppressed spontaneous mutations. They suggested that gingerol may be activated by the presence of certain kinds of mutagen and thus would not be suppressed by the antimutagenic components of the juice [92].

The same workers [93] used the same strain of *E. coli* to compare the mutagenicity of [6]-shogaol, zingerone, curcumin and [6]-gingerol. Curcumin had little or no effect, zingerone had only 4% of the mutagenicity of shogaol which in turn was 10^4 times less mutagenic than [6]-gingerol. Morimoto et al. [94] reported that ginger rhizome was negative in the *Bacillus subtilis* spore rec-assay but gave positive results in the Ames test using *Salmonella* strain TA100 in the presence and absence of S9 activation mixture. Tests using strain TA98 were negative. Yamamoto et al. [95] reported similar results with dried ginger rhizome.

Bhide's group [96] also found that ginger extract did not induce revertants in *Salmonella* strains TA98 and TA1538 with or without S9 activation. They did however confirm that it was mutagenic in strains TA100 and TA1535 in the presence of S9 mixture. Zingerone was again non-mutagenic in all four strains. Gingerol and shogaol however were mutagenic after activation in strains TA100 and TA1535 with gingerol the most potent and the effect being dose-dependent. The extract and the pure compounds were non-toxic to the bacteria. These workers also found that zingerenone suppressed the mutagenicity of co-administered shogaol and gingerol in a dose-dependent fashion. Yet again there was no reduction in bacterial survival. They concluded that the weak mutagenic effect of the plant extract was the result of the combined action of pro- and antimutagenic fractions present in the rhizome. Mahmoud and his colleagues [97] reported that ginger was strongly mutagenic (200–500 revertants per plate) when tested against strain TA102 while it was of intermediate mutagenicity in strain TA98.

Koba et al. [98] reported in 1988 that pre-treatment of yellowtail meat with ginger juice reduced mutagen production in meat baked at high temperatures as revealed in the Ames test (strains TA98 and TA100). Kuroda et al. [99] recorded oil of ginger as a positive in a rec-assay using *Bacillus* DNA repair test for genotoxicity. Backon [80] refers to his unpublished observations that ginger showed no toxic effect in the SOS Chromotest for genotoxicity.

Neither ginger nor its purified constituents have been subjected to systematic investigations in mammalian cell cultures. As indicated earlier ginger has reported antitumour effects in human and mouse cancer cells [10]. Hikino et al. [36] also refer to the fact that high doses (1 mg/ml) of various ginger components, e. g. gingerols, gingerdione and dehydrogingerdione showed cytotoxic effects in primary cultured rat hepatocytes.

References

1. Govindarajan VS (1982) Ginger – chemistry, technology and quality evaluation: part 1. CRC Crit Rev Food Sci Nutr 17: 1–96 and 189–258
2. Anonymous (1993) British Pharmacopoeia. London HMSO Volume 1:305
3. Connell DW (1970) The chemistry of the essential oil and oleoresin of ginger (*Zingiber officinale* Roscoe). Flavour Industry 1:677–693
4. Lawrence BM (1984) Major tropical spices-ginger (*Zingiber officinale* Rose.). Perfumer Flavorist 9:1–40
5. MacLeod AJ, Pieris NM (1984) Volatile aroma constituents of Sri Lankan ginger. Phytochemistry 23:353–359
6. Van Beek TA, Posthumus MA, Lelyveld GP, Phiet HV and Yen BT (1987) Investigation of the essential oil of Vietnamese ginger. Phytochemistry 26:3005–3010
7. Anonymous (1949) The British Pharmaceutical Codex. The Pharmaceutical Press London. p. 1239
8. Steinegger E, Stucki K (1982) Trennung und quantitative Bestimmung der Hauptscharfstoffe von Zingiberis Rhizoma mittels kombinierter DC/HPLC. Pharm Acta Helv 57:66–71
9. Connell DW, Sutherland MD (1969) A re-examination of gingerol, shogaol and zingerenone, the pungent principles of Ginger (*Zingiber officinale* Roscoe). Aust J Chem 22:1033–1043

10. Hikino H (1985) Recent research on oriental medicinal plants In: Wagner H, Hikino H, Farnsworth NR (red) Economic and Medicinal Plant Research: Vol 1. London Academic Press pp. 61–85
11. Connell DW, McLachlan R (1972) Natural pungent compounds. Examination of the gingerols, shogaols, paradols and related compounds by Thin-layer and Gas Chromatography. J Chromatogr 67:29–35
12. Endo K, Kanno E and Oshima Y (1990) Structures of antifungal diarylheptenones, gingerenones A B C and isogingerenone B, isolated from the rhizomes of *Zingiber officinale*. Phytochemistry 29:797–799
13. Huang Q, Iwamoto M, Aoki et al. (1992) Anti-5-hydroxytryptamine$_3$ effect of galanolactone, diterpenoid isolated from Ginger. Chem Pharm Bull 39:397–399
14. Yoshikawa M, Hatakeyama S, Taniguchi K, Matuda H, Yamahara J (1992) 6-Gingesulfonic acid, a new anti-ulcer principle, and gingerglycolipids A, B and C. Three new monoacyldigalactosylglycerols, from Zingiberis Rhizoma originating in Taiwan. Chem Pharm Bull. 40:2239–2241
15. Yoshikawa M, Hatakeyama S, Chatani M, Nishino Y, Yamahara J (1993) Qualitative and quantitative analysis of bioactive principles in Zingeribis Rhizoma by means of high performance liquid chromatography and gas liquid chromatography. On the evaluation of Zingeribis Rhizoma and chemical change of constituents during Zingeribis Rhizoma processing. Yakugaku Zasshi 113:307–315
16. Tanabe M, Chen Y-D, Saito K-I, Kono Y (1993) Cholesterol biosynthesis inhibitory component from *Zingiber officinale* Roscoe. Chem Pharm Bull 41:710–713
17. Leung AY (1980) Encyclopedia of common natural ingredients used in food, drugs and cosmetics. New York: Wiley-Interscience pp. 184–186
18. Pancho LR, Kimura I, Unno R, Kurino M and Kimura M (1989) Reversed effects between crude and processed ginger extracts on PGF$_2\alpha$ – induced contraction in mouse mesenteric veins. Jap J Pharmacol 50:243–246
19. Mascolo N, Jain R, Jain SC and Capasso F (1989) Ethnopharmacologic investigation of Ginger (*Zingiber officinale*). J Ethnopharmacol 17:129–140
20. Suekawa M, Ishige A, Yuasa K, Sudo K, Aburada M and Hosoya E (1984) Pharmacological studies on Ginger 1. Pharmacological actions of pungent constituents (6)-gingerol and (6)-shogaol. J Pharm Dyn 7:836–848
21. Kiuchi F, Iwakami S, Shibuya M, Hanaoka F and Sankawa U (1992) Inhibition of prostaglandin and leukotriene biosynthesis by gingerols and diarylheptanoids. Chem Pharm Bull 40:387–391
22. Srivastava KC (1984) Effect of aqueous extracts of onion, garlic and ginger on platelet aggregation and metabolism of arachidonic acid in the blood vascular system: In vitro study. Prostagland Leukotr Med 13:227–235
23. Srivastava KC (1984) Aqueous extracts of onion, garlic and ginger inhibit platelet aggregation and alter arachidonic acid metabolism. Biomed Biochem Acta 43:S 335–S 346
24. Srivastava KC (1986) Isolation and effects of some ginger components on platelet aggregation and eicosanoid biosynthesis. Prostagland Leukotr Med 25:187–198
25. Srivastava KC (1989) Effect of onion and ginger consumption on platelet thromboxane production in humans. Prostagland Leukotr Med 35:183–185
26. Backon J (1986) Ginger: Inhibition of thromboxane synthetase and stimulation of prostacyclin: relevance for medicine and psychiatry. Med Hypotheses 20:271–278
27. Srivastava KC and Mustafa T (1989) Ginger (*Zingiber officinale*) and rheumatic disorders. Med Hypotheses 29:25–28
28. Srivastava KC and Mustafa T (1992) Ginger (Zingiber officinale) in rheumatism and musculoskeletal disorders. Med Hypotheses 39:342–348
29. Wei Y (1986) Shengjiang. In: Chang H-M, But PP-H (red) Pharmacology and Applications of Chinese Materia Medica Vol 1. Singapore: World Scientific pp 366–369
30. Backon J (1987) Use of a novel thromboxane synthetase inhibitor in burns. Burns 13:252–254
31. Leung AY (1988) Fresh Ginger juice in treatment of kitchen burns. Herbalgram No 16:6

32. Yamahara J, Rong HQ, Iwamoto M, Kobayashi G, Matsuda H and Fujimura H (1989) Active components of Ginger exhibiting anti-serotonergic action. Phytotherapy Res 3:70–71
33. Marles RJ. Kaminski J. Arnason IT et al. (1992) A bioassay for inhibition of serotonin release from bovine platelets. J Nat Prod 55:1044–1056
34. Mustafa T and Srivastava KC (1990) Ginger (*Zingiber officinale*) in migraine headache. J Ethnopharmacol 29:267–273
35. Yamahara J. Miki K, Chisaka T et al. (1985) Cholagogic effect of Ginger and its active constituents. J Ethnopharmacol 13:217–225
36. Hikino H, Kiso Y, Kato N et al. (1985) Antihepatotoxic actions of gingerols and diarylheptanoids. J Ethnopharmacol 14:31–39
37. Gugral S, Bhumra H and Swaroop M (1987) Effect of Ginger (*Zingiber officinale* Roscoe) oleoresin on serum and hepatic cholesterol levels in cholesterol fed rats. Nutr Rep 17:183–184
38. Giri J. Devi TKS and Meerarani S (1984) Effect of Ginger on serum cholesterol levels. Ind J Nutr Diet 21:433–436
39. Sambaiah K and Srinivasan K (1989) Influence of spices and spice principles on hepatic mixed function oxygenase system in rats. Ind J Biochem Biophys 26:254–258
40. Srinivasan K and Sambaiah K (1991) The effects of spices on cholesterol 7α hydroxylase activity and on serum and hepatic cholesterol levels in the rat. Int J Vitam Nut Res 61:364–369 [through Chem Abstr 116:127559]
41. Babu PS, Srinivasan K (1993) Influence of dietary spices on adrenal steroidogenesis in rats. Nutr Res 13:435–444
42. Sakai K, Miyazaki Y, Yamane T, Taitoh Y, Ikawa C and Mishihata T (1989) Effect of extracts of Zingiberaceae herbs on gastric secretion in rabbits. Chem Pharm Bull 37:215–217
43. Yamahara J. Mochizuki M, Rong HQ, Matsuda H and Fujimura H (1988) The anti-ulcer effect in rats of Ginger constituents. J Ethnopharmacol 23:299–304
44. Kawai T, Kinoshita K, Koyama K, Takahashi K (1994) Antiemetic principles of Magnolia obovata bark and Zingiber officinale rhizome. Planta Med 60:17–20
45. Mowrey DB and Clayson DE (1982) Motion sickness, Ginger and psychophysics. Lancet i: 655–657
46. Grontved A and Hentzer E (1986) Vertigo-reducing effect of Ginger root. A controlled clinical study. J Oto-Rhinolaryngol 48:282–286
47. Grontved A, Brask T, Kambskard J and Hentzer E. (1988) Ginger root against seasickness. A controlled trial on the open sea. Acta Otolaryngol (Stockh) 105:45–49
48. Bone ME, Wilkinson DJ, Young JR, McNeil I, Charlton S (1990) Ginger root – a new antiemetic. The effect of Ginger root on postoperative nausea and vomiting after major gynaecological surgery. Anaesthesia 45:669–671
49. Fischer-Rasmussen W, Kjaer SK, Dahl C and Asping U (1990) Ginger treatment of hyperemesis gravidarum. Eur J Obstet Gynaecol Reprod Biol 35:19–24
50. Phillips S, Ruggier R, Hutchinson SE (1993) *Zingiber officinale* Ginger – an antiemetic for day case surgery. Anaesthesia 48:715–717
51. Stott JRR, Hubble MP, Spense MB (1985) A double blind comparative trial of powdered Ginger root, Hyoscine hydrobromide and Cinnarizine in the prophylaxis of motion sickness induced by cross coupled stimulation. Advisory Group for Aerospace Research and Development, Conference Proceedings 372, 39:1–6
52. Wood CD, Manno JE, Wood MJ, Manno BR, Mims ME (1988) Comparison of efficacy of Ginger with various antimotion sickness drugs. Clin Rès Pract Drug Reg Aff 6:129–136
53. Stewart JJ, Wood MJ, Wood CD, Mims ME (1991) Effects of Ginger on motion sickness susceptibility and gastric function. Pharmacology 42:111–120
54. Bradley P (red) (1992) British Herbal Compendium. Volume I. Bournemouth: British Herbal Medicine Association pp 114–116
55. Adewunmi CO, Ogantimein BO, Furu P (1990) Molluscicidal and antischistosomal activities of Zingiber officinale. Planta Med 56:374–376

56. Denyer CV, Jackson P, Loakes DM, Ellis MR, Young DAB (1994) Isolation of antirhinoviral sesquiterpenes from Ginger (*Zingiber officinale*). J Nat Prod 57:658–662
57. Kawada T, Sakabe S-I, Watanabe T, Yamamoto M, Iwai K (1988) Some pungent principles of spices cause the adrenal medulla to secrete catecholamine in anaesthesised rats. Proc Soc Exp Biol Med 188:229–233
58. Kims B, Kang IH, Park YH (1987) DNA damage of lipid oxidation products and its inhibition mechanism. Han'guk Susan Hah-heochi 20:419–430 [through Chem Abstr 109:5390]
59. Huang JK, Wang CS and Chang WH (1981) Studies on the antioxidative activities of spices grown in Taiwan I. Chung-Kuo Hung Yeh Hua Hsueh Hui Chi 19:200–207 [through Chem Abstr 97:143289]
60. Anonymous (1993) Drug products containing active ingredients offered over the counter (OTC) for use as a smoking deterrent. Fed Reg 58:31241
61. Ding G, Naora K, Hayashibara M, Katagiri Y, Kano Y, Iwamoto K (1991) Pharmacokinetics of [6]-gingerol after intravenous administration in rats. Chem Pharm Bull 39:1612–1614
62. Anonymous (1981) Flavouring Substances and Natural Sources of Flavourings. 3rd edn. Council of Europe Moulins-lès Mets, Maisonneuve
63. Emig HE (1931) The pharmacological action of Ginger. J Am Pharm Assoc 20:114–116
64. Opdyke DLJ (1979) Ginger Oil. Food Cosmet Toxicol 12:901–902
65. Scott PM, Kennedy BPC (1975) The analysis of spices and herbs for aflatoxins. Can Inst Food Sci Technol J 8:124–125
66. Smith MI, Elvove E, Valaer PJ, Frazier WH and Mallory CE (1930) Pharmacological and chemical studies of the cause of the so-called Ginger paralysis. Preliminary Report. US Public Health Reports 45:1703–1716
67. Shoji N, Iwasa A, Takemoto T, Ishida Y, Ohizumi Y (1982) Cardiotonic principles of Ginger (*Zingiber officinale* Roscoe). J Pharm Sci 71:1174–1175
68. Suekawa M, Aburada M, Hosoya E (1986) Pharmacological studies on Ginger II. Pressor action of (6)-shogaol in anaesthesised rats, or hindquarters, tail and mesenteric vascular beds of rats. J Pharmacobio-Dyn 9:842–852
69. Tulipan L (1938) Cosmetic irritants. Archs Derm Syph 38:906
70. Stäger J. Wüthrich B, Johansson SGO (1991) Spice allergy in celery-sensitive patients. Allergy 46:475–478
71. Futrell JM, Rietschel RL (1993) Spice allergy evaluated by results of patch tests. Cutis 52:288–290
72. Yamamato K (1960) Experimental study on Ginger ingestion: Dermatological study of spice ingestion. Igaku Kenkyu 30:207–210
73. Liu PHW, Ho HL (1983) Ginger and drug bezoar induced small bowel obstruction. J Roy Coll Surg Edinburgh 28:397–398
74. Awang DCV (1992) Ginger. Can Pharm J:309–311
75. Desai HG, Kalro RH, Choksi AP (1990) Effect of ginger and garlic on DNA content of gastric aspirate. Ind J Med Res 92:139–141
76. Haginawa J, Harada M, Morishita J (1963) Pharmacological studies on crude drugs VII. Properties of essential oil components of aromatics and their pharmacological effect on mouse intestine. Yakugaku Zasshi 93:624–628 [through Chem Abstr 60:999]
77. Huang Q, Matsuda H, Sakai K, Yamahara J, Tamai Y (1990) The effect of Ginger on serotonin-induced hypothermia and diarrhoea. Yakugaku Zasshi 110:936–942
78. Yamahara J. Huang Q, Li YH, Xul, Fujimura H (1990) Gastrointestinal motility enhancing effect of Ginger and its active constituents. Chem Pharm Bull 38:430–431
79. Phillips S, Hutchinson S, Ruggier R (1993) *Zingiber officinale* does not affect gastric emptying rate. A randomised, placebo controlled, crossover trial. Anaesthesia 48:393–395
80. Backon J (1990) Ginger as an antiemetic: possible side effects due to its thromboxane synthetase activity. Anaesthesia 46:705–706
81. Verma SK, Singh J, Khamesra R, Bordia A (1993) Effect of ginger on platelet aggregation in man. Ind J Med Res Section B 98:240–242

82. Lumb AB (1994) Effect of dried ginger on human platelet function. Thromb Haemostas 71:110–111
83. Meghal SK, Nath MC (1962) Effect of spice diet on the intestinal synthesis of thiamine in rats. Ann Biochem Exp Med 22:99–104 [through Chem Abstr 57:11625]
84. Rattanapanone V (1979) Antithiamin factor in fruits, mushrooms and spices. Chiang Mai Med Bull 18:9–16 [through Chem Abstr 91:191647]
85. Henry CJK, Piggott SM (1987) Effect of Ginger on metabolic rate. Hum Nutr Clin Nutr 41C:89–92
86. Madaus G (1979) Lehrbuch der biologischen Heilmittel. Band 1–111. Hildesheim: Georg Olms Verlag, p. 2870
87. Sakai K, Oshima N et al. (1986) Pharmaceutical studies on crude drugs 1. Effect of the Zingiberaceae crude drug extracts on sulfaguanidine absorption from rat small intestine. Yakugaku Zasshi 106:947–950
88. Perry LM (1980) Medicinal plants of East and Southeast Asia. MIT Press Cambridge, pp. 443–444
89. Kada T, Morita K, Inowe T (1978) Anti-mutagenic action of vegetable factor(s) on the mutagenic principle of tryptophan pyrolysate. Mutat Res 53:351–353
90. Morita K, Hara M, Kada T (1978) Studies on natural desmutagens: screening for vegetable and fruit factors active in inactivation of mutagenic pyrolysis products from amino acids. Agric Biol Chem 42:1235–1238
91. Mamoru A (1978) Experimental urinary bladder cancer by bladder implantation of pellets containing Mioga extract, 1-arginine and piperidine. Tokyo Iikeikae Ika Daigaku Zasshi 93:698–704 [through Chem Abstr 91:50849]
92. Nakamura H, Yamamoto T (1982) Mutagen and anti-mutagen in Ginger, Zingiber officinale. Mutat Res 103:119–126
93. Nakamura H, Yamamoto T (1983) The active part of the [6]-Gingerol molecule in mutagenesis. Mutat Res 122:87–94
94. Morimoto L, Watanabe F, Osawa T, Okibsu T (1982) Mutagenicity screening of crude drugs with *Bacillus subtilis* rec-assay and *Salmonella*/microsome reversion assay. Mutat Res 97:81–102
95. Yamamoto H, Mizutani T, Nomura H (1982) Studies on the mutagenicity of crude drug extracts. I. Yakugaku Zasshi 102:596–601
96. Nagabhushan AI, Amonkar AJ, Bhide SV (1987) Mutagenicity of Gingerol and Shogaol and antimutagenicity of Zingerenone in *Salmonella*/microsome assay. Cancer Lett 36:221–223
97. Mahmoud J, Alkafahi A, Abdelaziz A (1992) Mutagenic an toxic activities of several spices and some Jordanian medicinal plants. Int J Pharmacognosy 30:81–85
98. Koba H, Hasegawa Y, Matsuoka A et al. (1988) Mutagenicity and deactivation of yellowtail products produced by cooking. Nippon Kasei Gakkaishi pp. 1105–1110 [through Chem Abst 110:22440]
99. Kuroda K, Yoo YS, Ishibashi T (1989) *Rec*-Assay of natural food additives Part 2. Seikatsu Eisei 33:15–23 [through Chem Abstr 111:38126]

Notes Added in Proof

P.A.G.M. De Smet

Introduction

This book series is kept up to date by concluding every volume with additional notes. These notes are not meant to supplement the general introductory chapters nor do they cover all recent references on a certain herb. Instead, they focus on new and clinically relevant information about the adverse reaction profiles of the specific herbal drugs that have been reviewed in the form of a monograph.

Allium Sativum (Volume 1 pp. 73–77; Volume 2 p. 315)

There are recent case reports to suggest that non-dietary intake of garlic [1] and excessive dietary intake [2] may increase the risk of bleeding and postoperative hemorrhagic complications in patients undergoing surgery. It would thus seem prudent to enquire about the intake of garlic well before an operation and, if needs be, to advise its discontinuation.

Gupta et al. [3] reported on a case of myocardial infarction following excessive consumption of garlic. Circumstantial evidence and the lack of any risk factors in the patient raised the possibility of adverse haemodynamic effects following garlic overuse but an indisputable causal relationship was not documented.

Topical exposure to garlic can lead not only to allergic contact dermatitis but also to burn-like skin lesions [4,5].

Anthranoid Derivatives (Volume 2 pp. 105–139)

The German health authorities have restricted the indication of herbal anthranoid laxatives to constipation which has not responded to bulk-forming therapy, which rules out their inclusion in slimming aids. In addition, restrictions were imposed to the laxative use of anthranoid-containing herbs, e.g. not to be used for more than 1 to 2 weeks without medical advice, in children under 12 years of age, or during pregnancy and lactation [6,7]. See the additional notes on *Cassia* species for a deviation from these general rules.

Kleibeuker et al. [8] raised the question whether the reported association between the abuse of anthranoid derivatives and the development of colonic tumors might be related not only to their mutagenic properties but also to stimulation of colonic epithelial cell proliferation. They observed such stimulation following a high oral dose of sennosides A plus B (2 mg/kg with a maximum of 150 mg). They caution, however, that these results should not be extrapolated to chronic users, if only because recent animal studies suggest that long-term administration may lead to adaptation. In a reaction to Kleibeuker et al., Chapman [9] offers an alternative explanation for their suggestion that the observed increase of cell division was due to a direct stimulatory effect. In his opinion, senna could induce a relative lack of butyrate (which plays a part in controlling cell proliferation), because it can inhibit the growth of anaerobic butyrate-producing *Bacteroides* species.

See also the additional notes on *Rubia* species.

Arctium Species (Volume 2 pp. 141–146)

In Spanish folk medicine, burdock root (*Arctium* sp.) is often used in the form of infusions or plasters for its supposed anti-inflammatory properties. Three cases of contact dermatitis following the application of burdock root plasters have now been reported [10].

Aristolochia species (Volume 1 pp. 79–89)

As was already discussed in volume 1, the roots of *Aristolochia clematitis* yield a nephrotoxic substance called aristolochic acid which is a mixture of several nitrophenanthrene derivatives (mainly the aristolochic acids I and II). The nephrotoxic effects of aristolochic acid in the rat were recently reported in detail by Mengs and Stotzem [11]. Following single intragastric doses of 10, 50 or 100 mg/kg, renal lesions developed in a dose-dependent way within 3 days. Functionally, there were rises in plasma creatinine and urea together with increases in urinary glucose, protein, N-acetyl-beta-glucosaminidase, gammaglutamyl transferase and malate dehydrogenase. Histologically, there was evidence of necrosis of the epithelium of the renal tubules.

A human outbreak of renal toxicity of *Aristolochia* occurred in Belgium, where nephropathy was observed in more than 70 users of a slimming preparation that supposedly contained the Chinese herbs *Stephania tetrandra* and *Magnolia officinalis* [12,13]. Analysis of the incriminated material showed that the root of *Stephania tetrandra* (Chinese name "Fangji") had in all probability been substituted or contaminated with the root of *Aristolochia fangchi* (Chinese name "Guang fangji") [14]. In most cases, renal failure progressed despite the withdrawal of the slimming preparation, and 35 patients required renal replacement therapy. Renal biopsies showed extensive interstitial fibrosis with atrophy and loss of tubules [12,13,15,16]. The supposition that the renal interstitial fibrosis was immune-mediated was supported by the finding that the progression of the renal failure could be slowed by steroid therapy with prednisolone [17]. At least two of the patients exposed to the slimming preparation rapidly developed urothelial malignancy [18,19]. This should not come as a great surprise, because the aristolochic acids in *Aristolochia* plants are extremely potent rodent carcinogens (see volume 1). Further evidence of the implication of aristolochic acid was provided by Schmeiser et al. [20], who searched for aristolochic acid DNA adducts in renal tissue samples of five victims. The demonstration of the deoxyadenosine adduct of aristolochic acid I conclusively showed that aristolochic acid had been ingested in amounts sufficient to alter cellular DNA.

Remarkably, renal toxicity due to *Aristolochia* species was already reported in the Chinese literature in 1964, i.e. almost thirty years before the Belgian epidemic was described [21]. Also noteworthy is that the Belgian tragedy with *Stephania/Aristolochia* did not immediately result in a worldwide wave of restrictive measures. Two French victims were detected sixteen months after the first publication in The Lancet [22,23].

Since the morphological and clinical presentation of the Belgian patients was similar to that seen in Balkan endemic nephropathy, the possibility of a common etiological factor has been suggested [24]. Contamination of wheat flour from the endemic region with seeds of *Aristolochia clematitis* has been demonstrated but a causal role in Balkan nephropathy was not proven by determination of aristolochic acid in the blood, urine and kidney tissue of patients and unaffected controls [25].

Another *Aristolochia* species in traditional Chinese medicine is *Aristolochia manshuriensis*. Since there is evidence that aristolochic acid passes into human breast milk following maternal use (see volume 1), it is disturbing that this herb is recommended for the improvement of mammary gland growth and function [26]. Another area of concern is the possibility of substitution of *Akebia quinata* ("Mutong") by *Aristolochia manshuriensis* ("Guanmutong") [27]. In a recent pharmacognostic study of crude Chinese materials imported into the United Kingdom, one Mutong sample came from *Aristolochia manshuriensis* [28]. To this it may be added that not all practitioners of traditional Chinese medicine in the UK are experts in herb recognition [29].

Berberine (Volume 1 pp. 97–104 and 260)

According to a recent WHO overview, the Singapore government already prohibited the importation and sale of preparations containing the *Coptis* alkaloid berberine in 1979, following observations of jaundice and haemolytic anaemia in infants with glucose-6-phosphate-dehydrogenase (G6PD) deficiency [30]. While the incidence of kernicterus in Singapore dropped considerably after this ban, it remained high among Chinese infants in Hong Kong and in the southern region of China [31]. Because of reports that Chinese infants with G6PD deficiency developed severe haemolysis, often accompanied by kernicterus, within hours of taking a tea prepared from Chuen-Lin (*Coptis chinensis* or *Coptis japonicum*), Yeung et al. [32] tested such a tea in vitro. Addition of the tea to neonatal serum produced such a decrease in bilirubin protein binding that the investigators strongly discouraged further use during the perinatal period. Chan [31] subsequently reported that the bilirubin displacing effects of *Coptis chinensis* are, at least in part, due to its constituent berberine. This implies that neonates at risk of haemolytic jaundice should avoid not only Chuen-Lin but also other traditional herbal medicines rich in berberine.

Cassia **Species** (Volume 2 pp. 125–128)

Mutagenicity testing of sennosides has produced negative results in several bacterial and mammalian systems, except for a weak effect in *Salmonella typhimurium* strain TA102 [33,34]. A well-defined purified senna extract was not carcinogenic, when administered orally to rats in daily doses up to 25 mg/kg for two years [35]. No evidence of reproductive toxicity of sennosides has been found in rats and rabbits [36]. When a standardized preparation containing senna pods (providing 15 mg of sennosides per day) was given to breast-feeding mothers, the suckling infants were only exposed to a non-laxative amount of rhein, which remained a factor 10^{-3} below the maternal intake of this active metabolite [37]. With an eye on these findings, the German health authorities do not forbid the use of senna fruit during pregnancy and lactation [6].

See also the general entry on anthranoid derivatives.

Chamomilla Recutita (Volume 1 pp. 243-248; Volume 2 p.263)

As is evident from two Norwegian cases, appropriate caution is needed to avoid serious burns, when inhalation of steam from camomile tea is used in children as a home remedy for inflammation of the upper respiratory tract [38].

Eupatorium **Species** (Volume 2 pp. 171–194)

White snakeroot (*Eupatorium rugosum*) is a toxic plant which can produce livestock poisoning as well as milk sickness. This latter syndrome can occur when humans ingest the milk from animals with abudant access to the plant (see volume 2). Tremetol has long been considered to be the poisonous principle in white snakeroot but chemically this substance is a mixture of many different compounds, including the ketones tremetone, hydroxytremetone, and dehydrotremetone. To identify which constituent is the actual toxin, Beier et al. [39] submitted white snakeroot to fractionated extraction guided by in vitro toxicity testing in mammalian cell lines. Tremetone was isolated as the major toxic component but it only produced its toxicity after microsomal activation. Tremetone readily decomposes to dehydrotremetone, but this latter compound was not toxic, not even after microsomal activation. Tremetone was also isolated as toxic component of the rayless goldenrod (*Isocoma wrightii* syn. *Aplopappus heterophyllus*). This plant has the same poisonous effects in livestock and humans as the white snakeroot.

Ginkgo Biloba (Volume 3 pp.51–66)

Yagi et al. [40] determined serum levels of 4-O-methylpyridoxine (MPN) in a 21 month-sold child, who suffered from gin-nan food poisoning after taking about 50 ginkgo albumens. MPN concentrations were 0.09 micrograms/ml at 8.5 h after taking the ginkgo seeds and less than the detection limit of 0.05 micrograms/ml at 15.5 h.

Gossypol (Volume 2 pp. 195–208)

Flack et al. [41] examined the efficacy and toxicity of oral gossypol (30–70 mg/day) as a treatment for metastatic adrenal cancer. Xerostomia, transient transaminitis, dry skin, fatigue, intermittent nausea, vomiting, transient ileus and minor hair thinning were observed as side effects. One patient with pre-existing gynaecomastia showed an increased size and tenderness of breast tissue. The most serious side effect was abdominal ileus in some patients who had taken gossypol continuously for 3 months at a level of 40 mg/day or more. In all these patients, the ileus resolved when the drug was temporarily withheld and restarted at a lower dose.

Larrea Tridentata (Volume 2 pp. 231–240 and 316)

In addition to the three cases of hepatotoxicity, which were already discussed in the previous volume, six more cases have now been published [42–45]. The period of exposure to chaparral before the onset of symptoms varied from 6 weeks to 15 months, and in one case inadvertent rechallenge led to recurrence within 4 weeks [45]. In one of the patients, 160 mg of chaparral daily for approximately 2 months was followed by cholangiolithic hepatitis, characterized by severe cholestasis and hepatocellular injury [43]. In another patient, who had taken chaparral for 40 weeks (2 capsules daily, increased to 6 capsules daily approximately 3 weeks before hospitalization), the hepatitis was complicated by encephalopathy and progressed to end-stage liver failure requiring orthotopic liver transplantation. This latter patient also developed renal failure but the reporting physicians considered a causal relationship with the chaparral use unlikely [44].

Which component or components of chaparral may be responsible, remains to be seen. It has been suggested that the known estrogenic activity of chaparral may be involved, since it is known that women on birth control pills can have liver problems [46]. Obermeyer et al. [47] point out that there are close structural similarities between several lignan components of chaparral (e.g. nordihydroguaiaretic acid) and diethylstilbestrol. As most of the chaparral dietary supplements associated with toxic hepatitis were in capsule or tablet forms, they compared the lignan composition of a methanolic extract of chaparral with that of an infusion made by steeping an identical quantity of the same chaparral for 5 min. This indicated that exposure to many of the lignan components of chaparral would be mucher greater from the capsule or tablet forms than from a steeped tea. Capdevilla et al. [48] reported *in vitro* evidence that nordihydroguaiaretic acid inhibits the cytochrome *P*-450-dependent arachidonic acid metabolism in the liver.

As was pointed out in the previous volume, nordihydroguaiaretic acid is able to produce renal lesions, when given chronically in high doses to rodents. The first human case of renal disease associated with a history of consumption of chaparral tea has now been reported. The patient was a 56-year-old woman, who had taken 3–4 cups daily in a 3-month period approximately 1.5 years earlier; she had also consumed 5–6 cups daily of taheebo tea for 6 months. Computerized tomography revealed bilateral cystic renal disease with two complex renal cysts in the left kidney.

Postoperative examination of sections obtained at surgery showed low grade cystic clear cell carcinoma involving both cysts, which finding prompted left radical nephrectomy [49].

Medicago Sativa (Volume 1 pp. 161–170)

Because dietary alfalfa sprouts are tender, they are eaten raw so that potential pathogenic bacteria are viable. The seeds should therefore be pasteurised before sprouting or the sprouts should be sufficiently heated before consumption. Pönkä et al. [50] reported an epidemic due to *Salmonella bovismorbificans* in alfalfa sprouts, which occurred in Sweden (282 cases) and Finland (210 cases) and which could be traced to contamination of alfalfa seeds from Australia. Salmonellae could not be cultured from the seeds but only after sprouting.

Herbert and Kasdan [51] reported on a female patient, who developed systematic lupus erythematosus after prolonged use of alfalfa tablets (4-6 tablets daily for 7 years) and vitamin E supplements. Autoimmune-like symptoms were also observed in other members of the family (her mother, her sister, and two cousins), who had also adhered to a regimen of alfalfa and vitamine E. Chemical analysis of the alfalfa tablets revealed that they contained < 3–5 ppm of L-canavanine. In a reaction to this report, Whittam et al. [52] rightly pointed out that insufficient details about clinical course, exposure, and potentially confounding factors were reported.

Mentha Piperita and *Mentha Spicata* (Volume 1 pp. 171–178)

Jarvik et al. [53] compared regular cigarettes with mentholated cigarettes in 20 smokers and found that the latter increased exposure to the toxic effects of carbon monoxide, even though they decreased the volume of smoke inhaled.

As menthol combustion produces carcinogenic compounds such as benzo(a)pyrenes, the question has been raised whether mentholation of cigarettes increases the risk of developing cancer. Several case-control studies have been published in which the smoking of mentholated cigarettes versus non-mentholated cigarettes was not associated with an increased risk of oesophageal cancer [54], lung cancer [55], or oropharyngeal cancer [56]. A recent prospective study suggests, however, that mentholated cigarette use is associated with an increased risk of lung cancer in long-term male smokers, whereas there is no such association in long-term female smokers. The relative risk of mentholated versus non-mentholated cigarettes amounted to 1.45 in the men (95 % confidence interval 1.03 to 2.02) and to 0.75 in the women (95 % confidence interval 0.51 to 1.11) [57].

Panax Ginseng (Volume 1 pp. 179–192)

Ryu and Chien [58] observed cerebral arteritis in a 28-year-old woman from Taiwan, who had ingested approximately 200 ml of an extract prepared by stewing 25 g of ginseng root with 400 ml of rice wine. After 8 hours, she developed an explosive headache, nausea and vomiting, and chest tightness. She was referred to hospital 6 days later, where cerebral angiograms revealed multiple areas of alternating focal constriction and dilatation ("beading" appearance) in the anterior and posterior cerebral and superior cerebral arteries and in the superior cerebellar artery. The headache gradually resolved over the next 10 days. No known cause of cerebral arteritis (e.g. use of sympathicomimetics or cocaine, CNS infection or aneurysm) could be established.

Wilkie and Cordess [59] described five schizophrenic inpatients, all on maintenance depot neuroleptic medication, who became generally irritable, uncooperative with their treatment programmes, and overactive with disturbed sleep, after they had started to smoke ginseng cigarettes on a regular basis. When the smoking of these cigarettes stopped, their behaviour was noticed to improve. The authors add the cautionary note, however, that these observations do not demostrate an unequivocal role for ginseng in the genesis of mental deterioration.

González-Seijo et al. [60] reported on a woman with prior episodes of depression who suffered a manic episode some days after initiating ginseng consumption. They clearly state, however, that the woman interrupted her orthodox treatment with lithium carbonate and amitriptyline at the same time when she started to use ginseng and that her manic symptoms resolved after she resumed her treatment of lithium together with haloperidol. Consequently there is insufficient ground for their suggestion of a direct relationship between the manic episode and the use of ginseng.

As was already outlined in the first volume, the evaluation of case reports on ginseng is hampered by the variable quality of commercial ginseng preparations [61,62].

Pausinystalia Species (Volume 3 pp. 211–214)

Betz et al. [63] analysed 18 different yohimbe products on the US health food market and only recovered such low levels of yohimbine that the examined products would most likely pose little health risks when used as directed on the product label. Two of the preparations yielded 0.03% and 0.05%, whereas the remaining samples contained 0.001% or less. A question was raised about the exact origin of some yohimbe products, because their GC chromatograms only showed yohimbine and not the expected mixture of yohimbe alkaloids.

Phytolacca Americana (Volume 2 pp. 253–261)

Hamilton et al. [64] treated two patients who had ingested uncooked leaves of pokeweed (*Phytolacca americana*). One patient merely showed the classic symptoms of pokeweed poisoning (frequent vomiting, diarrhoea and lethargy). The other patient had more severe gastrointestinal symptoms and developed a type I Mobitz heart block. It was considered unlikely that this cardiac effect had been produced by a specific toxin, because both patients had reportedly taken similar amounts of the plant material, The diversity of cardiac manifestations in previous cases also argues against the presence of a specific cardiotoxin in pokeweed.

Pyrrolizidine Alkaloids (Volume 1 pp. 193–226 and 262–263; Volume 2 pp. 316–317)

Ortiz Cansado et al. [65] documented a fatal case of veno-occlusive liver disease in an elderly patient, who had continuously consumed a herbal tea from *Senecio vulgaris* for two years.

Sperl et al. [66] described a very young Austrian boy who developed veno-occlusive disease of the liver after long-term consumption of a tea prepared from *Adenostyles alliariae*. This herb had been erroneously gathered by the boy's parents instead of coltsfoot (*Tussilago farfara*) and its level of hepatotoxic pyrrolizidine alkaloids is much higher than the level in coltsfoot [67].

The Mexican herb *Packera candidissima* (Asteraceae) should be added to the list of medicinal plants which contain hepatotoxic pyrrolizidine alkaloids [68].

Rheum Species (Volume 2 pp. 133-136)

Since dietary rhubarb is rich in oxalate, its intake as a food can significantly increase urinary oxalate excretion, which effect might compromise treatments to reduce the risk of calcium oxalate kidney stones [69,70].

Rubia Species (Volume 2 pp. 137–139)

The German health authorities no longer permit the use of herbal medicines prepared from the root of *Rubia tinctorum* (madder root) [71].

Kawasaki et al. [72] tested 25 anthranoids for mutagenicity in *Salmonella typhimurium* and found that 13 gave positive results in strains TA98 and/or TA100. Eight of these mutagens had been isolated from *Rubia tinctorum*. The authors add the concern that six of these eight constituents as well as two additional mutagenic anthranoids not found in madder root have been isolated from other rubiaceous plants, which serve as Oriental medicines (*Morinda umbellata*, *Rubia cordifolia*, *Hymenodictyon excelsum* and *Damnacanthus indicus*).

Sassafras Albidum (Volume 3 pp. 123–127)

The German health authorities have recently proposed the withdrawal of *Sassafras*-containing medicines, including homoeopathic products up to D3, from the market [73].

Scutellaria Species (Volume 2 pp. 289–296 and 317)

As was pointed out in the previous volume, it is unclear whether the hepatotoxic reactions that have been associated with preparations containing skullcap should be attributed to *Scutellaria*, *Teucrium* or both. It has now become known that in at least one case the skullcap material did not come from *Scutellaria lateriflora* but from *Teucrium canadense* (see the monograph on *Teucrium chamaedrys* in the present volume).

Kim et al. [74] carried out animal studies to assess the teratogenicity of Scutellariae Radix (originating from the Oriental species *Scutellaria baicalensis*). Female rats were treated orally with concentrated aqueous extracts from day 7 to 17 of gestation at daily dose levels of 0.25, 12.5 and 25 g/kg. There were significant dose-dependent increases in the incidence of skeletal variations and in the incidence of abnormalities in the urinary system.

Teucrium Chamaedrys (Volume 2 p.317; Volume 3 pp. 137–144)

Further evidence that the hepatotoxicity of the wall germander (*Teucrium chamaedrys*) resides in one or more reactive metabolites of its furanoditerpenoid fraction has been provided by Kouzi et al. [75]. They found that one of the major diterpenoids in the herb, teucrin A, caused the same hepatocellular damage in mice after bioactivation as did crude extracts from the plant. The tetrahydrofuran analog of teucrin A was not active in this model, so a furan ring moiety is apparently needed for the hepatotoxic reactions.

Two new cases of germander hepatitis were reported from Canada [76], whereas a case of severe hepatitis associated with the use of *Teucrium polium* was recently observed in France [77]. This latter herb is valued as a traditional medicine in the Mediterrean region for its cicatrizant, antimicrobial and anti-inflammatory activites [77]. The occurrence of furanoditerpenoids in the aerial parts of its different varieties and subspecies is reviewed in the accompanying Table.

Table.1 Occurrence of furanoditerpenoids in aerial parts of *Teucrium polium*

Variety/subspecies (geographical origin)	Diterpenoid(s)
var. *album* (Egypt)	montanin C [78]
var. *polium* (Bulgaria)	19-acetylgnaphalin, montanins B and E, teucrin P_1, teupolins I, II, III, IV and V, teulamifin B and 19-deacetylteuscorodol [79-82]
ssp. *aureum* (Sicily, Spain)	teucrin P_1 (?) and gnaphalidin from Sicilian sample; 19-acetylgnaphalin and auropolin from Spanish sample [79]
ssp. *capitatum* (Spain)	teucjaponin B, picropolin, picropolinol, picropolinone, 19-acetylgnaphalin, 7-deacetylcapitatin, and 20-epi-isoeriocephalin [83]
ssp. *expansum* (Spain)	picropolinone, 19-acetylteulepicin, 3-*O*-deacetylteugracilin [84]
ssp. *pilosum* (Arabian Gulf)	19-acetylteupolin IV [85]
ssp. *vincentinum* (Portugal)	19-acetylgnaphalin, eriocephalin, isoëriocephalin, 3-deacetyl-20-*epi*-teulanigin, teuvincentins A, B and C [86]

Tripterygium **Species** (Volume 3 pp. 145–163)

New clinical evidence of the toxic potential of *Tripterygium wilfordii* was presented by Chiu and colleagues [87], who described a fatal human intoxication. A 36-year-old male developed severe vomiting and diarrhoea about 10 h after the ingestion of a fluid composed of self-collected plant material and tap water. Upon hospitalization on the 3rd day, he showed hypotension, leukopenia, thrombocytopenia, hypocalcemia, metabolic acidosis, prolongation of prothrombin time and of activated partial thromboplastin time, and anuria. Serial ECGs, elevated cardiac enzymes, and echocardiography suggested the possibility of cardiac damage. In spite of vigorous therapy, the patient's condition deteriorated and he died of shock 15 h after admission.

Chan and Ng [88] demonstrated that an aqueous extract of the peeled root of *Tripterygium wilfordii* had an embryotoxic effect *in vitro* on mouse embryos. This effect could be destroyed by heat treatment of the extract at 80° C for 6 hours.

Valeriana **Species** (Volume 3 pp. 165–180)

Willey et al. [89] treated a young woman with activated charcoal after she had ingested approximately 20 g of valerian root in a suicide attempt. Her clinical course was benign, with no other symptoms than fatigue, abdominal cramping, chest tightness, tremor of the hands and feet, lightheadedness and mydriasis.

References

1. German K, Kumar U, Blackford HN (1995) Garlic and the risk of TURP bleeding. Br J Urol 76:518
2. Burnham BE (1995) Garlic as a possible risk for postoperative bleeding. Plast Reconstruct Surg 95:213
3. Gupta MK, Mittal SR, Mathur AK, Bhan AK (1993) Garlic the other side of the coin. Int J Cardiol 38:333

5. Canduela V, Mongil I, Carrascosa M, Docio S, Cagigas P (1995) Garlic: always good for the health? Br J Dermatol 132:161–162
6. Kommission E (1993) Aufbereitungsmonographien. Dtsch Apoth Ztg 133:2791–2794
7. Anonymous (1994) Anthranoid-haltige Humanarzneimittel. Pharm Ztg 139:2432
8. Kleibeuker JH, Cats A, Zwart N, Mulder NH, Hardonk MJ, De Vries EG (1995) Excessively high cell proliferation in sigmoid colon after an oral purge with anthraquinone glycosides. J Nat Canc Inst 87:452–453
9. Chapman M (1995) Excessively high cell proliferation in sigmoid colon after an oral purge with anthraquinone glycosides. J Nat Canc Inst 87:1086–1087
10. Rodriguez P, Blanco J, Juste S, Garcés M, Pérez R, Alonso L, Marcos M (1995) Allergic contact dermatitis due to burdock (*Arctium lappa*). Contactdermatitis 33:134–135
11. Mengs U, Stotzem CD (1993) Renal toxicity of aristolochic acid in rats as an example of nephrotoxicity testing in routine toxicology. Arch Toxicol 67:307–311
12. Vanherweghem JL, Depierreux M, Tielemans C, Abramowicz D, Dratwa M, Jadoul M, Richard C, Vandervelde D, Verbeelen D, Vanhaelen-Fastre R, et al. (1993) Rapidly progressive interstitial renal fibrosis in young women: association with slimming regimen including Chinese herbs. Lancet 341:387–391
13. Vanherweghem JL (1994) Une nouvelle forme de nephropathie secondaire a l'absorption d'herbes chinoises. Bull Mem Acad Roy Med Belg 149:128–135
14. Vanhaelen M, VanhaelenFastre R, But P, Vanherweghem JL (1994) Identification of aristolochic acid in Chinese herbs. Lancet 343:174
15. Van Ypersele De Strihou C, Vanherweghem JL (1995) The tragic paradigm of Chinese herbs nephropathy. Nephrol Dial Transplant 10:157–160
16. Depierreux M, Van Damme B, Vanden Houte K, Vanherweghem JL (1994) Pathologic aspects of a newly described nephropathy related to the prolonged use of Chinese herbs. Am J Kidney Dis 24:172–180
17. Vanherweghem J-L, Abramowicz D, Tielemans C, Depierreux M (1996) Effects of steroids on the progression of renal failure in chronic interstitial renal fibrosis: a pilot study in Chinese herbs nephropathy. Am J Kidney Dis 27:209–215
18. Cosyns J-P, Jadoul M, Squifflet J-P, Van Cangh P-J, Van Ypersele De Strihou C (1994) Urothelial malignancy in nephropathy due to Chinese herbs. Lancet 344:188
19. Vanherweghem JL, Tielemans C, Simon J, Depierreux M (1995) Chinese herbs nephropathy and renal pelvic carcinoma. Nephrol Dial Transplant 10:270–273
20. Schmeiser HH, Bieler CA, Wiessler M, Van Ypersele De Strihou C, Cosyns J-P (1996) Detection of DNA adducts formed by aristolochic acid in renal tissue from patients with Chinese herbs nephropathy. Cancer Res 56:2025–2028
21. Zhu Y-P, Woerdenbag HJ (1995) Traditional Chinese herbal medicine. Pharm World Sci 17:103–112
22. Arzneimittelkommission der Deutschen Apotheker. Chinesisches Pflanzenpulver. Dtsch Apoth Ztg 1994;134:2212
23. Pourrat J, Montastruc JL, Lacombe JL, Cisterne JM, Rascol O, Dumazer Ph (1994) Néphropathie associée des herbes chinoises 2 cas. Presse Méd 23:1669
24. Cosyns J-P, Jadoul M, Squifflet J-P, De Plaen J-F, Ferluga D, Van Ypersele De Strihou C (1994) Chinese herbs nephropathy: a clue to Balkan endemic nephropathy? Kidney Int 45:1680–1688
25. Stefanovíc V, Polenakovíc MH (1991) Balkan nephropathy – Kidney disease beyond the Balkans? Am J Nephrol 11:1–11
26. Wu G, Yamamoto K, Mori T, Inatomi H, Nagasawa H (1995) Improvement by Guan-mutong (*Caulis aristolochiae manshuriensis*) of lactation in mice. Am J Chin Med 23:159–165
27. Quansheng C (1986) Mutong. In: Chang H-M, But PP-H, eds. Pharmacology and Applications of Chinese Materia Medica. Volume 1. World Scientific Publishing, Singapore, pp.195–198
28. Anonymous (1995) Drug development from natural products. Pharm J 255:430–431

29. Jin Y, Berry MI, Chan K (1995) Chinese herbal medicine in the United Kingdom. Pharm J 255:R37
30. Anonymous (1995) "Natural" medicines: a Pandora's box. WHO Drug Information 9:147–149
31. Chan E (1993) Displacement of bilirubin from albumin by berberine. Biol Neonate 63:201–208
32. Yeung CY, Lee FT, Wong HN (1990) Effect of a popular Chinese herb on neonatal bilirubin protein binding. Biol Neonate 58:98–103
33. Mengs U (1988) Toxic effects of sennosides in laboratory animals and in vitro. Pharmacology 36 (Suppl.1):180–187
34. Sandnes D, Johansen T, Teien G, Ulsaker G (1992) Mutagenicity of crude senna and senna glycosides in *Salmonella typhimurium*. Pharmacol Toxicol 71:165–172
35. Lydén-Sokolowski A, Nilsson A, Sjöberg P (1993) Two-year carcinogenicity study with sennosides in the rat: emphasis on gastro-intestinal alterations. Pharmacology 47(Suppl 1):209-15
36. Mengs U (1986) Reproductive toxicological investigations with sennosides. Arzneim Forsch 36:1355–1358
37. Faber P, Strenge-Hesse A (1988) Relevance of rhein excretion into breast milk. Pharmacology 36(Suppl.1):212–220
38. Balslev T, Moller AB (1990) Forbraendinger hos born forarsaget af kamillete. Ugeskr Laeg 152:1384
39. Beier RC, Norman JO, Reagor JC, Rees MS, Mundy BP (1993) Isolation of the major component in white snakeroot that is toxic after microsomal activation: possible explanation of sporadic toxicity of white snakeroot plants and extracts. Natural Toxins 1:286–293
40. Yagi M, Wada K, Sakata M, Kokubo M, Haga M (1993) Studies on the constituents of edible and medicinal plants. IV. Determination of 4-O-methylpyridoxine in serum of the patient with gin-nan food poisoning Yakugaku Zasshi 113:596–599
41. Flack MR, Pyle RG, Mullen NM, Lorenzo B, Wu YW, Knazek RA, Nisula BC, Reidenberg MM (1993) Oral gossypol in the treatment of metastatic adrenal cancer. J Clin Endocrinol Metab 76:1019–1024
42. Smith BC, Desmond PV (1993) Acute hepatitis induced by ingestion of the herbal medication chaparral. Aust NZ J Med 23:526
43. Alderman S, Kailas S, Goldfarb S, Singaram C, Malone DG (1994) Cholestatic hepatitis after ingestion of chaparral leaf: confirmation by endoscopic retrograde cholangiopancreatography and liver biopsy. J Clin Gastroenterol 19:242–247
44. Gordon DW, Rosenthal G, Hart J, Sirota R, Baker AL (1995) Chaparral ingestion. The broadening spectrum of liver injury caused by herbal medications. JAMA 273:489–490
45. Batchelor WB, Heathcote J, Wanless IR (1995) Chaparral-induced hepatic injury. Am J Gastroenterol 90:831–833
46. Blumenthal M (1993) Herb industry and FDA issue chaparral warning – Experts unable to explain possible links to five cases of hepatitis. HerbalGram No.28:38–39,53,59,63,69
47. Obermeyer WR, Musser SM, Betz JM, Casey RE, Pohland AE, Page SW (1995) Chemical studies of phytoestrogens and related compounds in dietary supplements: flax and chaparral. Proc Soc Exp Biol Med 208:6–12
48. Capdevilla J, Gil J, Orellana M et al. (1988) Inhibitors of cytochrome P-450-dependent arachidonic acid metabolism. Arch Biochem Biophys 261:257–263
49. Smith AY, Feddersen RM, Gardner Jr KD, Davis Jr CJ (1994) Cystic renal cell carcinoma and acquired renal cystic disease associated with consumption of chaparral tea: a case report. J Urol 152:2089–2091
50. Pönkä A, Andersson Y, Siitonen A, De Jong B, Jahkola M, Haikala O, Kuhmonen A, Pakkala P (1995) Salmonella in alfalfa sprouts. Lancet 345:462–463
51. Herbert V, Kasdan TS (1994) Alfalfa, vitamin E, and autoimmune disorders. Am J Clin Nutr 60:639–640

52. Whittam J, Jensen C, Hudson T (1995) Alfalfa, vitamin E, and autoimmune disorders. Am J Clin Nutr 62:1025–1026
53. Jarvik ME, Tashkin DP, Caskey NH, McCarthy WJ, Rosenblatt MR (1994) Mentholated cigarettes decrease puff volume of smoke and increase carbon monoxide absorption. Physiol Behavior 56:563–570
54. Hebert JR, Kabat GC (1989) Menthol cigarette smoking and oesophageal cancer. Int J Epidemiol 18:37–44
55. Kabat GC, Hebert JR (1991) Use of mentholated cigarettes and lung cancer risk. Cancer Res 51:6510–6513
56. Kabat GC, Hebert JR (1994) Use of mentholated cigarettes and oropharyngeal cancer. Epidemiol 5:183–188
57. Sidney S, Tekawa IS, Friedman GD, Sadler MC, Tashkin DP (1995) Mentholated cigarette use and lung cancer. Arch Intern Med 155:727–732
58. Ryu S-J, Chien Y-Y (1995) Ginseng-associated cerebral arteritis. Neurology 45:829–830
59. Wilkie A, Cordess C (1994) Ginseng a root just like a carrot? J Roy Soc Med 87:594–595
60. González-Seijo JC, Ramos YM, Lastra I (1995) Manic episode and ginseng: report of a possible case. J Clin Psychopharmacol 15:447–448
61. Cui J, Garle M, Eneroth P, Björkhem I (1994) What do commercial ginseng preparations contain? Lancet 344:134
62. Chuang W-C, Wu H-K, Sheu S-J, Chiou S-H, Chang H-C, Chen Y-P (1995) A comparative study on commercial samples of ginseng radix. Planta Med 61:459–465
63. Betz JM, White KD, Der Marderosian AH (1995) Gas chromatographic determination of yohimbine in commercial yohimbe products. J AOAC Int 78:1189–1194
64. Hamilton RJ, Shih RD, Hoffman RS (1995) Mobitz type I heart block after pokeweed ingestion. Vet Hum Toxicol 37:66–67
65. Ortiz Cansado A, Crespo Valades E, Morales Blanco P, Saenz de Santamaria J, Gonzalez Campillejo JM, Ruiz Tellez T (1995) Enfermedad venooclusiva hepatica por ingestion de infusiones de Senecio vulgaris. Gastroenterol Hepatol 18:413–416
66. Sperl W, Stuppner H, Gassner I, Judmaier W, Dietze O, Vogel W (1995) Reversible hepatic venoocclusive disease in an infant after consumption of pyrrolizidinecontaining herbal tea. Eur J Pediatrics 154:112–116
67. De Smet PAGM (1989) Drugs used in nonorthodox medicine. In: Dukes MNG, Beeley L, eds. Side Effects of Drugs Annual 13. Amsterdam: Elsevier, pp.442–473
68. Bah M, Bye R, Pereda-Miranda R (1994) Hepatotoxic pyrrolizidine alkaloids in the Mexican medicinal plant *Packera candidissima* (Asteraceae: Senecioneae). J Ethnopharmacol 43:19–30
69. Massey LK, Roman-Smith H, Sutton RA (1993) Effect of dietary oxalate and calcium on urinary oxalate and risk of formation of calcium oxalate kidney stones. J Am Diet Assoc 93:901–906
70. Hesse A, Siener R, Heynck H, Jahnen A (1993) The influence of dietary factors on the risk of urinary stone formation. Scanning Microscopy 7:1119–1127
71. BGA-Pressedienst (1993) Widerruf der Zulassung für Krappwurzelhaltige Arzneimittel angeordnet. Berlin: Bundesgesundheitsamt, 15/1993
72. Kawasaki Y, Goda Y, Yoshihira K (1992) The mutagenic constituents of *Rubia tinctorum*. Chem Pharm Bull 40:1504–1509
73. Arzneimittelkommission der Deutschen Apotheker (1995) Vorinformation Sassafras-haltige Arzneimittel. Dtsch Apoth Ztg 135:366–368
74. Kim S-H, Kim Y-H, Han S-S, Roh JK (1993) Teratogenicity studies of *Scutellariae* radix in rats. Reprod Toxicol 7:73–79
75. Kouzi SA, McMurtry RJ, Nelson SD (1994) Hepatotoxicity of germander (Teucrium chamaedrys L.) and one of its constituent neoclerodane diterpenes teucrin A in the mouse. Chem Res Toxicol 7:850–856
76. Laliberté L, Villeneuve J-P (1996) Hepatitis after the use of germander, a herbal remedy. Can Med Assoc J 154:1689–1692

77. Mattei A, Rucay P, Samuel D, Feray C, Reynes M, Bismuth H (1995) Liver transplantation for severe acute liver failure after herbal medicine (Teucrium polium) administration. J Hepatol 22:597
78. De La Torre MC, Rodriguez B, Rizk A-FM, Bruno M, Piozzi F (1988) Montanin C from *Teucrium polium* var. *album*. Fitoterapia 59:129–130
79. Piozzi F (1981) The diterpenoids of *Teucrium* species. Heterocycles 15:1489–1503
80. Malakov PY, Papanov GY, Ziesche J (1982) Teupolin III, a furanoid diterpene from *Teucrium polium*. Phytochemistry 21:2597–2598
81. Malakov PY, Papanov GY (1983) Furanoid diterpenes from *Teucrium polium*. Phytochemistry 22:2791–2793
82. Malakov PY, Boneva IM, Papanov GY, Spassov SL (1988) Teulamifin B, a neo-clerodane diterpenoid from *Teucrium lamiifolium* and *T. polium*. Phytochemistry 27: 1141–1143
83. Fernández P, Rodriguez B, Savona G, Piozzi F (1986) Neo-clerodane diterpenoids from *Teucrium-polium* subsp. *capitatum*. Phytochemistry 25:181–184
84. Alcázar R, De La Torre MC, Rodríguez B, Bruno M, Piozzi F, Savona G, Arnold NA (1992) *Neo*-clerodane diterpenoids from three species of *Teucrium*. Phytochemistry 31:3957–3960
85. De La Torre MC, Piozzi F, Rizk A-F, Rodriguez B, Savona G (1986) 19-Acetylteupolin IV, a neo-clerodane diterpenoid from *Teucrium polium* ssp. *pilosum*. Phytochemistry 25:2239–2240
86. Carreiras MC, Rodríguez B, Piozzi F, Savona G, Torres MR, Perales A (1989) A chlorine-containing and two 17β-*neo*-clerodane diterpenoids from *Teucrium-polium* subsp. *vincentinum*. Phytochemistry 28:1453–1461
87. Chou W-C, Wu C-C, Yang P-C, Lee Y-T (1995) Hypovolemic shock and mortality after ingestion of *Tripterygium wilfordii* hook F.: a case report. Int J Cardiol 49:173–177
88. Chan WY, Ng TB (1995) Adverse effect of *Tripterygium wilfordii* extract on mouse embryonic development. Contraception 51:65–71
89. Willey LB, Mady SP, Cobaugh DJ, Wax PM (1995) Valerian overdose: a case report. Vet Hum Toxicol 37:364–365

Subject Index

A
3'-acetoxyisosafrole 109
1'-acetoxysafrole 109, 111
acetoxyvalerenic acid 166
19-acetylgnaphalin 236
18-acetylmontanin D 141
acetylsalicylic acid 68
19-acetyltenlepicin 236
19-acetylteupolin IV 236
acevaltrate 166, 171, 173
aconitines 7, 8
Aconitum 7, 8
– *A. carmichaeli* 7, 8
– *A. japonicum* 7, 8
actinidine 167
Adenostylesalliariae 234
ague tree 123
ajmalicine 211
Ajuga
– *A. chamaepitys* 141
– *A. iva* 141
Akebia quinata 231
akuammigine 207
Alchornea floribunda 181
alchorneine 181
alchorneinone 181
alfalfa 233
algin 38
alginates 38, 40
alginic acid 38, 40
Allium sativum 229
alloyohimbine 182, 187, 199, 211
4- allylcatechol 106
aloe 8
amentoflavone 52
γ-aminobutyric acid 167
amiodarone 44
amsonine 182
β-amyrin 68, 137, 140
anacardic acids 53

anethole 72
anthocyanidins 90
anthranoids 8, 9, 229
aphrodine 182
apigenin 100, 137
– 4'-*O*-glucoside 100
Aplopappus heterophyllus 232
aporphine 123
apple, bitter 29
arbre aux quarante écus 51
Arctium 230
Aristolochia 230
– *A. clematitis* 230
– *A. fangchi* 230
– *A. manshuriensis* 230, 231
aristolochic acid 230
– I 230
– II 230
arnica 10
arsenic 41, 42, 44
arsenobetaine 42
Artemisia
– *A. absynthium* 15
– *A. alba* 15
– *A. brevifolia* 15
– *A. camphorata* 15
– *A. cina* 15–21
– *A. gallica* 15
– *A. kurramensis* 15
– *A. maritima* 15
– *A. mexicana* 15
– *A. mogoltavica* 15
– *A. monogyna* 15
– *A. neo-mexicana* 15
– *A. pauciflora* 15
– *A. wrightii* 15
artemisin 15
asarone 123
ascophyllan 38
Ascophyllum nodosum 37, 38

ascorbic acid 24, 52
aspalathin 23
Aspalathus
- *A. contaminatus* 23
- *A. corymbosus* 23
- *A. linearis* 23–27
Aspidosperma quebracho-blanco 181
Atherosperma moschatum 123
atropine 198
auropolin 236
avenasterol, Δ^3- 89

B
baldrinal 166, 167, 170, 174
- glucoronide 171
baldrinals 166–186, 172–174
barbotine 15
*benz(a)*anthracene 34
benziodarone 44
benzo(*a*)pyrene 34
benzo(*b*)fluoranthene 34
benzo(*j*)fluoranthene 34
benzoylaconines 7, 8
berberine 231
bilobalide 51, 53–55, 57
bilobanone 52
bilobetin 52
bilobal 57
bilobolol 52, 57
birdlime 99
bisabolene, β- 215
black-tang 37
blackwrack 37
bladderwrack 37
bois de sassafras 123
bois doux 67
boldine 123
Borbonia pinifolia 23
borneol 170, 215
bornyl
- acetate 168, 170
- isovalerate 168, 170
bough, golden 99
burdock root 230
Busch Tee, roter 23
bushtea, red 23

C
cadmium 94
caffeine 23
Caichongyao 145
calendula 10
calycanthine 212
camomile 231

campesterol 89
camphene 215
camphor 123, 124
carbenoxolone 69
carotene
- α 38
- β 38, 129
caryophyllene 137
cascara 8
Cassia 231
celabenzine 145
celacinnine 145
celafurine 145
celastrol 146, 149
Centranthus 166
chamaedroxide 138
Chamaedrys officinalis 137
chamomile 10
Chamomilla recutita 231
chaparral 232
Chlorella 132
chlorogenic acid 52, 137
chlorophyll 38, 129, 132
cholesterol 38, 89
choline 29, 137
Chuen-Lin 231
cicloxolone 69
Cinae anthodia 15
cineole 16, 215
cinnamolaurine 124
Cinnamomum
- *C. camphora* 105
- *C. micranthum* 105
cinnamon wood 123
cirsiliol 137
cirsimaritin 137
cis-sesquisabinene hydrate 215
citral 124
- α-citral 215
- β-citral 215
Citrillus colocynthis 29–36
cocaine 197
colocins 30, 31
- colocin 1 30
- colocin 2 30
colocynth 29–34
Colocynthis vulgaris 29
coloquinthe 29
coloside A 30
coltsfoot 234
coniferaldehyde 123
Coptis 231
- *C. chinensis* 231
- *C. japonicum* 231

Subject Index   243

Corynanthe   181, 207–209
C. johimbe   211
– *C. macroceras*   211
– *C. mayumbensis*   207
– *C. pachyceras*   207, 208, 211
– *C. paniculata*   207
– *C. yohimbe*   211
corynantheidine   182, 185, 188, 199, 207
corynantheine   182, 183, 207, 211
corynanthidine   182, 207
corynanthine   182, 183, 185, 187, 188, 192, 196, 199, 207, 211, 212
corynine   182
corynoxeine   182, 207
corynoxine   182, 207
coumaric acid   52
Crotalaria   24
cryptofauronol   165, 166
cucumber, bitter   29
cucurbitacins   29, 30
– B   29
– E   29
– E glycoside   29
– I   29
– J   29
– L   29
– T   29
curcumin   223
curcumene, α-   215
cut-weed   37, 38
cyanohydrins   93
cycloartenol   89

D
damascenone   24
Damnacanthus indicus   235
danthrone   8
daucosterol   89
3-deacetyl-20-epi-teulanigin   236
7-deacetylcapitatin   236
3-*O*-deacetyltengracilin   236
19-deacetylteuscorodol   236
dehydrogingerdione   216, 224
dehydrotremetone   231, 232
delphidenone   52
– glucoside   52
– tricetin   52
Delphinium consolida   7
desmethoxyashantin   124
desoxypseudosantonin   15
diaomaocao   145
didrovaltrate   166, 171, 173, 174
E-10,11-dihydroatlantone   52
Z-10,11-dihydroathlantone   52

dihydrocorynantheine   183, 207, 211
E-10,11-dihydro-b-oxo-atlantone   52
dihydrosafrole   113
dihydrositsirikine   211, 212
22,23-dihydrostigmasterol   68
dihydroteugin   138
dihydrovaltrate   174
1,8-dihydroxy-4-hydroxymethyl-anthraquinone   146
(+)-2,3-dihydroxy-1-(3,4-methylendioxy-phenyl)-propane   124
10,14-dimethyl-hexadecan-14-ol-2-one   30
11,14-dimethyl-hexadecan-14-ol-2-one   30
10,13-dimethyl-pentadec-13-en-1-al   30
diosmine   137
3,24-dioxo-friedelan-29-oic acid   146
Diplorhynchus condylocarpon   181
docosan-1-ol acetate   29
Doryphora sassafras   123
drift weed kelp   38
Dunaliella   131
dulcitol   146, 149, 152

E
echinacea   10
Edelgamander   137
EGb 761   52
α-elaterin glycoside   29
α-elaterin-2-D-glucopyranoside   30, 33
Elefantenohr   51
elemol   52
enterodiol   91
enterolactone   91
(epi)catechin   52
(epi)gallocatechin   52
epi-3-yohimbine   184
epi-3-α-yohimbine   182
epi-19 ajmalicine   207
3-epi-18-β-glycyrrhetic acid   70
3-epikatonic acid   146
epi-3-rauhimbine   182
6-epiteucrin A   138
12-epiteupolin II   141
20-epi-isoeriocephalin   236
13,14-epoxide 9,11,12-trihydroxytriptolide   146
eriocephalin   236
estragole   110
β-eudesmol   52
γ-eudesmol   52
eugenol   106, 123
euonine   145, 149
euonymine   146
Eupatorium   231
– *E. rugosum*   231

F

Fächerblattbaum 51
Fangchi 230
E,E-α-farnesene 215
faurinone 166
fauronyl acetate 166
Fenchelholz 123
Flachs 89
flax, common 89
flaxseed 89
fluoride 24, 25
frangula 8
fucinic acid 38
fucoidan 38, 44, 45
L-fucose 38
fucosterol 38
fucoxanthin 38
Fucus 37–40
– *F. nodosum* 37
– *F. serratus* 37, 38
– *F. spiralis* 37, 38
– *F. vesiculosus* 37–50

G

galanolactone 216
Gamander 137
Gan Cao 69
garlic 229
GBE 53–60
geranial 215
germander, common 137
gerany Pacetone 24
germandrée
– chamaedrys 137
– petit-chéne 137
gingediacetates 216
ginger 105, 215–224
gingerdiols 216
gingerdione 224
gingerenones 216
gingerglycolipids 216
gingerols 215, 216, 220, 221, 224
[6]-gingerol 216–220, 223
[6]-gingesulphonic acid 216, 217
ginkgo 52–60
ginkgobiloba 51–66, 232
ginkgol 52
ginkgols 52
– gastrointestinal reactions 59
ginkgolic acids 52, 53, 56, 58, 59
ginkgolides 51–56
– A 51, 53, 55, 57, 58
– B 51, 53–55, 57, 58
– C 51, 53, 58

– J 51, 53
– M 51
ginkgotoxin 58
ginkyo 51
gin-nan 53, 58
ginseng 233, 234
glabrolide 68
glicoricone 68
glisoflavone 68
glucan, 1-3 β 38
glycesterone 78
glycyramarin 68
glycyrin 68
glycyrrhetic acid 68
– 18-β- 70
glycyrrhetinic acid 68–78
– 18-β- 68
glycyrrhetol 68
Glycyrrhiza
– *G. glabra* 67–68
– *G. uralensis* 67, 69, 79
glycyrrhizic acid 67
glycyrrhizin 67–79
glycyrrhizinic acid 67
gnaphalidin 236
goldenrod, rayless 232
gossypol 232
gourd, bitter 29
GTW 147
guaiacol 24
Guang fangii 230
Guangmutong 231

H

hamamelis 10
hentriacontane 29
heptacosan-1-ol 29
2,4-heptadienal 24
herniarin 68
Heshi 16
1,26-hexacosan-diol 29
hexahydrocurcumin 216
hexanoate ester 166
(22-27)-hexanorcucurbitacin I 29
2-hexenal 52
histamine 42
Hokkai-Kisso 169
homobaldrinal 166, 170, 171, 174
homo-orientin 23
Hosome-kombu 38
Huangteng 145
humulene 137
hydrocyanic acid 92–94
hydroginkgolic acid 52

Subject Index 245

hydroginkgolinic acid 52
1-hydroxyanthraquinone 8
p-hydroxybenzoic acid 52
3'-hydroxyisosafrole 109
6-hydroxykynurenic acid 52
hydroxysafrole
– 1'- 106, 108, 109, 112, 113, 123
– 3'- 106
6α-hydroxyteuscordin 138
hydroxytremetone 231
16-hydroxytriptolide 146, 149
hydroxyvalerenic acids 166
hydroxyvaleric acid 166
hydroxywilfordic acid 145
10-hydroxy-yohimbine 186
11-hydroxy-yohimbine 186
Hymenodictyon excelsum 235
hypodiolide 146
hypolaetin 137

I
Illicium
– *I. anisatum* 105
– *I. verum* 105
iodine 38–45
iso-3 epi-19 ajamalicine 207
iso-3 rauniticine 207
isoalchorneine 181
isoboldine 123
isoborneol 170
isobornyl acetate 170
Isocoma wrightii 232
isoeriocephalin 236
isoferulic acid 167
(iso)ginkgetin 52
isoglabrolide 68
isoliquiritigenin 68, 79
isoliquiritin 68
isoliquiritoside 68
isomagnolol 124
isoneotriptophenolide 146
iso-orientin 90
isoquercetin 137
isoquercitrin 23
isorauhimbine 182
isorhamnetin 52
isosafrole 107, 109, 113
isoschaftoside 100
isoscutellarein 137
isoteuflidin 138
isoteuflin 141
isovalerate ester 166
isovaleric acid 166
isovaleroxyhydroxydidrovaltrate 166

isovaltrate 166, 170, 174
iso-vitexin 90
isoyohimbine 182

J
Japanbaum 51
jatamansone 166
Juzentaibo-gan 4

K
kaempferol 52, 56
Kaigen 4
Keimeigashin-san 4
Keishi-bukuryo-gan 4
kelp 37–44
– kelp-ware 37
kessan 166
kessoglycol 169
kessyl
– acetate 166
– – 2-acetate 169
– – 8-acetate 169
– – diacetate 169
– glycol 171
Kinshigan 4
Kinshigyoku 4
knobbed-wrack 37
Koloquinthe 29
kombu 43
kung sun shu 51
Kunmingshanhaitang 145

L
Lakritzenwurzel 67
laminaran 38, 45
Laminaria 37–40, 42, 45
– *L. cloustoni* 37
– *L. digitata* 37, 38
– *L. japonica* 37
– *L. longissima* 38
– *L. ochotensis* 38
– *L. religiosa* 44
– *L. saccharina* 37, 38
laminine 42
lanarine isovalerianate 167
larkspur, forking 7
Larrea tridentata 232
lecitine, β- 52
Lei Gong Teng 145
Lein 89
licoarylcoumarin 68
licochalcone A 69
licoflavonol 68
licofuranone 68

licopyranocoumarin 68
licoric acid 68
licorice 67–79
licoricidin 68
licoricone 68
lignin 68
lin 89
linalool 215
linamarase 92, 93
linamarin 90
linase 92
linatine 90, 92, 93, 95
linen flax 89
linin 92
linocinnamarin 89
linoleic acid 89
linolenic acid 89, 91, 92
– α 129
– γ 129
linseed 89–95
Linum
– *L. album* 90
– *L. alpinum* 90
– *L. altaicum* 89
– *L. arboreum* 90
– *L. campanulatum* 90
– *L. capitatum* 90
– *L. catharticum* 89, 90, 92, 94
– *L. chamissonis* 89
– *L. elegans* 90
– *L. flavum* 90
– *L. gallicum* 90
– *L. grandiflorum* 90
– *L. humile* 89
– *L. kingii* 90
– *L. lewisii* 90
– *L. marginale* 90
– *L. maritimum* 90
– *L. pallescens* 89
– *L. pamphylicum* 90
– *L. perenne* 89
– *L. strictum* 89
– *L. tauricum* 90
– *L. thracicum* 90
– *L. usitatissimum* 89–98
– *L. vulgare* 89
linusitamarin 89
linustatin 90
liqcoumarin 68
liquiritiae radix 67
liquiritigenin 68
liquiritin 68
liquiritoside 68
liquirizia 67

liquirtic acid 68
liquorice 67
lithium carbonate 145
Liufangteng 145
Lochnera lancea 181
lotaustralin 90
Lotononis 24
lucein-1 90
lucein-2 90
luteolin 23, 52, 137
Lyngbya majuscala 42

M
maaliol 166
Macassar oil 125
mace 105, 107
Macrocystis pyrifera 37, 39
madder root 235
Magnolia officinalis 230
magnolol 124
maidenhair tree 51
Makombu 38
Mang Cao 145
mannitol 38, 68
Massai tee 23
Matricaria 10
mayumbine 207
Medicago sativa 233
Mentha
– *M. piperita* 233
– *M. spicata* 233
menthol 233
mercury 131
mesoyohimbine 182
4-methoxy-8-pentyl-1-naphtolic acid 167
8- methoxyactinidine 167
5- methoxyeugenol 123
Mespilodaphne sassafras 123
5-methoxypodophyllotoxin 90, 92
24-methylene cycloartenol 89
methyleugenol 110
[6]- methylgingediol 216
6-methyl-3,5-heptadien-2-one 24
6-methyl-5-hepten-2-one 24
4-O-methylpyridoxine (MPN) 52, 57, 58, 232
methylsalicylate 68
mibulactone 15
mistletoe 99–101
– American 99–101
– European 99
– false 99
mixoxanthophyll 129
MKsan 4

Subject Index 247

monogynin 15
montanin
– B 236
– C 236
– E 236
Morinda umbellata 235
MPN 52, 57, 232
Mutong 231
myricetine 54
myristic acid 89
Myristica fragrans 105

N

Nagakombu 38
naphthyridylmethylketone 167
Nardostachys jatamansi 169
nekombu 42
neoisoliquiritin 68
neolinustatin 90
neotriptonolide 146
neotriptonoterpene 146
neotriptophenolide 146
neral 215
nicotinamide 89
norboldine 123
norcinnamolaurine 124
nordihydroguaiaretic acid 232
noyer du Japon 51
nutmeg 105, 107

O

Ocotea
– *O. cymbarum* 105, 124
– *O. pretiosa* 123
n-octacosanol 29
oleanolic acid 140
oleic acid 89
orientin 23, 90
orthosphenic acid 146, 149
1'-oxosafrole 109
oxysantonin 17

P

Packera candidissima 234
palmitic acid 89
Panax ginseng 233
paniculatine 207
paradols 216
pastis 72
patchouli alcohol 166

Pausinystalia 181, 211–214, 234
– *P. angolensis* 212
– *P. johimbe* 211
– *P. macroceras* 211, 212
– *P. pachyceras* 207
– *P. trillesii Beille* 212
– *P. yohimbe* 211–213
pei kuo 51, 53
(ZZ)-4,4-(1,4'-pentadiene-1,5-diyl)diphenol 52
pepper, black 105
phellandrene 123, 124
phenylalanine 131
β-phenylethylalcohol 24
pheophorbide-a 132
Phoradendron
– *P. flavescens* 99–103
– *P. leucarpum* 99
– *P. serotinum* 99
– *P. tomentosum* 99, 100
phoratoxin 99–101
– B 99
Phytolacca americana 234
picropolin 236
picropolinol 236
picropolinone 236
pinene 16
– α 123, 137
pinitol 52
Piper nigrum 105
piperonyl acrolein 123, 124
podophyllin resin 32
podophyllotoxin 95
pokeweed 234
polpunonic acid 146
polyprenols 52
potassium chloride 38
potassium sulphate 38
primisterine 146
proanthocyanidins 52, 53
prodelphinidins 52
protocatechuic acid 52
Pseudocinchona
– *P. africana* 207
– *P. mayumbensis* 207
– *P. pachyceras* 207
pseudosantonin 15
pseudoyohimbine 182, 183, 211, 212
Psoralea linearis 23
Pterophyllus salisburensis 51
pyrrolizidine alkaloids 3, 23, 234

Q

quebrachine 182
quercetin 23–25, 52, 54
Quercus marina 37
quinic acid 52

R

raubasine 181–183, 185–187, 190, 192, 194–196, 199, 200, 211, 212
rauhimbine 182
rauniticine 207
Rauwolfia 181
- *R. canescens* 181
- *R. serpentina* 181
rauwolscine 181–183, 185, 187, 192, 193, 196, 199, 207, 211, 212
regaliz 67
regelide 146
regelin 146, 150
- C 146
- D 146
regelindiol
- A 146
- B 146
regelinol 146, 150
reglisse 67
reserpine 182, 197, 198
reticuline 124
rhamnoisoliquiritin 68
rhamnoliquiritin 68
Rheum 234
rhubarb 8, 234
ricin 30
Rikkunshi-to 4
Rishiri kombu 38
rooibos tea 23–25
rooitea 23
„roter Busch Tee" 23
Rubia 235
- *R. cordifolia* 235
- *R. tinctorum* 235
rutin 23

S

safrole 105–127
Saiboku-to 4, 71
Saiko-keishi-to 4
Sairei-to 4
Sakaki Gachyagi 4
salaspermic acid 146, 150
salicylic acid 68
Salisburia adiantifolia 51
saloop 123
santogenin 17
santolactone 15
santonica 15, 16, 20
santonin 15–20
- α-santonin 15
- β-santonin 17
- L-santonin 15

Sassafras 123–126
- Australian 123
- Brazilian 123, 124
- New Caledonian 123
Sassafras
- *S. albidum* 105, 123–127, 235
- *S. officinale* 123
- *S. randaiense* 124
- *S. variifolium* 123
sassafrid 123
saxifrax 123
schaftoside 100
sciadopitysin 52
Scutellaria 235
- *S. baicalensis* 235
- *S. lateriflora* 140
sea mugwort 15
sea-girdle 37
sea-tangle 37
secoisolariciresinol diglucoside 89
secoisolariciresol diglucoside 91
semencine 15
Senecio vulgaris 234
senna 229, 231
sennosides 229, 231
sequoyitol 52
D-(+)-sesamine 124
sesquiphellandrene, β- 215
shikimic acid 52
shogaols 215, 216, 221
[6]-shogaol 216, 219, 220, 223
Sho-saiko-to 4
sitosterol 52, 89, 100, 140
- glycoside 52
- β-sitosterol 68, 124, 137
skullcap 140, 172
snakeroot, white 233
sodium carbonate 38
spartein 23
Spirulina 129–135
- *S. fusiformis* 129
- *S. maxima* 129, 131, 133
- *S. platensis* 129, 133
star anise 105
stearic acid 89
Stephania tetrandra 230
stigmasterol 52, 68, 89, 100, 137, 140
Stronger-Neo-Minophagen C® 4, 75, 76
1'-sulfo-oxysafrole 113
Süssholz 67
(-)-syringaresinol 146

T

T2 147

Subject Index 249

Tanakan 53
tannin 23, 38, 100, 137
tea, red 23
Tebonin® 58, 59
terpinene 16
terpineol 16
tetrahydroalstonine 207
teuchamaedrin C 138
teuchamaedryn A 138
teuchamaedryn B 138
teucjaponin B 236
teucrin
– A 137, 138, 235
– B 138
– E 138
– F 138
– G 138
– H1 138
– H2 138
– P1 236
teucrioside 137
Teucrium 137 ff.
– *T. africanum* 141
– *T. aureum* 141
– *T. botrys* 141
– *T. canadense* 141
– *T. canadense* 140
– *T. capense* 141
– *T. chamaedrys* 8, 137–144, 235
– *T. chamaepitys* 141
– *T. creticum* 141
– *T. cubense* 141
– *T. flavum* 141
– *T. fruticans* 141
– *T. incanum* 141
– *T. inflatum* 141
– *T. iva* 141
– *T. maritimum* 141
– *T. marum* 141
– *T. montanum* 141
– *T. officinale* 137
– *T. polium* 141, 235
– *T. riparium* 141
– *T. scordium* 141
– *T. scorodonia* 141
– *T. stocksianum* 141
– *T. villosum* 141
teucroxide 138
teucvidin 138, 141
teucvin 138
teuflidin 138
teuflin 138, 141
teugin 138
teulamifin B 236

(12R)-teupolin I 141
teupolins 236
teuscorodal 141
teuvincentins 236
theaflavins 23
thunder god vine 145
tocopherol 90
tremetol 231
tremetone 231, 232
$2\alpha, 3\alpha$-trihydroxy-Δ^{12}-ursene-28-oic acid 146
tripchlorolide 146, 149, 158
tripdiolide 145, 146, 149, 150, 157, 158
tripdioltonide 146
tripterifordin 146, 150
tripterine 146
Tripterygium 145–163, 236
– *T. hypoglaucum* 145, 146, 150, 152, 153, 158, 159
– *T. regelii* 145, 146, 150
– *T. wilfordii* 145, 159, 236
– *T. wilfordii var. regelii* 145, 146, 150
tripterygone 146
triptodihydroxy acid methyl ester 146
trytoditerpenic acid 146
triptofordins 146, 150
– F-2 150
triptofordinine
– A-1 145
– A-2 145
triptogelins 146
– A-1 150
triptolide 145, 146, 149, 150, 152, 153, 157
– chlorohydrin 146
triptolidenol 146, 149
triptonide 145, 146, 149, 150
triptonodiol 146
triptonolide 146
triptonoterpene 146
triptonoterpenol 146
triptophenolide 146, 149, 152
triptotriterpenic acid 146
– A 146
– B 146, 149
triptotriterpenoidal lactone A 146
triptriolide 146, 149
Tussilago farfara 234
tyramine 100

U
umbelliferone 68
ursolic acid 137

V
valepotriates 166–174

Subject Index

valeranone 165, 166, 168, 169, 172
valerenal 165, 166, 169
valerenic acid 166–172
– methylester 166
valerenol 168
– acetate 166
Valerian 165–173, 236
Valeriana 165–167, 236
– *V. alternifolia* 165
– *V. collina* 165
– *V. edulis* 165–167
– *V. exaltata* 165
– *V. excelsa* 165
– *V. jatamansi* 165
– *V. mexicana* 165
– *V. officinalis* 165–167, 169, 170
– *V. pratensis* 165
– *V. procurrens* 165
– *V. sambucifolia* 165
– *V. sylvestris* 165
– *V. wallichii* 165–168, 170
valerianine 167
valerianol 165
valeric acid 166
valerosidate 166
valtrate 166, 170, 171, 173, 174
vanillic acid 52
vicenin
– 1 90
– 2 90
Vinca 181
– *V. rosea* 181
viscotoxin(s) 99, 101
Viscum 101
– *V. album* 99
– *V. flavescens* 99
vitamin B_{12} 129, 130, 132
vitexin 90, 100

W

wall germander 8, 137, 235

wilfordic acid 145
wilfordine 145, 146
wilforgine 145, 146
wilforine 145, 146
wilforlide
– A 146
– B 146
wilfornine 145
wilforonide 146
wilfortrine 145, 146
wilforzine 145, 146
wood, sweet 67
Wurmsaamen 15
Wurmsaat 15

Y

ya chio 51
yin-hsing 51
Yohimbe 183–204, 234
yohimbehe 211
yohimbic acid 211
yohimbine 181–200, 207, 211, 212, 234
– α- 182, 207, 211, 212
– β- 182, 183, 187, 196, 199, 207, 211, 212
– φ- 182
yohimbinic acid 186
yo-yo" 184

Z

zingerenone 218
zingerone 216, 223
Zingiber
– *Z. mioga* 223
– *Z. officinale* 105, 215–228
zingiberene 217
– α- 215
zingiberenol 215
zingiberol 215
Zitwerbeifuß 15
Zitwersamen 15
ZT 216, 219

Herbal remedies and plant-derived drugs

The second volume contains a general introductory chapter on the legislation of herbal remedies in different countries, which is followed by twenty-six plant-oriented monographs.

Contents:
- Legislatory Outlook on the Safety of Herbal Remedies.
- Abies, Picea and Pinus Species.
- Anthranoid Derivatives (Aloe, Cassia, Rhamnus, Rheum, Rubia).
- Arctium Species.
- Borago Officinalis.
- Caulophyllum Thalictroides.
- Eleutherococcus Senticosus.
- Eupatorium Species.
- Gossypol.
- Hedera Helix.
- Juniperus Species.
- Larrea Tridentata.
- Lithospermum Species.
- Lycopus Species.
- Phytolacca Americana.
- Podophyllum Species.
- Polygala Species.
- Quillaja Saponaria.
- Scutellaria Species.
- Taraxacum Officinale.
- Tilia Species.
- Vaccinium myrtillus.
- Notes Added in Proof.
- Subject Index.

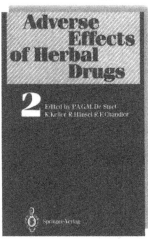

Adverse Effects of Herbal Drugs
Volume 2
Edited by P. A. G. M. de Smet (Managing Editor), K. Keller, R. Hänsel, R. F. Chamdler
In collaboration with the Pharmaceuticals Programme of the World Health Organization, Regional Office for Europe
With contributions by numerous experts
1993. XIV, 348 pages. 9 tables.
ISBN 3-540-55800-4

Price subject to change without notice.
In EU countries the local VAT is effective.

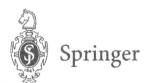

Please order by
Fax: +49 30 8207 301
e-mail: orders@springer.de
or through your bookseller

Springer-Verlag, P. O. Box 31 13 40, D-10643 Berlin, Germany.